The Year in
Endocrinology

1975-1976

The Year in Endocrinology

Editor-in-Chief: SIDNEY H. INGBAR • Boston, Massachusetts

The Year in Endocrinology

1975-1976

Edited by

Sidney H. Ingbar, M. D.

Professor of Medicine, Harvard Medical School
Director, Thorndike Laboratory
of Harvard Medical School
at the
Beth Israel Hospital
Boston, Massachusetts

PLENUM MEDICAL BOOK COMPANY
NEW YORK AND LONDON

Library of Congress Cataloging in Publication Data

Main entry under title:

The Year in endocrinology, 1975-1976.

Includes bibliographical references and index.
1. Endocrinology. I. Ingbar, Sidney H. [DNLM: 1. Endocrinology—Yearbooks.
W1 YE39]
QP187.Y44   612'.4   76-46325

ISBN-13: 978-1-4615-8845-0   e-ISBN-13: 978-1-4615-8843-6
DOI: 10.1007/978-1-4615-8843-6

© 1976 Plenum Publishing Corporation
Softcover reprint of the hardcover 1st edition 1976
227 West 17th Street, New York, N. Y. 10011

Plenum Medical Book Company is an imprint of Plenum Publishing Corporation

Contributors

Louis V. Avioli, M.D.
Schoenberg Professor of Medicine; Director, Division of Bone and Mineral Metabolism, Washington University School of Medicine, St. Louis, Missouri

Edward G. Biglieri, M.D.
Chief of Endocrinology Division of the Medical Service and Director of the Clinical Study Center, San Francisco General Hospital; and Professor of Medicine, University of California, San Francisco, California

Lewis E. Braverman, M.D.
Professor of Medicine; Director of Endocrinology and Metabolism, University of Massachusetts Medical School, Worcester, Massachusetts

Richard E. Buller, Ph.D.
Department of Cell Biology, Baylor College of Medicine, Houston, Texas

William H. Daughaday, M.D.
Professor of Medicine; Director, Metabolism Division, Department of Medicine, Washington University School of Medicine, St. Louis, Missouri

Daniel D. Federman, M.D.
Arthur L. Bloomfield Professor and Chairman, Department of Medicine, Stanford University Medical Center, Stanford, California

v

Dorothy T. Krieger, M.D.
Professor of Medicine; Director, Division of Endocrinology and Metabolism, The Mount Sinai School of Medicine of the City University of New York, New York, New York

Lewis Landsberg, M.D.
Assistant Professor of Medicine, Harvard Medical School; and Associate Chief, Department of Medicine, Beth Israel Hospital, Boston, Massachusetts

Mortimer B. Lipsett, M.D.
Director, Clinical Center, National Institutes of Health, Bethesda, Maryland

Robert L. Ney, M.D.
Professor and Chairman, Department of Medicine, University of North Carolina School of Medicine, Chapel Hill, North Carolina

Bert W. O'Malley, M.D.
Professor and Chairman, Department of Cell Biology, and Director, Baylor Center for Population Research and Reproductive Biology, Baylor College of Medicine, Houston, Texas

Griff T. Ross, M.D.
Deputy Director, Clinical Center, National Institutes of Health, Bethesda, Maryland

Louis M. Sherwood, M.D.
Physician-in Chief and Chairman, Department of Medicine, Michael Reese Hospital and Medical Center; and Professor of Medicine, Pritzker School of Medicine, University of Chicago, Chicago, Illinois

Kenneth A. Woeber, M.D.
Professor of Medicine, University of California; Chief of Medicine, Mount Zion Hospital and Medical Center, San Francisco, California

Preface

It is unclear, and really no longer relevant, whether the information explosion that we now contend with has been fostered by the growth of specialization and subspecialization in medicine, or vice versa. What is clear is that the two are mutually supportive and constitute what would be in endocrine parlance a short-loop positive feedback system. As a result, for most areas of medicine, even the subspecialist in that area has a problem in maintaining currency, the more general specialist has substantial difficulty in doing so, and the generalist is tempted to abandon the effort altogether.

Nevertheless, for all, both the internal pressures of conscience and self-esteem and the external pressures generated by peer review, recertification, and subspecialty boards create the need for continuous self-education. We are, therefore, in an era in which the means of dissemination of new information deserves as much creative attention as does its acquisition.

Because of the complexity of their underlying physiology and biochemistry and the diversity of disease entities that they encompass, the
fields of endocrinology and metabolism have been prone to subspecialization as much as or more than any others. To meet the problems attendant
upon this fact, two major approaches, apart from traditional journals and
textbooks, have been developed; both generally appear on an annual
basis. In the first, abstracts of the preceding year's key papers in a given
area are presented. What this format gains in detail and comprehensive-
ness, it necessarily gives up with respect to integration, despite accompa-
nying insightful editorial comment. Another type of annual publication
presents authoritative, in-depth reviews of selected topics within one or
more specialty or subspecialty areas. What this format gains in compre-
hensiveness and integration, it necessarily loses in breadth of subject
matter.

The present companion volumes, *The Year in Endocrinology* and *The
Year in Metabolism,* reflect our effort to approach the problem of information acquisition in these fields, and to bridge the gap between the foregoing types of annual publication, in a still different manner. In our idealized vision, they would represent a transposition into the written word of
what might have been the content of several evenings' discussion of each
topic with an acknowledged authority in that area, who would, in a
relaxed and relaxing manner, describe what has appeared in the field
during the past year that he or she considers important, why it is important, how it relates to what has gone before, and how it might influence
what will come in the future. Although we hope that these volumes can be
turned to by readers who are seeking a particular recent reference or a
discussion of a highly specific topic, our principal aim is to provide a
source that readers would turn to with the thought that an evening's
reading of a particular chapter would provide them with a quite comprehensive, integrated overview of recent findings and trends within that
topic area.

Most authors have accepted five-year appointments to the Editorial
Board. Such continuity should not only permit comprehensive coverage
in succeeding years of any aspects that have been slighted in a single year,
but should also facilitate the kind of fine-tuning of the product from year
to year that would increase its value and interest. Most importantly, the
continuity of authorship should maximize the likelihood that the faithful
reader will, over time, come to perceive the implicit or explicit philosophi-
cal approach of each author to his field. In a few cases, where it appears
appropriate, pairs of topics will be covered every other year in an alternat-
ing manner. Moreover, the intention is to include, when appropriate, a
special chapter on some subject of broad general interest and immediacy.

Idealized visions never come entirely to pass, particularly in the early efforts to bring them to fruition, and we recognize that this is true of both volumes in this new series, since errors of both omission and commission have quite clearly occurred. It is our hope that these "teething troubles" will diminish and disappear as the series gains maturity. The Editors also hope that the series will achieve its own popularity, without encroaching upon the deserved popularity of existing publications. It is our desire instead that *The Year in Endocrinology* and *The Year in Metabolism* provide an efficient and enjoyable bridge between those who are creating new knowledge at the bench or at the bedside and the professional consciousness of those for whom such knowledge is ultimately intended.

Sidney H. Ingbar, M.D.
Norbert Freinkel, M.D.

Contents

Chapter 1
Neuroendocrinology
Dorothy T. Krieger

Chapter 2
Anterior Pituitary
William H. Daughaday

Chapter 3
The Thyroid
Kenneth A. Woeber and Lewis E. Braverman

Chapter 4
The Ovary
Mortimer B. Lipsett and Griff T. Ross

Chapter 5
The Testis
Daniel D. Federman

Chapter 6
The Adrenal Cortex
Robert L. Ney

Chapter 7
Aldosterone and the Renin–Angiotensin System
Edward G. Biglieri

Chapter 8
Catecholamines and the Sympathoadrenal System
Lewis Landsberg

Chapter 9
Calcitonin
Louis V. Avioli

Chapter 10
Ectopic Hormone Syndromes
Louis M. Sherwood

Chapter 11
Current Concepts in Steroid Hormone Action
Bert W. O'Malley and Richard E. Buller

Neuroendocrinology

Dorothy T. Krieger

1.1. Introduction

In recent years, the field of neuroendocrinology has been greatly expanded. Earlier emphasis was on (1) the isolation and characterization of hypothalamic "hypophysiotropic" factors; (2) the localization of discrete and unique sites of production of such "factors," and of the neuroanatomical pathways converging on such sites; and (3) neuropharmacological manipulations designed to investigate the role of specific neurotransmitters on specific hypophysiotropic factors. During this time, there has been growing realization that there are extrahypothalamic sites of production of these factors and extrapituitary "behavioral" actions of these factors, possibly mediated via changes in CNS chemistry. It is also evident that there is a lack of specificity of many of the neuropharmacological agents employed in the investigation of neurotransmitter action; there is also the

---

DOROTHY T. KRIEGER • Division of Endocrinology and Metabolism, The Mount Sinai School of Medicine of the City University of New York, New York, New York.

additional realization that different species may utilize different neuro-transmitters and anatomical pathways for the regulation of a given hypo-physiotropic factor, making extrapolation to the human less than precise.

This chapter is designed to cover only selected aspects of developments in neuroendocrinology that have occurred over the past year, wherever possible stressing newer concepts and newer experimental approaches that may be applicable at the present time only to selected hypophysiotropic factors. Specific references will in the main be given only to articles appearing in the past year. General background information and a literature survey through 1974 are provided in specific sections of the *Handbook of Physiology*.[1,2]

1.2. Neural Regulation of Endocrine Function

1.2.1. Characterization of CNS Factors Acting on the Anterior Pituitary Gland

In the past seven years, three such factors have been isolated and definitively characterized: thyrotropin-releasing factor (TRF); gonadotropin-releasing factor (GnRF)—though there is still controversy as to whether there is one such factor modulating synthesis and release of both follicle-stimulating hormone (FSH) and luteinizing hormone (LH) or separate factors for each of these pituitary hormones; and growth hor-mone release–inhibiting factor or somatotropin release–inhibiting factor (somatostatin; SRIF). In the case of both TRF and SRIF, it has become apparent that these substances affect more than one pituitary hormone. In normal human subjects, SRIF, in addition to inhibiting growth-hor-mone release, also inhibits TRF-induced release of TSH, while TRF administration is associated with the release of both thyroid-stimulating hormone (TSH) and prolactin.

No other pituitary releasing or inhibiting factors have yet been characterized, although the existence of growth hormone–releasing fac-tor (GRF), prolactin-releasing factor (PRF), prolactin release–inhibiting factor (PIF), corticotropin-releasing factor (CRF), and MSH*-releasing and release–inhibiting factors have long been postulated. The observed effect of TRF on prolactin release raises the question whether it is necessary to postulate an additional prolactin-releasing factor. Addition-ally, in view of the demonstration of a direct pituitary action of dopamine in inhibiting prolactin release, there have been questions whether it is necessary to postulate the existence of an additional prolactin release–inhibiting factor. To date, there are no conclusive answers with regard to either of these questions.

*Melanocyte-stimulating hormone.

In the past year, there has been additional evidence from three laboratories of the existence of a GRF. This factor has been isolated from ovine hypothalami[3] and porcine stalk–median eminence preparations,[4,5] following purification on Sephadex G-25 columns. GRF has been assayed by measuring the increase of immunoreactive growth hormone (GH) following injection of "GRF" into a hypophyseal portal vein of a rat,[4] following *in vitro* incubation of rat pituitary tissue with "GRF,"[3] and following intravenous injection of "GRF" into estradiol-primed rats.[5] Such assays are more valid than the previously utilized "pituitary depletion" assay, in which animals showing a positive response by this assay failed to exhibit an elevation of immunoreactive GH in their plasma. The *in vivo* studies[5] also demonstrated that SRIF inhibits the GRF effects of median-eminence extracts.

1.2.2. Anatomical Localization of Hypophysiotropic Factors

The availability of purified TRF, GnRF, and SRIF, and antibodies thereto, has made possible the demonstration and measurement of these substances in nervous tissue by either radioimmunoassay or immunohisto-chemistry. Such analyses have been performed either on discrete CNS areas or on discrete CNS nuclei, the latter made possible by the availability of a simple and reproducible method for removing such nuclei. These studies have indicated that localization of TRF and SRIF is not confined to the hypothalamus. Additionally, hypothalamic deafferentation has demonstrated that the hypothalamus is not the source of production of hypophysiotropic factors found in extrahypothalamic sites. As a general statement, it appears that while each hypophysiotropic factor thus far studied has a different pattern of distribution within the CNS, in each instance, the highest concentrations are found in the median eminence.

Demonstration of hypophysiotropic factors in ependymal cells lining the third ventricle, if corroborated, raises questions concerning the direction of transport of such factors from these cells (i.e., whether they are eventually transported from extrahypothalamic areas to the hypothalamus, or whether they move from the hypothalamus retrograde into the CSF for transport to the extrahypothalamic areas).

The combined assay of neurotransmitter and hypophysiotropic factors in the same area of the CNS can give some indication of whether or not a given neurotransmitter is involved in the final step of release of a given hypophysiotropic hormone, although such studies will obviously not yield information with regard to other neurotransmitters that may be involved in the multisynaptic pathways impinging on the nerve cell producing the hypophysiotropic factor. All such localization studies to date have been performed on rodent brain; it is possible that studies in different species will yield different patterns of distribution (see Sections 1.2.2.1–4 and Table I).

Before reported observations on each of the hypophysiotropic factors are considered, several methodological considerations should be stressed. Radioimmunoassay will detect the substance being measured without indicating its cellular content or subcellular localization, whereas immunohistochemistry at the light- or electron-microscopic level will give such details with regard to perikaryal or axonal localization, or both, as well as possible nonneural, i.e., ependymal, localization. The nature of the results obtained with either method obviously depends on the specificity of the antisera employed. In the case of immunohistochemistry, nonspecific tissue-binding with either rabbit anti-BSA (used for conjugation), rabbit IgG, or endogenous peroxidase (depending on the technique employed) may lead to erroneous interpretations with regard to localization. Additionally, the method of preparation of tissues for microscopy (dehydration and embedding) leads to major losses of hypophysiotropic factors,[6] so that it is not surprising that studies using radioimmunoassay reveal more sites in which such factors are found than those using immunohistochemistry.

1.2.2.1. Thyrotropin-Releasing Factor

The distribution of TRF has been studied by radioimmunoassay.[7–9] Higher concentrations are present in the median eminence (38.4 ng/mg protein) than in other hypothalamic areas (Table I). Additional studies have indicated small but significant concentrations in other brain areas— i.e., approximately 1.08 ng/mg protein in the preoptic area, 0.85 ng/mg protein in the septal area, and 0.18 ng/mg protein in the medulla.[7,8] These amounts become significant when it is considered that hypothalamic weight is only $\frac{1}{100}$ of the total weight of the brain in the rat. Deafferentation[9] decreases only hypothalamic, not extrahypothalamic, TRF concentrations, indicating that extrahypothalamic TRF is not produced by hypothalamic neurosecretory cells. The decrease in hypothalamic TRF might be considered secondary to: (1) removal of stimulatory neural inputs to TRF-producing cells in the hypothalamus (hypothalamic norepinephrine and serotonin levels decrease following deafferentation,[10] although enzymes involved in norepinephrine synthesis are not affected[11]); (2) transection of axons carrying TRF from areas outside the hypothalamus; or (3) operative disruption of CSF flow, thereby interfering with transport of TRF from extrahypothalamic areas to the hypothalamus. The possibility of such transport has been demonstrated in studies in which intraventricularly injected TRF was found in hypophyseal portal plasma, and in which such injection also occasioned a rise in serum TSH levels.[12]

Table I. Luteinizing Hormone–Releasing Hormone (LH–RH), Thyroptropin-Releasing Hormone (TRH), and Somatostatin in the Hypothalamus of the Rat[a]

Region	LH–RH (ng/mg protein)	TRH (ng/mg protein)	Somatostatin (ng/mg protein)
Medial preoptic nucleus	<0.05	2.0±0.1	14.0±2.5
Periventricular nucleus	<0.05	4.2±0.7	23.7±9.0
Suprachiasmatic nucleus	trace (<0.1)	1.8±0.2	8.0±0.6
Supraoptic nucleus	trace (<0.1)	0.9±0.2	3.2±0.6
Anterior hypothalamic nucleus	<0.05	0.8±0.3	8.6±1.5
Lateral anterior nucleus	<0.05	0.7±0.2	4.9±1.1
Paraventricular nucleus	<0.05	2.6±0.7	4.4±1.8
Arcuate nucleus	2.9±0.8	3.9±0.9	44.6±6.1
Ventromedial nucleus	—		14.6±2.1
lateral part	0.6±0.5	3.0±0.6	—
medial part	trace (<0.1)	9.0±3.3	—
Dorsomedial nucleus	<0.05	4.0±0.8	5.4±2.1
Perifornical nucleus	<0.05	2.0±0.7	3.8±0.7
Lateral posterior area	<0.05	1.2±0.5	3.5±0.7
Posterior hypothalamic nucleus	trace (<0.1)	1.8±0.2	3.8±0.8
Dorsal premamillary nucleus	<0.05	1.5±0.2	4.3±0.7
Ventral premamillary nucleus	<0.05	1.3±0.3	17.3±4.4
Median eminence	22.4±2.2	38.4±8.3	309.1±60.8
Organum vasculosum	16.6±1.7	—	—

[a]From Brownstein et al.[24]

Other studies with deafferentation have also confirmed decreases in TRF in median eminence and anterior hypothalamus,[13] and have additionally demonstrated the presence of normal TSH responsiveness to administration of propylthiouracil and subsequent triiodothyronine replacement, and normal but reduced responsiveness to cold exposure in such animals.[13] Electrolytic destruction of the median eminence reduced these responses, which would indicate that the pool of TRF within the arcuate nucleus median eminence area, even following transection, is capable of maintaining normal feedback and pituitary responsiveness, albeit at lower levels.

1.2.2.2. Gonadotropin-Releasing Factor

In contrast to the extrahypothalamic as well as the hypothalamic localization of TRF, GnRF has been demonstrated (by immunoassay) to be contained almost solely in median eminence and organum vasculosum, with lesser concentrations detected in arcuate and ventromedial nuclei (Table I). Immunocytochemistry has demonstrated nerve fiber systems that contain GnRF that can be traced to the region of the retrochiasmatic area and arcuate nucleus[14] and the organum vasculosum.[15] The GnRF-containing axons that terminate in amygdalum, habenular ganglion, and the reticular formation of the mesencephalon have been less well studied. It has been suggested that these latter pathways[15] may be involved in the behavioral effects of GnRF. There has been some disagreement as to whether GnRF is synthesized in cell bodies, in view of the inability to demonstrate perikaryal localization of GnRF. Such localization, however, has been demonstrated following colchicine administration, which leads to proximal accumulation of immunoreactive material through inhibition of axoplasmic transport.[15]

Within the median eminence, GnRF has been observed only in neuronal elements, occurring in small, dense granules 75–90 nm in diameter.[16] This finding has been confirmed by sucrose-gradient studies in which LH release (measured *in vitro*) occurred only following incubation with a fraction containing electron-dense vesicles.[17]

There is disagreement concerning the effect of deafferentation on GnRF content within and without the hypothalamus. In diverse studies, deafferentation has been reported to decrease hypothalamic GnRF[18,19] and have no effect on GnRF content in the supraoptic crest[20] or organum vasculosum,[19] whereas another study demonstrated no change in median eminence or hypothalamic content, but increased GnRF in cerebrospinal fluid and in the pineal.[21] The only apparent difference among these studies is the size of the hypothalamic island obtained; the first three studies[18-20] include median eminence, arcuate, ventromedial, and dorsomedial nuclei, as well as premamillary and anterior hypothalamic areas; the fourth study[21] includes only arcuate nucleus and median eminence.

The report of increased CSF concentrations of GnRF after deafferentation again raises the question of the physiological role of CSF transport of hypophysiotropic hormones in the regulation of pituitary hormone release. Although localization of GnRF, following third ventricular administration, is seen in ependymal cell bodies and processes, portal capillaries, and pituitary sinusoids and parenchymal cells,[22] it is not clear whether this represents a physiological or scavenger function of the ependymal cell. GnRF has not been detected in CSF under a number of experimental conditions known to elevate LH release.[23]

1.2.2.3. Somatostatin

Although the highest concentrations are found in median eminence (see Table I), somatostatin is also found in appreciable concentrations in other hypothalamic areas. Significant concentrations (by immunoassay) are also found in thalamus, cortex, septum, preoptic area, and midbrain,[24] as well as in spinal cord (Guillemin, personal communication). Immunocytochemical techniques do not show so widespread a distribution, probably because of destruction during fixation. With these techniques, localization to organum vasculosum and pineal has been described, but in different

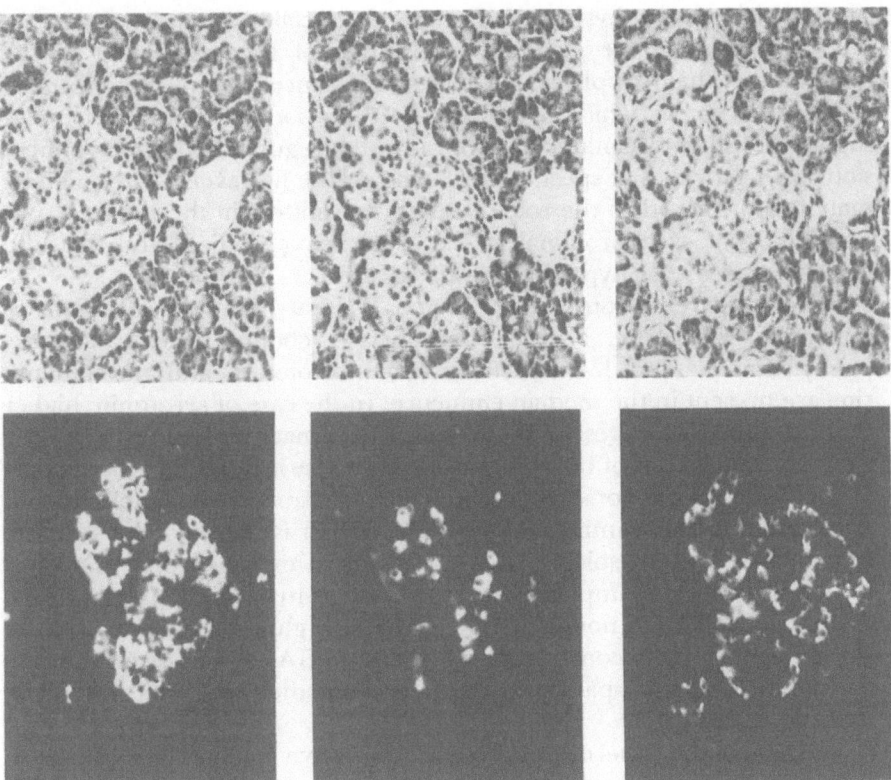

Fig. 1. Human pancreas–immunofluorescence reactions on the same islet (homologous fields of three contiguous serial sections) with antisera: (a) antiinsulin; (b) antisomatostatin; (c) antiglucagon. Each section is seen in normal light (above) and ultraviolet light (below). x 560. Autopsy material, male, 65 years old.[Reproduced from Dubois[26] of the Institut National de la Recherche Agronomique (France), with permission.]

nerve endings than those in which GnRF has been located.[25] The demonstration of somatostatin in nonneural tissue—pancreas[26,27] (see Fig. 1) and gastrointestinal tract[28,29]—and the physiological demonstration of its effectiveness on such tissue make it evident that somatostatin cannot be considered solely a hypophysiotropic factor. This may also be true for the other "hypophysiotropic" factors (see Section 1.3.3.3).

1.2.2.4. Neurotransmitter Localization

In the past few years, extensive mapping of CNS localization of putative neurotransmitters and enzymes involved in their metabolism has been performed, utilizing both biochemical and histochemical techniques.[10] Demonstration of localization of a given neurotransmitter at a site in which a hypophysiotropic factor is also localized would support, but not provide definitive evidence for, a role of the transmitter in the regulation of the hypophysiotropic factor. Absence of a given neurotransmitter at a site in which a hypophysiotropic factor is localized would suggest that the transmitter has no role in the regulation of the hypophysiotropic factor at that specific site. Such studies, however, yield no information with regard to the role of neurotransmitters in the multisynaptic pathways that exist proximal to the areas being studied, and that also modulate release of hypophysiotropic factors.

It is apparent from Tables II and III that high concentrations of dopamine, histamine, tyrosine hydroxylase, choline acetyltransferase, phenylethanolamine N-methlytransferase, serotonin, and norepinephrine are present in the median eminence. In the case of serotonin, higher concentrations are present in the suprachiasmatic and arcuate nuclei, while concentrations of norepinephrine in the periventricular, paraventricular, ventro- and dorsomedial and retrochiasmatic nuclei, are higher than in the median eminence (see Table II). It is not yet clear whether histamine is present solely in nerve cells or in extraneuronal elements. GABA has also been implicated in regulation of hypophysiotropic factors. Although GABA has not been assayed directly, glutamic acid decarboxylase, the enzyme that converts glutamic acid to GABA, has been found in the suprachiasmatic, paraventricular, dorsomedial, and anterior hypothalamic nuclei.

These studies, therefore, provide supportive evidence for the possibility of specific neurotransmitter interactions with cells producing the hypophysiotropic factors.

1.2.3. Neurotransmitter Regulation of Releasing Factors

Previous studies of neurotransmitter regulation of the release of hypophysiotropic factors have generally been based on *in vivo* CNS implantation of neurotransmitter agents or administration of neuropharmacological agents known to affect central neurotransmitter concentration or action. More recently, *in vitro* studies have been performed using coincubation of neurotransmitters and hypothalamus, with assay of medium for releasing-factor activity[30] or study of the effect of neurotransmitters on the release of hypophysiotropic factors from synaptosomes derived from different hypothalamic regions.[31]

1.2.3.1. Corticotropin-Releasing Factor

Previous *in vivo* studies had indicated a stimulatory role for ACh and GABA.[32] There has been controversy as to whether norepinephrine and

Table II. Biogenic Amines in the Hypothalamus of the Rat[a]

Region	Norepinephrine (ng/mg protein)	Dopamine (ng/mg protein)	Serotonin (ng/mg protein)	Histamine (ng/mg protein)
Periventricular nucleus	33.5±3.3	7.1±0.9	10.9±4.1	3.7±0.4
Supraoptic nucleus	23.6±5.0	3.7±0.6	9.5±2.8	3.0±0.6
Paraventricular nucleus	51.0±6.4	10.0±1.5	13.5±3.1	2.4±0.5
Anterior hypothalamic nucleus	16.2±4.6	5.0±0.9	10.2±2.3	3.3±0.8
Suprachiasmatic nucleus				
internal	20.5±4.0	8.5±2.4	37.2±4.7	—
external	29.2±3.9	9.5±1.3	17.0±1.3	—
Retrochiasmatic area	48.0±7.9	15.1±1.1	15.9±2.3	—
Arcuate nucleus				
I	35.9±3.4	28.2±3.7	—	—
II	18.9±3.0	18.7±4.4	—	—
III	21.2±4.1	12.0±2.6	36.4±9.8	6.2±0.7
IV	12.5±1.1	7.1±2.1	—	—
V	12.0±1.5	7.0±1.7	—	—
Ventromedial nucleus				
anterior	16.1±1.8	5.7±0.8	—	—
anterior medial	16.3±2.6	6.0±1.1	—	—
anterior lateral	22.5±2.0	7.0±1.1	8.5±3.9	3.6±0.8
posterior medial	38.2±3.6	10.0±1.1	—	—
posterior lateral	17.9±2.0	5.1±0.5	—	—
Dorsomedial nucleus				
dorsal	21.8±3.3	8.5±0.7	—	—
ventral	54.6±12.9	11.9±2.4	13.6±5.3	4.0±0.5
Perifornical nucleus	17.9±3.8	6.0±1.1	30.0±10.9	2.2±0.6
Dorsal premamillary nucleus	14.2±4.2	3.9±1.2	22.9±8.8	2.9±0.5
Ventral premamillary nucleus	16.3±6.2	3.4±0.9	18.3±8.2	8.1±0.8
Hypothalamic nucleus (posterior)	13.9±2.2	4.3±1.0	24.5±7.6	4.6±0.7
Medial forebrain bundle				
anterior	16.9±1.9	6.1±0.9	21.6±5.8	2.7±0.5
posterior	20.2±2.7	11.0±1.5	30.7±8.0	—
Median eminence	29.5±4.0	65.0±6.1	15.3±3.2	17.8±2.2

[a]From Brownstein et al.[11]

Table III. Levels of Enzymes Involved in the Synthesis of Neurotransmitters in the Hypothalamus of the Rat[c]

Region	Tyrosine hydroxylase[a]	Dopamine-β-hydroxylase[a]	Phenylethanolamine N-methyl transferase[b]	Tryptophan hydroxylase[a]	Choline acetyl transferase[a]
Periventricular nucleus	4.55±0.70	4.19±0.45	4.2±0.3	0.44±.05	8.0±0.9
Supraoptic nucleus	0.92±0.14	1.83±0.36	8.3±1.1	0.31±.04	5.2±1.3
Paraventricular nucleus	3.14±0.82	3.55±0.82	7.7±0.8	0.32±.05	15.0±2.5
Anterior hypothalamic nucleus	1.46±0.20	0.68±0.08	7.4±0.3	0.68±.12	5.9±1.3
Suprachiasmatic nucleus	1.83±0.33	0.79±0.14	5.0±0.9	0.55±.08	5.6±0.7
Arcuate nucleus	4.33±0.43	0.83±0.32	4.3±0.7	0.29±.04	10.3±2.0
Ventromedial nucleus	1.83±0.61	1.00±0.33	3.6±0.5	0.43±.07	8.3±1.6
Dorsomedial nucleus	2.10±0.32	3.06±0.93	8.4±1.2	0.47±.07	10.9±3.2
Dorsal premamillary nucleus	0.42±0.10	0.51±0.09	11.1±0.8	0.24±.02	4.1±0.5
Ventral premamillary nucleus	0.90±0.20	0.58±0.13	4.0±1.0	0.33±.07	4.9±1.4
Posterior hypothalamic nucleus	1.46±0.30	0.59±0.06	13.7±1.3	0.35±.05	5.1±1.0
Periformical nucleus	4.50±0.71	0.46±0.07	7.9±0.8	1.16±.17	8.1±1.6
Medial forebrain bundle	—	—	—	—	—
anterior	5.70±1.04	0.88±0.16	11.1±0.9	—	6.2±0.5
posterior	7.20±0.80	0.83±0.18	—	1.13±.19	5.3±1.2
Median eminence	18.03±1.04	1.26±0.31	19.5±0.6	0.41±.03	15.6±3.0

[a] Results are expressed in nmole product/mg protein per hr and represent the means ± S.E.M. for groups of 6–8 animals.
[b] Results are expressed in pmole product/mg protein per hr and represent the means ± S.E.M. for groups of 6–8 animals.
[c] From Brownstein et al.[11]

serotonin have inhibitory[33,34] or excitatory roles,[32] these discrepancies perhaps being in part species-related and in part a function of whether basal or stress-induced release is being studied. Recent *in vitro* studies indicate a dose-dependent release of CRF following administration of ACh (blocked by atropine) or serotonin (blocked by both hexamethonium and methysergide[30]). The latter studies suggest that serotonin may act via a cholinergic interneuron. While GABA, norepinephrine, dopamine, and histamine had no effect on basal CRF release in this system, norepinephrine and GABA were able to inhibit ACh-stimulated release.

1.2.3.2. Gonadotropin-Releasing Factor

Evidence that monoamines (dopamine or norepinephrine) exert a stimulatory effect on gonadotropin release in the rat has been extended by newer studies indicating that the synapse involved may lie in the preoptic area,[35] in which significant concentrations of GnRF are present (see Section 1.2.2.2). The results with isolated sheep synaptosomes prepared from median eminence indicate a stimulatory effect of dopamine, but not of norepinephrine or epinephrine, on GnRF release. No effect was noted with synaptosomes prepared from the periventricular region or the remainder of the hypothalamus (see Table I re relative GnRF concentrations). ACh is ineffective in this system, as is the *in vivo* intraventricular administration of carabachol.[36] This finding is in contrast to previous *in vivo* studies in which blockade of ovulation occurred following pharmacological doses of cholinergic blocking agents, and is also in contrast to recent *in vitro* studies (employing higher than physiological concentrations of ACh) that also suggest a stimulatory role.[37] The effect of other neurotransmitters, i.e., serotonin, histamine, and GABA, on GnRF release has still not been clarified.

1.2.3.3. Prolactin

The inhibitory role of dopamine on prolactin secretion is well established, although some question remains as to whether or not an additional hypothalamic prolactin-inhibitory factor exists. Recent evidence suggests that serotonin may stimulate prolactin release. Systemic administration of serotonin[38] or 5-hydroxytryptophan (5-HTP)[39] increases serum prolactin concentration, while *p*-chlorophenylalanine (an inhibitor of serotonin synthesis) blocks estrogen-induced prolactin release.[40] *p*-Chloroamphetamine, which also inhibits serotonin synthesis, decreases prolactin levels in estrogen-primed ovariectomized animals. Since these last two compounds also have effects on catecholaminergic systems, the report that administration of 5-HTP with Lilly 110140, which appears to be a specific inhibitor of serotonin uptake, leads to a marked increase in serum prolactin concentrations gives further support for a stimulatory role of serotonin on prolactin release.[41]

ACh has been reported to have both stimulatory and inhibitory effects on prolactin secretion under different physiological conditions. Pseudopregnant rats exhibit a circadian rhythm of plasma prolactin concentrations. This circadian rise is reported to be blocked by atropine, and this inhibition is reversed by eserine,[42] suggesting cholinergic involvement in this aspect of prolactin secretion.

1.2.3.4. Thyrotropin-Releasing Factor

Studies with the sheep median eminence–synaptosome preparation used to study GnRF release (see Section 1.2.2.2) have demonstrated serotoninergic inhibition of TRF release, and stimulation of such release by dopamine. Administration of pimozide, a specific dopaminergic receptor blocking agent, decreases serum TSH levels in humans.[43] In this study, an inhibitory effect of dopamine on human prolactin levels and a stimulatory effect on LH levels were confirmed, but no effect on GH or cortisol concentrations was noted.

1.2.4. Role of Prostaglandins in the Regulation of Hypophysiotropic Factors and Pituitary Hormones

In view of the ubiquitous distribution of prostaglandins (including their demonstration in nervous tissue), and their role in adenylate cyclase regulation (including that in pituitary), numerous studies have been performed to elucidate their role in the regulation of adenohypophyseal secretion, since releasing factors have also been reported to increase pituitary AMP accumulation. Prostaglandins have been reported to directly antagonize norepinephrine effects on cerebellar Purkinje cells[44]; hence, it is possible that any described endocrine effects may be mediated via an effect on neurotransmitters. Feedback effects of hormones may also be modulated partly via alterations in CNS prostaglandin concentration.[45] In this discussion, only those studies in which direct effects of prostaglandins on either hypothalamus or pituitary were studied will be cited, since prostaglandins administered systemically have widespread effects on other tissues.

A pituitary locus of action of the PGE series on hormone synthesis and release has been established in the case of growth hormone.[46] A stimulatory hypothalamic locus of action of the PGE series has been demonstrated with regard to the release of prolactin,[47] ACTH,[48] and LH.[49,50] The stimulatory effect on prolactin concentrations is blocked by

L-DOPA.[51] It has been suggested that the PGE_2 acts intraneuronally to effect GnRF release, since α-adrenergic, dopaminergic, serotoninergic, and cholinergic receptor-blocking agents are ineffective in modifying such PGE_2-induced release.[52]

1.2.5. Brain and Pituitary Growth Factors

It has long been assumed that the pituitary tropic hormones regulate both the size and secretory function of their target glands. The existence of separate weight-maintaining factors, i.e., an adrenal weight-maintaining factor, separate from ACTH, has been suggested, but not rigorously demonstrated. Recent studies report the presence of ovarian growth factor and fibroblast growth factor (FGF) in extracts of bovine pituitary glands[53]; FGF has also been identified in brain extracts. FGF from bovine pituitary has been purified[54] and shown to be a polypeptide of 13,300 mol. wt., homogeneous on analysis by polyacrylamide gel electrophoresis, carboxymethyl Sephadex gradient elution chromatography, and Sephadex G-50 chromatography. It is different from ovarian growth factor in both amino acid composition and mobility on polyacrylamide gel electrophoresis. Brain FGF has not yet been characterized. FGF is a mitogenic agent for cells as diverse as fibroblasts, chondrocytes, the Yl adrenal cell line, and glial or endometrial cells obtained from murine, bovine, and human sources.[54] It is also similar to a neurotropic factor demonstrated in brain that affects the appearance and mitotic rate of regenerative cells following amputation. Future developments in this field should be of importance in understanding the regulation of the growth of both endocrine and nonendocrine tissues.

1.3. Hormone–Nervous System Interactions

1.3.1. Catechol Estrogens

Specific cytoplasmic and nuclear uptake, as well as autoradiographic localization, of estradiol in preoptic area, hypothalamus, and amygdala has been well documented. Increased norepinephrine turnover in hypothalamus and midbrain has also been noted in ovariectomized rats. Rat hypothalamic tissue, unlike cortex, has now been shown to be capable of converting estradiol and estrone to 2-hydroxyestrone, a catechol estrogen.[55] Catechol estrogens have been reported to be competitive inhibitors of O-methylation of catecholamines by catechol-o-methyltransferase.[56] They also compete with estradiol for estrogen-binding sites in pituitary and hypothalamus, with association constants within one order of magnitude of those of the parent compounds.[57] Since, in humans, ⅓ of an injected dose of estradiol has been shown to undergo C-2 hydroxylation,[58] and the capability of such transformation has now been demonstrated in nervous tissue, either of the two mechanisms noted above (in addition to others) may be involved in the neural effects of estrogen.

1.3.2. CNS Uptake of Steroids

1.3.2.1. Corticosteroids

Many studies to investigate the various feedback aspects of CNS–pituitary–adrenal function have utilized potent synthetic glucocorticoids, especially dexamethasone, because of methodological considerations. It is now apparent that in the rat, the native glucocorticoid, corticosterone, and the synthetic glucocorticoid, dexamethasone, exhibit different cytosol and nuclear binding capacities in hippocampus, hypothalamus, and anterior pituitary.[59] Dexamethasone and corticosterone both exhibit greater *in vitro* cytosol binding in hippocampus than in hypothalamus; nuclear binding of dexamethasone is equal in both areas, whereas that of corticosterone exhibits the same variation as seen in cytosol. In the pituitary, dexamethasone exhibits greater binding to pituitary nuclei than does corticosterone, while the reverse is found with regard to cytosol binding. These findings suggest the existence of more than one population of corticosteroid-binding sites in brain and anterior pituitary, which may be involved in different mechanisms of regulation.

1.3.2.2. Androgens

Androgens are known to influence both sexual behavior and gonadotropin secretion. One area of active investigation is the nature of the androgen or its metabolite, or both, mediating these separate actions, i.e., whether testosterone, dihydrotestosterone (DHT), or estrogen (arising from aromatization of testosterone) is the effective agent. Cytosol receptors for androgen have previously been described in ventral prostate, testis, and epididymis. Recent studies[60] indicate that cytosol fractions of anterior pituitary, hypothalamus, preoptic area, and cortex possess similar specific androgen-binding proteins, greater amounts of radioactivity being bound per milligram of cytosol protein in anterior pituitary than in hypothalamus or preoptic area, and only small amounts being bound by cortex. Unaltered testosterone accounted for the major part of radioactivity present, although the affinity of testosterone and DHT for binding proteins was of similar magnitude (unlike the greater affinity of DHT for receptors in other androgen-sensitive tissues).

Further characterization[61] of the anterior pituitary cytosol receptor

by mobility in acrylamide gels and isoelectric focusing revealed characteristics with regard to steroid specificity, equilibrium constant, binding
capacity, and isolelectric point similar to those seen in androgen receptors
in other tissues. It is of interest that 17-β-estradiol had little affinity for the
pituitary androgen receptor. Subsequent conversion of testosterone to
estrogen within the cytosol could still occur, however, and could be
responsible for any effects noted after testosterone administration.

1.3.3. Peptide Hormone–Nervous System Interactions

1.3.3.1. Effect of Peptide Fragments on Learning and Memory

A long series of studies, originally concerned with investigation of the
role of vasopressin as a CRF, has culminated in the finding that vasopressin, vasopressin fragments, ACTH, and ACTH fragments have marked
effects on rat learning and behavior in the absence of either the pituitary
or the adrenals.[62] The parameters tested were rate of acquisition of
avoidance behavior (memory retention) and inhibition of extinction of
avoidance behavior (i.e., persistence of a learned response).

The smallest effective fragment with regard to learning is the 4–7
amino-acid sequence of the ACTH molecule; effects on memory can also
be elicited with the 4–10 fragment. It has been suggested that these
compounds affect learning and memory by increasing the state of arousal
of the animal. Similar results with regard to increased mental alertness
and increased visual memory have been reported in human subjects
following $ACTH_{4-10}$ administration.[63] The neurotransmitter basis for the
effects of these peptides is a matter of question; $ACTH_{4-10}$ increases
catecholamine turnover and synthesis in brains of intact rats, but does not
do so in hypophysectomized or adrenalectomized animals,[64] although
$ACTH_{4-10}$ is not steroidogenic *per se*.

The effects of vasopressin are similar to those reported for ACTH
fragments. Oxytocin is inactive,[65] although its C-terminal tripeptide, Pro-
Leu-Gly-amide, is active.

1.3.3.2. Effect of Peptides on Opiate Receptors

The demonstration in 1973 of opiate receptors in brain led to further
investigation to uncover the naturally occurring endogenous material that
would bind to such receptors. At least four different types of peptides
reported to possess such activity have been isolated from brain or pituitary. Of these, one is a morphinelike factor of mol. wt. approximately

1000 daltons. [66,67] Another, "enkephalin," is a mixture of 2 pentapeptides, methionine–enkephalin and leucine–enkephalin, of mol. wt. 800 daltons, methionine–enkephalin being identical to the 61–65 residues in β-lipotropin, a pituitary lipid mobilizing peptide. [68] The final group is that of the endorphins, [69] of which one, α-endorphin, has the same sequence as the 61–76 fragment of β-lipotropin, and obviously includes the amino acid sequence described for methionine–enkephalin.

A peptide, named the pituitary-opioid-peptide, has also been obtained from whole bovine pituitary gland. [70] Subsequently characterized as being more concentrated in posterior than in anterior pituitary gland, it behaves as an opiate agonist, but has different enzyme sensitivities, molecular weight (approximately 1800 daltons), and ionic properties than the peptides isolated from brain. A similar substance has also been isolated from a crude porcine ACTH preparation.

Concentration-dependent inhibition of dihydromorphine-binding to rat brain membrane preparations by $ACTH_{4-10,7-16}$ and $ACTH_{11-24}$ has been described. [71] The structural relationships among β_h-lipotropin, β_h-MSH (sequences 37–58 of β_h-lipotropin), and ACTH (the 4–10 sequence is the 47–53 sequence of β_h-lipotropin) are well known; the cited studies now suggest a precursor role of β_h-lipotropin for peptides with opiate-receptor activity as well. Further dissection of the site of production of the endogenous opiate-receptor binding material, factors regulating its synthesis and secretion, its physiological role, and its relationship to the peptide effects on learning and memory described above will add entirely new dimensions to the understanding of hormone–CNS relationships.

1.3.3.3. Effect of Releasing Factors on Brain Excitability and Behavior

The widespread distribution of at least some of the releasing factors within the CNS, the demonstration that concentrations of these factors in extrahypothalamic sites persist following hypothalamic deafferentation (see Section 1.2.2), and the demonstrated presence of TRF in the brain of primitive vertebrates that lack a pituitary or thyroid[72] is consistent with the possibility that such releasing factors may have a direct effect on CNS function.

Clinical and neurophysiological evidence is accumulating in support of such a possibility. The initial reports of alleviation of depressive states by TRF administration have not been confirmed. There is, however, evidence that TRF is a CNS stimulant. It has been demonstrated that TRF lessens the duration of pentobarbital anesthesia, [73] increases the LD_{50} of pentobarbital and decreases the LD_{50} of strychnine, [74] and potentiates the behavioral effects of dopamine and of serotonin.[75] Many of these effects are observed in hypophysectomized and thyroidectomized animals, supporting the concept of a direct effect on the CNS.

Somatostatin, in contrast, appears to be a CNS depressant. It lengthens pentobarbital anesthesia time,[73] decreases the LD_{50} of pentobarbital, and increases the LD_{50} of strychnine. Both it[76] and 1-prolyl-1-leucylglycine amide,[77] which has MSH inhibitory activity, also potentiate the behavioral effects of L-DOPA, sharing that attribute with TRF. It remains to be seen whether such potentiation can be extended clinically in the treatment of parkinsonism.

1.4. Releasing Factors

1.4.1. Interrelationships

Major consideration of the effects of releasing factors will be found in Section 1.2.2. It is now becoming evident both that all the characterized releasing factors have actions on multiple hormones and that a given releasing factor may modify the response to another releasing factor.

In humans, concomitant infusion of dopamine, which may be considered to be a prolactin-inhibitory factor, blocks both the TSH and prolactin response to TRF.[78] TRF also blocks the increases in human plasma growth hormone levels seen following L-DOPA administration.[79] In animal studies, TRF blocks GH release induced by morphine and pentobarbital, but does not block GH release produced by prostaglandin.[80] Studies of structurally modified TRF indicate a correlation between its effect on TSH release and its effectiveness in blocking GH release. Last, in animal studies, somatostatin blocks TRF-induced secretion of TSH, but not of prolactin.[81]

These relationships are obviously in need of further clarification, and raise a number of questions as to the locus of the reported effects. The effects of dopamine may be considered to take place at a pituitary level. The cited effects of TRF on suppression of GH release may perhaps best be interpreted as occurring at a CNS locus, in keeping with other CNS actions of TRF, since the release of GH induced by L-DOPA, morphine, and pentobarbital appears to be mediated via the CNS. An effect of TRF on possible pituitary GRF receptors cannot be excluded, and would also be compatible with the effects of structural modifications of TRF, cited above. Inhibition by somatostatin of the effect of TRF on release of TSH, but not of prolactin, would imply either that the TRF receptors on the two types of cells are different or that the effect occurs beyond the receptor. Cortisone has effects similar to those of somatostatin on the TSH and prolactin responses to TRF, blocking the former, with no effect on the latter. Such steroid effects are believed to be modulated via intracellular receptors.

1.4.2. Therapeutic Uses of Gonadotropin-Releasing Factor

GnRF has been employed in cases of anovulatory infertility, anorexia nervosa perhaps being a special example, which will be considered subsequently (see Section 1.5.4).

1.4.2.1. Anovulation

There are practical and theoretical advantages in the use of synthetic GnRF in the treatment of anovulation. It is to be hoped that stimulation of the pituitary to release a "normal" ovulatory amount of LH will prevent the hyperstimulation syndrome seen with administration of human chorionic gonadotropin (HCG). Additionally, preparations currently available for induction of follicular growth, such as human menopausal gonadotropin or human pituitary gonadotropin, are relatively expensive and difficult to come by for large-scale use. Studies in anovulatory females have been concerned either with the induction of ovulation in amenorrheic women in whom follicular maturation was spontaneous or had been stimulated with prior GnRF, clomiphene, or HMG,[82,83] or with the induction of follicular growth and maturation in clomiphene-unresponsive women, with subsequent induction of ovulation with either HCG or additional larger doses of GnRF.[82–84] Interpretation of results is clouded because of the use of differing amounts, doses, routes of administration, and duration of administration of GnRF in these studies. Reported results also have to be compared with regard to the effect of placebo alone in inducing ovulation. Overall success rates with regard to ovulation have varied from approximately 25 to 75%; the incidence of pregnancy following induced ovulation varied from 50 to 70%.

To define the specific indications for the use of GnRF in the treatment of anovulatory infertility, it is apparent that additional studies, more clearly assessing the endocrine milieu of the subjects and using longer-acting preparations, are necessary. Such studies are presently ongoing.

1.4.2.2. Hypogonadism

As experience has accumulated with the use of GnRF in diagnostic testing, it has become apparent that lack of responsiveness to an acute injection does not necessarily confirm a pituitary etiology of hypogonadism. Such lack of responsiveness may also be due to chronic deprivation of endogenous GnRF. It has been possible to convert absent responsiveness to normal responsiveness with prolonged administration of GnRF[85] (Fig. 2). Of 9 patients with isolated gonadotropin deficiency (5 males, 4 females) previously unresponsive to 100 μg GnRF, 5 responded normally to this dose following daily infusion of 400 μg GnRF for 7 or more days. Absent responses to a second acute dose were seen only in those patients treated for less than 5 days. Similarly, of 9 patients with organic hypothalamic disease (histiocytosis X, tuberculous meningitis, ectopic pinealmoa, craniopharyngioma), 5 also showed restoration of responses following 5–7 days of GnRF therapy.

These findings suggest that in such patients, effective responses may be achieved by long-term therapy with GnRF. In 2 prepubertal patients (1 with isolated gonadotropin deficiency, 1 with craniopharyngioma) in whom growth had slowed sufficiently to justify an attempt at induction of

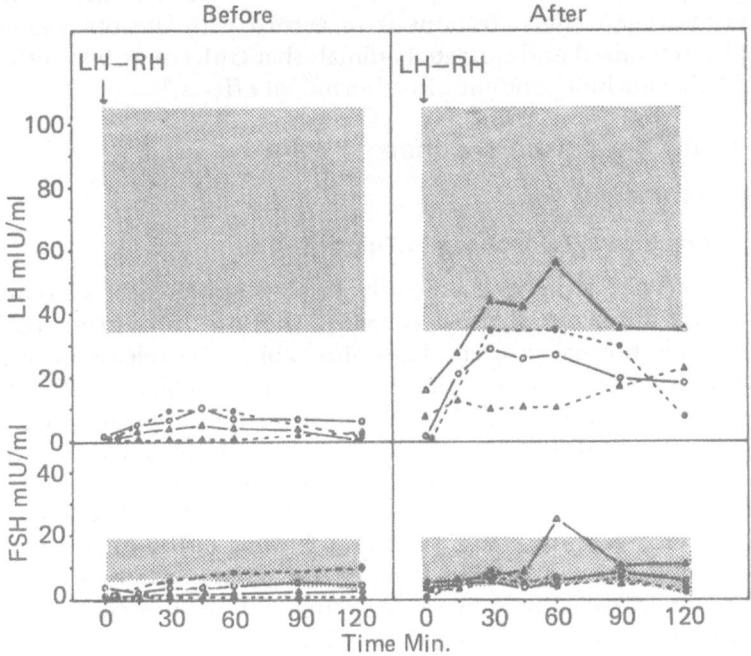

Fig. 2. Responses of plasma luteinizing hormone (LH) and follicle-stimulating hormone (FSH) to 100 μg LH–RH, before and after treatment with LH–RH, 400 μg daily, in representative cases of isolated gonadotropin deficiency. Each symbol (solid or open circle or triangle with solid or dashed line) in the left (Before) and right (After) panels represents the results of the test in the same patient. Shaded areas represent the peak ranges of plasma hormones after the injection of 100 μg LH–RH in normal subjects. (Reproduced from Yoshimoto et al.[85] with permission.)

puberty, self-administration of 500 μg GnRF subcutaneously at 8-hr intervals for 8 weeks led to increased pubic hair and testicular volume, and to spontaneous erections. Serum gonadotropin concentrations became normal, but plasma androgens (testosterone plus dihydrotestosterone) increased only slightly.[86] In this same study, similar treatment of 7 adult patients (4 with isolated gonadotropin deficiency and 1 each after treatment of craniopharygioma, acromegaly, and hypothalamic tumor) resulted in increased potency, noted 7–14 days following onset of therapy, and increased, but still subnormal, levels of plasma androgens. In 4 of the adults in whom treatment was continued for 26–52 weeks, the total sperm count increased from zero to maximum values of 7.8, 36.7, 60.8, and 432×10^6. The need for prolonged therapy is evident from an additional report in which 5 patients with isolated hypogonadism treated with 200 μg/day for 21 days showed increased serum gonadotropin levels, but no change in serum testosterone levels or improvement in azoospermia.[87]

The prompt increase in potency noted in the absence of normal plasma androgen concentrations is in accord with the observations in hypophysectomized and castrated animals that GnRF may have effects on sexual behavior independent of its hormonal effects.[88]

1.5. Neuroendocrine Disease

1.5.1. Acromegaly

1.5.1.1. Anomalous Responses to Testing

Acromegalic patients frequently display paradoxical responses to agents that stimulate (hypoglycemia, L-DOPA) or depress (glucose) GH release in normal subjects. They also exhibit GH release in response to stimuli that have no effect on release in normal subjects (TRF). It now appears that L-DOPA and TRF tests permit at least two groups of acromegalic patients to be distinguished: Of 29 acromegalic patients, 15 had a rise in plasma GH levels following TRF administration and a fall following L-DOPA administration. Of the remaining 14 subjects, 12 exhibited no significant change in plasma GH levels following either of these stimuli, while 2 had a significant fall following L-DOPA and no response to TRF.[89] There was no correlation in these subgroups with the presence or absence of paradoxical responses to other stimuli (i.e., insulin, glucose, arginine), and at present, the prognostic or functional significance of such paradoxical responses is unclear.

There is one report of an acromegalic patient who had reversal of such paradoxical responses following transphenoidal removal of a pituitary adenoma.[90] In a larger series of acromegalic patients treated with hypophysectomy,[91] 7 of 11 still had positive responses to TRF administration, although basal GH levels were now normal in 4 of the 7. Response to L-DOPA administration was not determined in these patients. Although the locus of action of TRF in causing an increase in plasma GH levels in acromegalics is unknown, the persistence of this abnormal response following successful treatment has been cited as further support of the suggestion that an underlying defect in the hypothalamic regulation of GH exists in some acromegalic subjects. From the limited information available, one cannot yet tell whether two subclasses of acromegalics will be defined—one with a primary pituitary, the other with a hypothalamic, etiology. It is of interest that GH release is also stimulated by TRF in patients with depression,[92] which might also suggest a CNS locus of action. Depressed patients have previously been reported to show decreased GH responsiveness to L-DOPA.

Another anomalous response that has been reported in acromegalic patients is enhanced suppressability by dexamethasone of the plasma cortisol response to insulin-induced hypoglycemia.[93] The mechanism of this effect is unknown. The effect of dexamethasone on other stimuli that influence the CNS–pituitary–adrenal axis in these patients has not been studied, nor has a possible effect of the acromegalic state on the metabolic clearance of dexamethasone been evaluated.

1.5.1.2. Response to Medical Therapy

1.5.1.2a. Somatostatin. With the demonstration of the marked effect of SRIF on GH release, a possible therapeutic effect in acromegaly was sought. To date, only preliminary acute studies are available, either with infusion[94,95] or with subcutaneous administration of SRIF mixed with protamine zinc insulin.[95] These studies indicate that suppression of elevated GH levels can be achieved for the duration of the infusion period, and that there is partial suppression for 4–5 hr following administration of the long-acting compound. Eventual therapeutic use will depend on either or both the availability of longer-acting preparations and the development of analogues that will influence only GH release, and not that of the other hormones that somatostatin has been shown to affect.

1.5.1.2b. Bromocryptine. When suppression of GH levels following L-DOPA administration was noted in acromegalic patients, attempts were made to use L-DOPA therapeutically; however, a stable reduction in plasma GH levels was not obtained.[96] Bromocryptine is an ergot alkaloid that also acts as a dopaminergic agonist, is active when given orally, and has a longer-lasting effect in lowering GH levels in those patients who exhibit a decrease following L-DOPA.[89] To date, there are reports of its use in 31 patients.[97–99] Excluding one regimen in which lower doses (7.5 mg/day) were employed,[99] 16 of 23 patients receiving 10–20 mg/day exhibited reduction of GH levels to normal. In the only series in which clinical manifestations were evaluated,[98] improvement was noted in all 11 subjects treated. Side effects of gastrointestinal discomfort, headache, or hypotension could be minimized by slow increments in dose. Thus far, the longest reported duration of treatment has been 11 weeks. It will be of interest to see whether permanent improvement will be reported after discontinuation of therapy.

1.5.2. Galactorrhea

It is now well recognized that spontaneous hyperprolactinemia, with or without associated galactorrhea, and usually accompanied by amenorrhea, occurs in association with micro- or macroadenomata of the pituitary, craniopharyngiomas, hypothalamic tumors, Cushing's disease, and both hypo- and hyperthyroidism. It has been estimated that 13% of patients with secondary amenorrhea unassociated with other endocrine disease have elevated serum prolactin levels, together with normal or decreased basal serum gonadotropin levels and absence of the normal pulsatile fluctuation of such levels.[100] Such patients are also clomiphine-unresponsive. Normal, impaired, or increased gonadotropin responsiveness to GnRF has been reported in hyperprolactinemic patients.[100–102] With suppression of the elevated prolactin levels, normal gonadal function returns.

Optimal treatment of the hyperprolactinemic state is now the subject of active study in several centers. Ergocryptine has been demonstrated to decrease serum prolactin levels in all species tested, presumably by a direct action on the pituitary. Its efficacy has now been well demonstrated in patients with idiopathic galactorrhea and amenorrhea,[100,103,104] in whom resumption of cyclic ovarian function occurs within 1–2 months following initiation of therapy. Several cases of successful pregnancy have also been reported. Treatment has been carried out for as long as 28 months with no side effects. Discontinuation of medication, however, is usually associated with rather prompt return of galactorrhea and amenorrhea. Ergocryptine has also been used successfully in the treatment of galactorrhea associated with pituitary disease.[102,105] There is one report of improvement of bitemporal visual field impairment while the patient received medication.[105] The comparative efficacy of medical treatment vs. transsphenoidal hypophysectomy, especially in the case of microadenomata, has not yet been adequately evaluated.

1.5.3. Cushing's Disease

As noted in Section 1.2.3.1, there is evidence for a stimulatory serotoninergic mechanism with regard to ACTH release. Cyproheptadine is a drug with definite antiserotonin effects, although it also possesses antihistaminic and anticholinergic properties. The normal rise in plasma cortisol concentration following insulin-induced hypoglycemia is blocked by prior cyproheptadine administration,[106] as is the exaggerated metyrapone response seen in patients with carcinoid tumors.[107]

Initially, 3 patients with Cushing's disease were treated with cyproheptadine.[108] Administration of 24 mg/day was associated with a relatively prompt return to normal of elevated corticosteroid levels, together with subjective and objective evidence of clinical improvement. One patient became pregnant on therapy; discontinuance of medication, thus far for 6 months, has resulted in only slight elevation of urinary cortisol concentrations. In a patient treated for 1 year, normal circadian periodicity of plasma corticosteroid concentrations, normal cortisol responsiveness to insulin-induced hypoglycemia, and return of previously absent sleep stages III and IV have also been noted.

Since this initial report, approximately 50 patients with Cushing's disease have been treated by ourselves and others, with a remission rate of approximately 60%. This may indicate the presence of two subgroups of patients with Cushing's disease, each representing a different etiology: pituitary in the one instance and hypothalamic in the other. Only the latter group would be expected to respond to cyproheptadine. The longest treatment interval to date has been 18 months, accompanied by sustained remission. Discontinuance of the drug has invariably been associated with relapse. Cyproheptadine therapy has also been effective in reducing plasma ACTH concentrations in 3 of 4 patients with Nelson's Syndrome, such reduction being accompanied by visible skin lightening in 2 of these patients.

1.5.4. Anorexia Nervosa

It is still unclear whether the endocrine disturbances seen in anorexia nervosa are secondary to chronic malnutrition or to primary hypothalamic dysfunction. The observed elevation of plasma GH concentrations appears to be correlated with the extent and duration of malnutrition.[109] Studies of thyroid function (low serum T_4 and T_3, a decreased serum T_3:T_4 ratio, and a delayed but normal TSH response to TRF[110]) are compatible with the decreased conversion of T_4 to T_3 seen in prolonged illness and starvation,[111] and with the altered pituitary responsiveness to TRF seen in hypothalamic hypothyroidism. Basal glucocorticoid function and ACTH reserve appear normal.[112]

The onset of amenorrhea prior to that of weight loss has been cited as evidence of a hypothalamic etiology of anorexia nervosa. Reports on the nature of alteration(s) in gonadotropin secretion vary. Decreased basal serum gonadotropin concentrations and absent responsiveness to an acute dose of GnRF have been reported in patients with anorexia nervosa or self-induced weight loss, in contrast to the normal responsiveness seen in patients with secondary amenorrhea without a history of self-imposed dieting or weight loss.[113] These decreased responses have no relation to observed estradiol concentrations. In other studies, either responses of FSH and LH to GnRF were absent to normal,[112] or a "prepubertal" type of response was noted, that of FSH being relatively greater than that of LH.[114] The 24-hour secretory patterns of plasma LH concentrations in 17- to 23-year-old women with anorexia nervosa were inappropriate to the patients' ages, resembling those seen in normal prepubertal or pubertal premenstrual girls, returning to an adult pattern in 1 patient who had a spontaneous remission.[115] It has been suggested[116] that the onset of menarche is related to the attainment of a "critical" body weight (about 48.6 kg), which may in some unknown manner influence hypothalamic–pituitary sensitivity to gonadal hormones. The observation of "prepubertal" patterns of response to GnRF in association with prepubertal LH secretory patterns in anorexia nervosa might represent a secondary reversal of the hypothalamic–pituitary–gonadal axis to a prepubertal or early pubertal state, perhaps engendered by the psychological mechanisms responsible for the disease.

Successful induction of follicular maturation and ovulation has been achieved in amenorrheic women with anorexia nervosa by long-term (500 μg at 8-hr intervals for 30 days) treatment with GnRF.[114]

1.6. The Pineal Gland

1.6.1. Regulation of Gonadotropic Function

Although antigonadotropic activity of the pineal gland has been demonstrated, the question as to what specific compound or compounds are responsible for such an effect is unresolved. Previously, melatonin had been the chief candidate for mediating such an effect. Subsequent studies, however, have demonstrated either antigonadal or progonadal effects, or no effect at all, of melatonin on the mammalian reproductive system. Antigonadotropic effects of melatonin-free pineal extracts have also been found. The diversity of such effects may be related in part to the species and dose employed,[117] and in part to the index of gonadal function measured (e.g., growth vs. endocrine function). Moreover, other compounds that are most likely peptide in nature, including arginine vasotocin, have been identified in mammalian pineal glands and shown to have antigonadotropic properties.

In hamsters, prolonged low-dose treatment with melatonin[117,118] or 5-methoxytryptophol[118] prevented the gonadal involution and decrease in pituitary LH concentrations[2] usually seen when animals are exposed to short daily photoperiods, whereas larger doses were ineffective.[117] In mice, melatonin also inhibited the antigonadotropic effect, as measured by the effect on compensatory ovarian hypertrophy, of one of two antigonadotropic fractions obtained from bovine pineal gland.[119] Systemically administered arginine vasotocin inhibited HCG-induced stimulation of uterine growth in mice,[120] and also retarded gonadal growth when administered early in sexual development.[121] Whether or not melatonin and arginine vasotocin modulate each other's secretion remains to be proven.

1.6.2. Neurotransmitter–Receptor–Enzyme Interactions

The basic observations demonstrating the presence of melatonin in the pineal; elucidation of the enzymatic steps involved in its synthesis from tryptophan; the demonstration that the level of the enzyme involved in the critical regulatory step, namely, serotonin N-acetyl transferase (NAT), could be altered by superior cervical ganglionectomy; and that, under influence of environmental lighting, there was a circadian variation of pineal melatonin concentration, as well as of the enzymes and intermediates involved in its biosynthesis—all laid the groundwork for fundamental investigations of regulation of circadian periodicity and of neurotransmitter–receptor–intracellular messenger interaction.

It had previously been shown that the nocturnal increase in NAT is secondary to increased β-adrenergic activity, the presence of light inhibiting the rate of firing of the postganglionic sympathetic fibers innervating the pineal. Such β-adrenergic activation is probably mediated via the adenylate cyclase–cAMP system. It has recently been shown that this nocturnal rise in NAT is secondary to stimulation of both transcription and translation, since it is blocked by both actinomycin[122] and cyclohexamide administration. There is also a circadian variation in sensitivity to stimulation by β-adrenergic agents. Exposure to low levels of neurotransmitters (e.g., lights-on or chronic denervation) is associated with rapid development both of hypersensitivity of NAT and cAMP to induction by β-adrenergic agonists and of hypersensitivity of NAT to induction by dibutyryl-cAMP.[123] Such hypersensitivity is manifested by requirement of lessened amounts of agonist to produce half-maximal NAT induction, by increases in the maximum enzyme activity achieved, and by decreases in the lag period preceding enzyme induction. A most recent finding has been the demonstration that the hypersensitive state is also associated with an increased number of β-adrenergic binding sites, an effect that does not require translation, i.e., that is not blocked by cyclohexamide,[124,125] and is not accompanied by changes in receptor binding affinity.

These findings suggest that there are several components that may be responsible for the changes seen in the hypersensitive state. Among these components could be a change in the coupling of the receptor to intracellular mechanisms (e.g., adenylate cyclase) or an increase in the effectiveness of such intracellular mechanisms (as mediated via cAMP) to synthesize or activate NAT. The findings may well be applicable to hormone–receptor interactions in other systems.

References

1. *Handbook of Physiology, Section 7: Endocrinology*, Vol. IV, *The Pituitary Gland and Its Neuroendocrine Control*, Part 1, Morphology of the hypothalamo–hypophyseal complex, pp. 1–102, American Physiological Society, Washington, D.C., 1974.

2. *Handbook of Physiology, Section 7: Endocrinology*, Vol. IV, *The Pituitary Gland and its Neuroendocrine Control*, Part 2, Secretion and regulation of adenohypophyseal hormones, pp. 367–588, American Physiological Society, Washington D.C., 1974.

3. Wilson, M. C., Steiner, A. L., Dhariwal, A. P., and Peake, G. T., 1974, Purified ovine growth hormone releasing factor: Effects on growth hormone secretion and pituitary cyclic nucleotide accumulation, *Neuroendocrinology* **15**:313–327.

4. Takahara, J., Arimura, A., and Schally, A. V., 1975, Assessment of GH releasing hormone activity in Sephadex-separated fractions of porcine hypothalamic extracts by hypophyseal portal vessel infusion in the rat, *Acta Endocrinol.* **78**:428–434.

5. Szabo, M., and Frohman, L. A., 1975, Effects of porcine stalk median eminence and prostaglandin E_2 on rat growth hormone secretion *in vivo* and their inhibition by somatostatin, *Endocrinology* **96**:955–961.

6. Goldsmith, P. C., and Ganong, W. F., 1975, Ultrastructural localization of luteinizing hormone–releasing hormone in the median eminence of the rat, *Brain Res.* **97**:181–193.

7. Jackson, I., and Reichlin, S., 1974, Thyrotropin releasing hormone distribution in the brain, blood and urine of the rat, *Life Sci.* **14**:2259–2266.

8. Brownstein, M., Palkovits, M., Saavedra, J. M., Bassiri, R. M., and Utiger, R. D., 1974, Thyrotropin releasing hormone in specific nuclei of the brain, *Science* **185**:267–269.

9. Brownstein, M. J., Utiger, R. D., Palkovits, M., and Kizer, J. S., 1975, Effect of hypothalamic deafferentation on thyrotropin releasing hormone levels in rat brain, *Proc. Nat. Acad. Sci. U.S.A.* **72**:4177–4179.

10. Weiner, R. I., 1973, Hypothalamic monoamine levels and gonadotropin secretion following deafferentation of the medial basal hypothalamus, *Prog. Brain Res.* **39**:165–170.

11. Brownstein, M. J., Palkovits, M., Saavedra, J. M., and Kizer, J. S., 1976, Distribution of hypothalamic hormones and neurotransmitters within the diencephalon, *in*: *Frontiers in Neuroendocrinology*, Vol. 4 (L. Martini and W. Ganong, eds.), Raven Press, New York (in press).

12. Oliver, C., Ben-Jonathan, N., Mical, R. S., and Porter, J. C., 1975, Transport of thyrotropin-releasing-hormone from cerebrospinal fluid to hypophysial portal blood and the release of thyrotropin, *Endocrinology* **97**:1138–1143.

13. Hefco, E., Krulich, L., and Aschenbrenner, J. E., 1975, Effect of hypothalamic deafferentation on the secretion of thyrotropin during thyropoid blockade and exposure to cold in the rat, *Endocrinology* **97**:1234–1240.

14. Setalo, G., Vigh, S., Schally, A. V., Arimura, A., and Flerko, B., 1975, LH–RH-containing neural elements in the rat hypothalamus, *Endocrinology* **96**:135–142.

15. Barry, Julien, 1976, Immunohistochemical localization of hypothalamic hormones (especially LRF) at the light microscopy level, *in*: *Hypothalamus and*

Endocrine Functions (F. Labrie, J. Meites, and G. Pelletier, eds.), pp. 451–473, Plenum Press, New York.

16. Goldsmith, P. C., and Ganong, W. F., 1975, Ultrastructural localization of luteinizing hormone–releasing hormone in the median eminence of the rat, *Brain Res.* **97:**181–193.

17. Taber, C. A., and Karavolas, H. J., 1975, Subcellular localization of LH releasing activity in the rat hypothalamus, *Endocrinology* **96:**446–452.

18. Brownstein, M. J., Arimura, A., Schally, A. V., Palkovits, M., and Kizer, J. S., 1976, The effect of surgical isolation of the hypothalamus on its luteinizing hormone–releasing hormone content, *Endocrinology* **98:**662–665.

19. Weiner, R. I., Pattou, E., Kerdelhue, B., and Kordon, C., 1975, Differential effects of hypothalamic deafferentation upon luteinizing hormone–releasing hormone in the median eminence and organum vasculosum or the lamina terminalis, *Endocrinology* **97:**1597–1600.

20. Brownstein, M. K., Palkovits, M., and Kizer, J. S., 1975, On the origin of luteinizing hormone–releasing hormone in the supraoptic crest, *Life Sci.* **17:**679–682.

21. Morris, M., Tandy, B., Sundberg, D. K., and Knigge, K. M., 1975, Modification of brain and CSF LH–RH following deafferentation, *Neuroendocrinology* **18:**131–135.

22. Uemura, H., Asai, T., Nozaki, M., and Kobayashi, H., 1975, Ependymal absorption of luteinizing hormone–releasing hormone injected into the third ventricle of the rat, *Cell Tiss. Res.* **160:**443–452.

23. Cramer, O. M., and Barraclough, C. A., 1975, Failure to detect luteinizing hormone–releasing hormone in third ventricle cerebral spinal fluid under a variety of experimental conditions, *Endocrinology* **96:**913–921.

24. Brownstein, M., Arimura, A., Sato, H., Schally, A. V., and Kizer, J. S., 1975, The regional distribution of somatostatin in the rat brain, *Endocrinology* **96:**1456–1461.

25. Pelletier, G., 1976, Immunohistochemical localization of hypothalamic hormones at the electron microscopic level, *in: Hypothalamus and Endocrine Functions* (F. Labrie, J. Meites, and G. Pelletier, eds.), pp. 433–450, Plenum Press, New York.

26. Dubois, M. B., 1975, Immunoreactive somatostatin is present in discrete cells of the endocrine pancreas, *Proc. Nat. Acad. Sci. U.S.A.* **72:**1340–1343.

27. Goldsmith, P. C., Rose, J. C., Arimura, A., and Ganong, W. F., 1975, Ultrastructural localization of somatostatin in pancreatic islets of the rat, *Endocrinology* **97:**1061–1064.

28. Hokfelt, T., Johansson, O., Efendic, S., Luft, T., and Aremura, A., 1975, Are there somatostatin-containing nerves in the rat gut? Immunohistochemical evidence for a new type of peripheral nerves, *Experientia* **31:**852–854.

29. Arimura, A., Sato, H., Dupont, A., Nishi, N., and Schally, A. V., 1975, Somatostatin: Abundance of immunoreactive hormone in rat stomach and pancreas, *Science* **189:**1007–1009.

30. Jones, M., Hillhouse, J., and Burden, J., 1976, The secretion of corticotropin-releasing hormone *in vitro*, *in: Frontiers in Neuroendocrinology*, Vol. 4 (L. Martini and W. F. Ganong, eds.), Raven Press, New York (in press).

31. Bennett, G. W., Edwardson, J. A., Holland, D., Jeffcoate, S. L., and White, N., 1975, Release of immunoreactive luteinizing hormone–releasing hormone and thyrotropin-releasing hormone from hypothalamic synaptosomes, *Nature* **257:**323–324.

32. Krieger, D. T., 1973, Neurotransmitter regulation of ACTH release, *Mt. Sinai J. Med. N.Y.* **40:**302–314.
33. Ganong, W. F., 1972, Evidence for a central noradrenergic system that inhibits ACTH secretion, *in: Brain Endocrine Interaction, Median Eminence: Structure and Function,* pp. 254–266, Karger, Basel.
34. Telgedy, G., and Vermes, I., 1973, The role of serotonin in the regulation of the hypophyseal–adrenal system, *in: Brain–Pituitary–Adrenal Interrelationships* (A. Brodish and E. S. Redgate, eds.), pp. 332–333, Karger, Basel.
35. Kalra, S. P., and McCann, S. M., 1973, Effect of drugs modifying catecholamine synthesis on LH release induced by preoptic stimulation in the rat, *Endocrinology* **93:**356–362.
36. McCann, S. M., and Moss, R. L., 1975, Putative neurotransmitters involved in discharging gonadotropin-releasing neurohormones and the action of LH releasing hormone on the CNS, *Life Sci.* **16:**833–852.
37. Fiorindo, P., and Martini, L., 1975, Evidence for a cholinergic component in the neuroendocrine control of luteinizing hormone secretion, *Neuroendocrinology* **18:**322–332.
38. Lawson, D. M., and Gala, R. R., 1975, The influence of adrenergic, dopaminergic, cholinergic and serotoninergic drugs on plasma prolactin levels in ovariectomized, estrogen-treated rats, *Endocrinology* **96:**313–318.
39. Caligaris, L., and Taleisnik, S., 1974, Involvement of neurones containing 5-hydroxytryptamine in the mechanism of prolactin release induced by oestrogen, *J. Endocrinol.* **62:**25–33.
40. Chen, H. J., and Meites, J., 1975, Effects of biogenic amines and TRH on release of prolactin and TSH in the rat, *Endocrinology* **96:**10–14.
41. Clemens, J. A., 1976, Neuropharmacological aspects of the neural control of prolactin secretion, *in: Hypothalamus and Endocrine Functions* (F. Labrie, J. Meites, and G. Pelletier, eds.), pp. 283–301, Plenum Press, New York.
42. McLean, B. K., and Nikitovitch-Winer, M., 1975, Cholinergic control of the nocturnal prolactin surge in the pseudopregnant rat, *Endocrinology* **97:**763–770.
43. Collu, R., Jequier, J. C., Leboeuf, G., Letarte, J., and Ducharme, J. R., 1975, Endocrine effects of pimozide, a specific dopaminergic blocker, *J. Clin. Endocrinol. Metab.* **41:**981–984.
44. Hoffer, B. J., Siggins, G. R., and Bloom, F. E., 1969, Prostaglandins E_1 and E_2 antagonize norepinephrine effects on cerebellar Purkinje cells: Microelectrophoretic study, *Science* **166:**1418–1420.
45. Roberts, J. S., and McCracken, J. A., 1975, Prostaglandin F_2 α production by the brain during estrogen-induced secretion of luteinizing hormone, *Science* **190:**894–896.
46. Labrie, F., DeLean, A., Barden, N., Ferland, L., Drouin, J., Borgeat, P., Beaulieu, M., and Morin, O., 1976, New aspects of the mechanism of action of hypothalamic regulatory hormones, *in: Hypothalamus and Endocrine Functions* (F. Labrie, J. Meites, and G. Pelletier, eds.), pp. 147–169, Plenum Press, New York.
47. Ojeda, S. R., Harms, P. G., and McCann, S. M., 1974, Central effect of prostaglandin E_1 (PGE_1) on prolactin release, *Endocrinology* **95:**613–618.
48. Hedge, G. A., 1972, The effects of prostaglandins on ACTH secretion, *Endocrinology* **91:**925–933.
49. Eskay, R. L., Warberg, L. J., Mical, R. S., and Porter, J., 1975, Prostaglandin E_2 induced release of LHRH into hypophyseal portal blood, *Endocrinology* **97:**816–824.

50. Chobsieng, P., Naor, A., Koch, Y., Zor, U., and Lindner, H. R., 1975, Stimulatory effect of prostaglandin E_2 on LH release in the rat: Evidence for hypothalamic site of action, *Neuroendocrinology* **17:**12–17.
51. Ojeda, S. R., Harms, P. G., and McCann, S. M., 1974, Possible role of cyclic AMP and prostaglandin E_1 in the dopaminergic control of prolactin release, *Endocrinology* **95:**1694–1703.
52. McCann, S. M., Ojeda, S. R., Harms, P. G., Wheaten, J. E., Sundberg, D. K., and Fawcett, C. P., 1976, Role of prostaglandins (PGS) in the control of adenohypophyseal hormone secretion, *in: Hypothalamus and Endocrine Functions* (F. Labrie, J. Meites, and G. Pelletier, eds.), pp. 21–35, Plenum Press, New York.
53. Gospodarowicz, D., 1974, Localization of a fibroblast growth factor and its effect alone and with hydrocortisone on $3T_3$ cell growth, *Nature* **249:**123–127.
54. Gospodarowicz, D., 1975, Purification of a fibroblast growth factor from bovine pituitary, *J. Biol. Chem.* **250:**2512–2520.
55. Fishman, J., and Norton, B., 1975, Catechol estrogen formation in the central nervous sytem of the rat, *Endocrinology* **96:**1054–1059.
56. Ball, P., Knuppen, R., Haupt, M., and Breuer, H., 1972, Interactions between estrogens and catechol amines: III. Studies on the methylation of catechol estrogens, catechol amines, and other catechols by catechol-*o*-methyltransferase of human liver, *J. Clin. Endocrinol. Metab.* **34:**736–746.
57. Davies, I. J., Naftolin, F., Ryan, K. J., Fishman, J., and Siu, J., 1975, The affinity of catechol estrogens for estrogen receptors in the pituitary and anterior hypothalamus of the rat, *Endocrinology* **97:**554–557.
58. Fishnan, J., Guzik, H., and Hellman, L., 1970, Aromatic ring hydroxylation of estradiol in man, *Biochemistry* **9:**1593–1598.
59. DeKloet, R., Wallach, G., and McEwen, B., 1975, Differences in corticosterone and dexamethasone binding to rat brain and pituitary, *Endocrinology* **96:**598–609.
60. Naess, O., Attramadal, A., and Aakvaag, A., 1975, Androgen binding proteins in the anterior pituitary, hypothalamus, preoptic area and brain cortex of the rat, *Endocrinology* **96:**1–9.
61. Naess, O., Hansson, V., Djoeseland, O., and Attramadal, A., 1975, Characterization of the androgen receptor in the anterior pituitary of the rat, *Endocrinology* **97:**1355–1363.
62. DeWied, D., 1974, Pituitary–adrenal system: Hormones and behavior, *in:* *The Neurosciences Third Study Program* (F. O. Semnitt and F. G. Worden, eds.), pp. 653–666, MIT Press, Cambridge, Massachusetts.
63. Miller, L. H., Kastin, A. F., Sandman, C. A., Fink, M., and VanWeen, W., 1974, Polypeptide influences on attention, memory and anxiety in man, *Pharmacol. Biochem. Behav.* **2:**663–668.
64. Versteeg, D. H. G., and Wurtman, R. J., 1975, Effect of $ACTH_{4-10}$ on the rate of synthesis of [^3H] catecholamines in the brains of intact, hypophysectomized and adrenalectomized rats, *Brain Res.* **93:**552–557.
65. Walter, R., Hoffman, P. L., Flexner, J. B., and Flexner, L. B., 1975, Neurohypophyseal hormones, analogs and fragments: Their effect on puromycin-induced amnesia, *Proc. Nat. Acad. Sci. U.S.A.* **72:**4180–4184.
66. Pasternak, G. W., Goodman, R., and Snyder, S. H., 1975, An endogenous morphine like factor in mammalian brain, *Life Sci.* **16:**1765–1769.
67. Terenius, L., Gispen, W. H., and DeWied, D., 1975, ACTH-like peptides and opiate receptors in the rat brain: Structure–activity studies, *Eur. J. Pharmacol.* **33:**395–399.

68. Hughes, J., Smith, T. W., Kosterlitz, H. W., Fothergill, L. A., Morgan, B. A., and Morris, H. R., 1975, Identification of two related pentapeptides from the brain with potent opiate agonist activity, *Nature (London)* **258**:577–579.

69. Guillemin, R., Ling, N., and Burgus, R., 1976, Endorphins. Hypothalamic and neurohypophysial peptides with morphinomimetic activity. Isolation and primary structure of α-endorphin, *C. R. Acad. Sci. Paris Ser. D.* **282**: 783–785.

70. Cox, B. M., Opheim, K. E., Teschemacher, H., and Goldstein, A., 1975, A peptide-like substance from pituitary that acts like morphine, *Life Sci.* **16**:1777–1782.

71. Terenius, L., and Wahlstrom, A., 1975, Search for an endogenous ligand for the opiate receptor, *Acta Physiol. Scand.* **94**:74–81.

72. Jackson, I. M. D., and Reichlin, S., 1974, Thyrotropin releasing hormone: Distribution in hypothalamic and extrahypothalamic brain tissue of mammalian and submammalian chordates, *Endocrinology* **95**:854–862.

73. Prange, A.J., Breese, G. R., Cott, J. M., Martin, B. R., Cooper, D. R., Wilson, I. C., and Plotnikoff, N. P., 1974, Thyrotropin releasing hormone: Antagonism of pentobarbital in rodents, *Life Sci.* **14**:447–455.

74. Brown, M., and Vale, W., 1975, Central nervous system effects of hypothalamic peptides, *Endocrinology* **96**:1333–1336.

75. Plotnikoff, N. P., Breese, G. R., and Prange, A. J., 1975, Thyrotropin releasing hormone (TRH): DOPA potentiation and biogenic amine studies, *Pharmacol. Biochem. Behav.* **3**:665–670.

76. Plotnikoff, N. P., Kastin, A. J., and Schally, A. V., 1974, Growth hormone release inhibiting hormone: Neuropharmacological studies, *Pharmacol. Biochem. Behav.* **2**:693–696.

77. Barbeau, A., 1975, Potentiation of levodopa effect by intravenous l-prolyl-l-leucyl-glycine amide in man, *Lancet* **i**:683–684.

78. Besses, G. S., Burrow, G. N., Spaulding, S. W., and Donabedian, R. K., 1975, Dopamine infusion acutely inhibits the TSH and prolactin response to TRH, *J. Clin. Endocrinol. Metab.* **41**:985–988.

79. Maeda, K., Kato, Y., Chihara, K., Ohgo, S., Iswasaki, Y., and Imura, H., 1975, Suppression by thyrotropin-releasing hormone of human growth hormone release induced by L-DOPA, *J. Clin. Endocrinol. Metab.* **41**:408–411.

80. Brown, M., and Vale, W., 1975, Growth hormone release in the rat: Effects of somatostatin and thyrotropin-releasing factor, *Endocrinology* **97**:1151–1156.

81. Vale, W., Rivier, C., Brazeau, P., and Guillemin, R., 1974, Effects of somatostatin on the secretion of thyrotropin and prolactin, *Endocrinology* **95**:968–977.

82. Casas, P. R. F., Badano, A. R., Aparicio, N., Lencioni, L. J., Berli, R. R., Badana, H., Biccoca, C., and Schally, A. V., 1975, Luteinizing hormone–releasing hormone in the treatment of anovulatory infertility, *Fertil. Steril.* **26**:549–553.

83. Nillius, S. J., 1976, Therapeutic use of luteinizing hormone–releasing hormone in the human female, *in: Hypothalamus and Endocrine Functions* (F. Labrie, J. Meites, and G. Pelletier, eds.), pp. 93–112, Plenum Press, New York.

84. Zarate, A., Canales, E. S., Soria, J., Gonzalez, A., Schally, A. V., and Kastina, A. J., 1974, Further observations on the therapy of anovulatory infertility with synthetic luteinizing hormone–releasing hormone, *Fertil. Steril.* **25**:3–10.

85. Yoshimoto, Y., Moridera, K., and Imura, H., 1975, Restoration of normal pituitary gonadotropin reserve by administration of luteinizing hormone–releasing hormone in patients with hypogonadotropic hypogonadism, *N. Engl. J. Med.* **292:**242–245.

86. Mortimer, C. H., McNeilly, A. S., Fisher, R. A., Murray, M. A. F., and Besser, G. M., 1974, Gonadotrophin-releasing hormone therapy in hypogonadal males with hypothalamic or pituitary dysfunction, *Br. Med. J.* **4:**617–621.

87. Hashimoto, T., Miyia, K., Onishi, T., Matsumoto, K., and Kumahara, Y., 1975, Comparison of short and long term treatment with synthetic LH-releasing hormone and clomiphene citrate in male hypothalamic hypogonadism, *J. Clin. Endocrinol. Metab.* **41:**905–910.

88. Moss, R., and McCann, S. M., 1973, Induction of mating behavior in rats by luteinizing hormone–releasing factor, *Science* **181:**177–179.

89. Liuzzi, A., Chiodini, P. G., Botalla, L., Silvestrini, F., and Muller, E. E., 1974, Growth hormone (GH)–releasing activity of TRH- and GH-lowering effect of dopaminergic drugs in acromegaly: Homogeneity in the two responses, *J. Clin. Endocrinol. Metab.* **39:**871–876.

90. Hoyte, K. M., and Martin, J. B., 1975, Recovery from paradoxical growth hormone responses in acromegaly after transphenoidal selective adenomectomy, *J. Clin. Endocrinol. Metab.* **41:**656–659.

91. Samaan, N. A., Leavens, M. D., and Jesse, R. H., 1974, Serum growth hormone and prolactin response to thyrotropin-releasing hormone in patients with acromegaly before and after surgery, *J. Clin. Endocrinol. Metab.* **38:**957–963.

92. Maeda, K., Kato, Y., Ohgo, S., Chihara, K., Yoshimoto, Y., Yamaguchi, N., Kuromaru, S., and Imura, I., 1975, Growth hormone and prolactin release after injection of thyrotropin-releasing hormone in patients with depression, *J. Clin. Endocrinol. Metab.* **40:**399–401.

93. Hofeldt, F. D., Levin, S. R., Von Werder, K., Becker, N., Schneider, V., Hane, S., Seymour, R., Adams, J. E., and Forsham, P. H., 1975, Altered hypothalamic–pituitary–adrenal responsiveness to dexamethasone–insulin tolerance test in active acromegaly, *J. Clin. Endocrinol. Metab.* **41:**309–401.

94. Yen, S. S. C., Siler, T. M., and DeVane, G. W., 1974, Effect of somatostatin in patients with acromegaly, *N. Engl. J. Med.* **290:**935–938.

95. Besser, G. M., Mortimer, C. H., McNeilly, A. S., Thorner, M. O., Batistoni, G. A., Bloom, S. R., Kastrup, K. W., Hanssen, K. F., Hall, R., Coy, D. H., Kastin, A. J., and Schally, A. V., 1974, Long term infusion of growth hormone release inhibiting hormone in acromegaly: Effects on pituitary and pancreatic hormone, *Br. Med. J.* **4:**622–627.

96. Chiodini, P. G., Liuzzi, A., Botalla, L., Cremascoli, G., and Silvestrini, F., 1974, Inhibitory effect of dopaminergic stimulation on GH release in acromegaly, *J. Clin. Endocrinol. Metab.* **38:**200–206.

97. Chiodini, P. G., Liuzzi, A., Botalla, L., Oppizzi, G., Muller, E. E., and Silvestrini, F., 1975, Stable reduction of plasma growth hormone (hGH) levels during chronic administration of 2-Br-α-ergocryptine (CB-154) in acromegalic patients, *J. Clin. Endocrinol. Metab.* **40:**705–708.

98. Thorner, M. O., Chait, A., Aitken, M., Benker, G., Bloom, S. R., Mortimer, C. H., Sanders, P., Mason, A. S., and Besser, G. M., 1975, Bromocryptine treatment of acromegaly, *Br. Med. J.* **1:**299–303.

99. Summers, V. K., Hipkin, L. J., Diver, M. J., and Davis, J. C., 1975, Treatment of acromegaly with bromocryptine, *J. Clin. Endocrinol. Metab.* **40:**904–906.

100. Bohnet, H. G., Dahlen, H. G., Wuttke, W., and Schneider, H. P. G., 1976, Hyperprolactinemic anovulatory syndrome, *J. Clin. Endocrinol. Metab.* **42:**132–143.

101. Bohnet, H. G., and Friesen, H. G., 1976, Control of prolactin secretion in man, *in: Hypothalamus and Endocrine Functions* (F. Labrie, J. Meites, and G. Pelletier, eds.), pp. 257–281, Plenum Press, New York.

102. Thorner, M., McNeilly, A. S., Hagan, C., and Besser, G. M., 1974, Long term treatment of galactorrhea and hypogonadism with bromocryptine, *Br. Med. J.* (May 25): 419–422.

103. DelPozo, E., Varga, L., Wyss, H., Tolis, G., Friesen, H., Wenner, R., Vetter, L., and Uettwiller, A., 1974, Clinical and hormonal response to bromocryptine (CB-154) in the galactorrhea syndromes, *J. Clin. Endocrinol. Metab.* **39:**18–26.

104. Seki, K., Seki, M., and Okumura, T., 1975, Effect of CB-154 (2-Br-α-ergocryptine) on serum follicle stimulating hormone, luteinizing hormone and prolactin in women with the amenorrhea–galactorrhea syndrome, *Acta Endocrinol.* **79:**25–33.

105. Corenblum, B., Webster, B. R., Mortimer, C. B., and Ezrin, C., 1975, Possible anti-tumor effect of 2 bromo-ergocryptine (CB-154 Sandoz) in 2 patients with large prolactin-secreting pituitary adenomas, *Clin. Res.* **23:**614A.

106. Plonk, J. W., Bivens, C. H., and Feldman, J. M., 1974, Inhibition of hypoglycemia-induced cortisol secretion by the serotonin antagonist cyproheptadine, *J. Clin. Endocrinol. Metab.* **38:**836–840.

107. Plonk, J. W., and Feldman, J. M., 1975, Adrenal function in the carcinoid syndrome, *Program of the 57th Meeting of the Endocrine Society,* p. 514.

108. Krieger, D. T., Amorosa, L., and Linick, F., 1975, Cyproheptadine-induced remission of Cushing's Disease, *N. Engl. J. Med.* **293:**893–896.

109. Garfinkel, P. E., Brown, G. M., Stancer, H. C., and Moldofsky, H., Hypothalamic–pituitary function in anorexia nervosa, *Arch. Gen. Psychiatry* **32:**739–744.

110. Miyai, K., Yamamoto, T., Azukizawa, M., Ishibashi, K., and Kumahara, Y., 1975, Serum thyroid hormones and thyrotropin in anorexia nervosa, *J. Clin. Endocrinol. Metab.* **40:**334–338.

111. Reichlin, S., Bollinger, J., Nejad, I., and Sullivan, P., 1973, Tissue thyroid hormone concentration of rat and man determined by radioimmunoassay: Biologic significance, *Mt. Sinai J. Med. N.Y.* **40:**502–510.

112. Mecklenburg, R. S., Loriaux, D. L., Thompson, R. H., Andersen, A. E., and Lipsett, M. B., 1974, Hypothalamic dysfunction in patients with anorexia nervosa, *Medicine* **53:**147–159.

113. Warren, M. P., Jewelewicz, R., Dyrenfurth, I., Ans, R., Khalaf, S., and VandeWiele, R. L., 1975, The significance of weight loss in the evaluation of pituitary response to LHRH in women with secondary amenorrhea, *J. Clin. Endocrinol. Metab.* **40:**601–611.

114. Nillius, S. J., and Wide, L., 1975, Gonadotrophin-releasing hormone treatment for induction of follicular maturation and ovulation in amenorrheic women with anorexia nervosa, *Br. Med. J.* (August 16):405–408.

115. Boyar, R. M., Katz, J., Finkelstein, J. W., Kapen, S., Weiner, H., Weitzman, E. D., and Hellman, L., 1974, Anorexia nervosa–immaturity of the 24 hour luteinizing hormone secretory pattern, *N. Engl. J. Med.* **291:**861–865.

116. Frisch, R. E., 1974, Critical weight at menarche and the initiation of the

adolescent growth spurt and control of puberty, *in: Control of the Onset of Puberty* (M. Grumbach, G. Grave, and F. Mayer, eds.), pp. 403–423, John Wiley and Sons, New York.

117. Turek, F. W., Desjardins, C., and Menaker, M., 1975, Melatonin: Antigonadal and progonadal effects in male golden hamsters, *Science* **190:**280, 281.

118. Reiter, R. J., Vaughan, M. K., Blask, D. E., and Johnson, L. Y., 1975, Pineal methoxyindoles: New evidence concerning their function in the control of pineal-mediated changes in the reproductive physiology of male golden hamsters, *Endocrinology* **96:**206–213.

119. Orts, R. J., Kocan, K. M., and Wilson, I. B., 1975, Inhibitory action of melatonin on a pineal antigonadotropin, *Life Sci.* **17:**845–850.

120. Vaughan, M. K., Vaughan, G. M., and Reiter, R. J., 1975, Inhibition of human chorionic gonadotropin induced ovarian and uterine growth in the mouse by synthetic arginine vasotocin, *Experientia* **31:**862, 863.

121. Vaughan, M. K., Vaughan, G. M., and Klein, D. C., 1974, Arginine vasotocin; effects on development of reproductive organs, *Science* **186:**938, 939.

122. Romero, J. A., Zatz, M., and Axelrod, J., 1975, β-Adrenergic stimulation of pineal *n*-acetyl-transferase: Adenosine 3′, 5′-cyclic monophosphate stimulates both RNA and protein synthesis, *Proc. Nat. Acad. Sci. U.S.A.* **72:**2107–2111.

123. Romero, J. A., and Axelrod, J., 1975, Regulation of sensitivity to β-adrenergic stimulation in induction of pineal *n*-acetyl-transferase, *Proc. Nat. Acad. Sci. U.S.A.* **72:**1661–1665.

124. Romero, J. A., Zatz, M., Kebabian, J. W., and Axelrod, J., 1975, Circadian cycles in binding of ³H-alprenolol to β-adrenergic receptor sites in rat pineal, *Nature* **258:**435, 436.

125. Kebabian, J. W., Zatz, M., Romero, J. A., and Axelrod, J., 1975, Rapid changes in rat pineal β-adrenergic receptor: Alterations in 1-[³H]alprenolol binding and adenylate cyclase, *Proc. Nat. Acad. Sci. U.S.A.* **72:**3735–3739.

Anterior Pituitary

William H. Daughaday

2.1. Introduction

Investigation of pituitary function in health and disease was active in 1975. The availability of radioimmunoassays for all pituitary hormones and for the separate subunits of the glycoprotein hormones have given investigators the basic tools for studying the responses to a great variety of physiological stimuli and hypophysiotropic hormones—thyrotropin-releasing hormone (TRH), luteinizing hormone–releasing hormone (LH–RH), and growth hormone–releasing factor or somatotropin release–inhibiting factor (SRIF, somatostatin)—in health and disease. This review, which makes no claim for completeness, focuses on clinical research. No attempt is made to consider the rapidly developing field of the somatomedins and other tissue growth factors.

WILLIAM H. DAUGHADAY • Metabolism Division, Department of Medicine, Washington University School of Medicine, St. Louis, Missouri 63110.

2.2. Corticotropin and Melanocyte-Stimulating Peptides

The radioimmunoassay for corticotropin has given valuable information concerning the regulation of secretion of this hormone, but there is doubt that the immunoassayable corticotropin can be considered equivalent to biologically active corticotropin in all situations. Liotta and Krieger[1] have described an improved bioassay for ACTH that is applicable for specimens of human plasma, facilitating direct comparisons between immunological and biological activity in individual samples: Corticotropin in plasma is purified by adsorption into silicic acid with subsequent desorption with aqueous acetone. The purified extract is added to primary cultures of rat adrenal cortical cells. The procedure has sufficient sensitivity to detect the ACTH in normal plasma, and appropriate diurnal changes in activity were observed. Plasma from patients with endocrine diseases had the expected changes. The ratio of immunoassayable to bioassayable ACTH in normal individuals under basal conditions was 1.10:1.64. In a later study, Krieger and Allen[2] measured immunoassayable and biologically active ACTH in normal subjects throughout a 24-hr period. Again, a good general correlation between these two methods of detection was observed. Increased levels of both indices of plasma ACTH were found in 3 patients with Cushing's disease, suggesting that there was no abnormality in the secreted hormone.

Evidence continues to accrue that the peptide in plasma that cross-reacts with antibodies raised against β-melanocyte-stimulating hormone (β-MSH) is of larger molecular size than is β-MSH itself. Gilkes and co-workers[3] have characterized the immunological specificity of two antibodies used for radioimmunoassay. One antibody cross-reacted with synthetic β_h-MSH, and also with the larger pituitary peptides, β_h- and α_h-lipotropin. Another antibody cross-reacted well with β_h-MSH and α_h-lipotropin, but had little cross-reactivity with β_h-lipotropin. Unlike synthetic β_h-MSH, which is highly unstable in plasma, the endogenous cross-reactive peptides in the β-MSH assay were stable in plasma at room temperature over 24 hr. The mean normal 09:00 level of "β_h-MSH" was 21 pg/ml (range 13–38 pg/ml), and at 21:00 it was 12 pg/ml (range 6–20 pg/ml). After induction of hypoglycemia, "β-MSH" rose in parallel with ACTH, and the results were much higher when the antiserum reactive with both β- and α-lipotropin was used. The expected rises of "β-MSH" in Cushing's disease, Nelson's syndrome, Addison's disease, and the ectopic ACTH syndrome were observed. Some of the conflicting evidence that has been obtained indicating nonparallel secretion of ACTH and MSH in response to certain stresses may be explained by the use of antisera with different specificities. For instance, Hirata et al.[4] found that the "MSH" response to ACTH was quite small, and no response to lysine vasopressin was observed, whereas a parallel response of "β-MSH" and ACTH to metyrapone was observed. The antisera used by these authors probably lacked full reactivity with β_h-lipotropin.

Genazzani and co-workers[5] have provided new evidence in support of the long-held hypothesis that the placenta secretes a corticotropinlike hormone. They found that the displacement of labeled ACTH by plasma of pregnant women did not parallel that produced by authentic ACTH. Cross-reactive material was also found in placental extracts. Such extracts also possessed demonstrable adrenal-stimulating activity when assayed *in vivo* by the Lipscomb and Nelson method. In order to establish that an ACTH-like material was actually being formed by placental tissue, the authors made primary cultures of placental tissue, and detected increased amounts of ACTH-like immunoactivity. These observations have led the authors to postulate that the human placenta makes and secretes a chorionic corticotropin that may contribute to the regulation of the adrenal during pregnancy.

2.3. Thyrotropin

Interest in the study of thyrotropin remains high. Pekary *et al.*[6] have reported an improved radioimmunoassay for human thyrotropin. They have developed in rabbits a highly specific antibody against human TSH. The equilibrium affinity constant for labeled human TSH was 4 times greater than the antibody previously distributed by the National Pituitary Agency. No cross-reactivity with bovine thyroid-stimulating hormone (TSH) or human chorionic gonadotropin (HCG) was observed, and the reactivity with monkey pituitary homogenates was nonparallel. The main advantage of this antibody is that it permits measurement of the normal level of TSH in human plasma on a workable part of the displacement curve. The authors report that the mean normal serum TSH concentration was 1.5 ± 1.0 μU/ml. With this assay, it may now be possible to study experimental and clinical conditions in which the normal level of TSH is suppressed.

There has been a continued interest in the thyrotropin subunits present in serum in various conditions. Golstein-Golarie and Vanhaelst[7] have reported their findings from gel filtration of the sera of 5 myxedematous patients. The effluents from the column were assayed using separate radioimmunoassays specific for the whole thyrotropin molecule and for α- and β-subunits. An interesting high-molecular-weight immunoactive material was detected with the β-subunit assay. In addition, there was free β-subunit immunoactivity in 4 of the 5 sera tested in a concentration from 4.5 to 40 ng/ml. An unusual feature of this study was the finding of free α-subunits in only 2 of the 5 sera. Of course, all sera contained greatly increased amounts of reactive material detected by the TSH radioimmunoassay in the expected location for TSH monomer.

Kourides and co-workers[8] searched for free α- and β-subunits of TSH in hypothyroid patients and normal subjects under basal conditions and after the administration of TRH. In the normal subjects, TSHβ was not detected either before or after TRH, and only low levels of α-subunits were found in men and premenopausal women. Greater amounts of free α-subunits were present in sera in postmenopausal women. It is likely that the free α-subunit in the latter case was associated with the increased secretion of gonadotropins, because no increase in α concentration followed the administration of TRH. The mean level of serum TSHβ in 20 patients with primary hypothyroidism was 1.3 ng/ml, and increased to 3.7 ng/ml after TRH. The α-subunit concentration in hypothyroid patients averaged 4.8 ng/ml under basal conditions, and increased to 7.5 ng/ml after TRH. Patients with Graves' disease and hyperfunctioning thyroid nodules had no detectable TSHβ in their plasma. When 3 hypothyroid women were given an injection of ^{125}I-labeled TSH, there was no radioactivity in the areas of elution of α- and β-subunits from gel filtration columns. It was concluded that the TSH subunits in serum were not derived by peripheral metabolism of thyrotropin, but were secreted as such by the pituitary. Similar conclusions were reached by Edmonds et al.,[9] who injected highly purified human TSH into euthyroid volunteers. Even though serum TSH concentrations reached 36 μU/ml, the concentration of α subunit did not increase. When the same individuals received TRH, a marked increase in their α-subunit concentration occurred.

Correlation between the biological activity of circulating thyrotropin and its radioimmunological assay is now possible with a highly sensitive *in vitro* histochemical method.[10] Explants of guinea pig thyroid are exposed to thyroid-stimulating substances. After incubation, sections of thyroid are cut on the cryostat and exposed to a naphthylamidase substrate. Enzyme activity is quantitated by a scanning and integrating microdensitometry. This method has remarkable sensitivity, and the correlation with radioimmunoassay of serum is surprisingly good. Reduced levels of bioactive TSH were observed in hyperthyroid patients. If the incubation of the thyroid slice continued for a longer time, increased thyroid-stimulating immunoglobulins could be demonstrated.

A possible dissociation of biological and radioimmunological activity in pituitaries of patients with atrophic thyroiditis was found by Vanhaelst et al.[11] Pituitaries from 22 cases of thyroiditis were homogenized and assayed by the familiar McKenzie method, and the results were compared with those yielded by radioimmunoassay. Increased amounts of pituitary thyrotropin were demonstrable by bioassay, but were not evident on radioimmunoassay. Moreover, the slopes of the dilution curves with pituitary were not parallel to TSH standards. The authors speculate that there may be a species of the TSH molecule in the pituitary with a much higher relative biological activity than heretofore recognized.

Certain observations in patients with hypothalamic hypopituitarism also suggest the possibility of altered biological activity of circulating thyrotropin. Illig et al.[12] found that basal TSH levels were slightly elevated in 6 patients with documented growth hormone (GH) deficiency and clinical hypothyroidism. After the administration of TRH, there was an exaggerated TSH response. That TRH administration to these children was followed by a rise in plasma T_4 suggested that TRH not only potentiated the secretion of TSH, but also increased the secretion of molecules of higher biological activity. This interesting speculation could be tested using the newly reported highly sensitive in vitro bioassay techniques for TSH.

Kuku and co-workers[13] have reinvestigated the metabolism of TSH in man. Following the intravenous infusion of 2 U hTSH over a 3-hr period, serum levels of TSH reached about 200 μU/liter. When the infusion was stopped, disappearance of the TSH was measured by radioimmunoassay. The mean half-life of disappearance was 77 min, and the metabolic clearance rate was 40 ml/min. It was calculated that the mean production rate of TSH in man is about 100 mU/day. The observed half-life following administration of exogenous TSH agreed closely with a value of 80 min observed following the infusion of TRH in 2 normal subjects. The urinary clearance of TSH in these experiments was extremely small. It is unexplained why the recovery of TSH from the urine is much less than that of gonadotropins.

While it has been difficult to establish an inhibitory effect of somatostatin on basal TSH secretion in normal subjects during daytime hours, Weeke et al.[14] were successful in inhibiting the elevated TSH levels that occur during the nighttime hours. Also, Lucke et al.[15] found that somatostatin could inhibit the high levels of TSH found in patients with primary hypothyroidism.

An interesting alteration of TSH secretion has been reported in patients with pituitary disease (4 patients with enlarged sella: 3 with GH deficiency and 1 with idiopathic hypopituitarism).[16] Induction of hypoglycemia by insulin was followed by a rise in plasma TSH from 4.3 to 28.6 μU/ml. No similar rise in TSH occurred in 7 normal subjects and 2 patients with acromegaly. The absence of GH inhibition of TSH release may be one factor responsible for the unusual response. It is as yet unknown how general this pattern of TSH secretion will prove to be.

Vinik et al.[17] have examined the effect of 12- and 36-hr fasts on TSH secretion. It was observed that the longer period of fasting lowered both the basal and the TRH-induced secretion of TSH.

Because of the great usefulness of TSH measurements in clinical diagnosis, it is important to determine the factors that modify the basal and TRH-induced levels of the hormone. Ramey et al.[18] found that contraceptive drugs did not alter basal TSH levels, but did increase the mean response to TRH (30 μU/ml, as compared with 19 μU/ml). It is becoming more evident that the adjustments of TSH secretion to decreased thyroid hormone levels may be considerably delayed if TSH secretion has been previously suppressed. Harada et al.[19] observed in patients with treated Graves' disease that basal TSH levels and response to TRH may remain low even after 6 months of euthyroidism. A similar delay in recovery was observed in rats after termination of large doses of thyroxine and desiccated thyroid. The kinetics of recovery of normal TSH–thyroid balance after stopping long-term thyroid therapy was studied in normal, euthyroid goitrous, and hypothyroid patients.[20] In the normal subjects, 16 days was required to regain normal TSH responses to TRH. The recovery of TSH secretion in the euthyroid goitrous patients was similarly delayed, with greater individual variation. In the hypothyroid individual, 16 days was required to reach a supranormal response to TRH. In evaluating patients after discontinuation of thyroxine therapy, it is well to remember that low levels of T_4 and T_3 may occur in euthyroid individuals during the first 4 weeks. Basal plasma TSH measurements may not reliably distinguish between normal persons and patients with primary hypothyroidism for 35 days. The authors did not believe that the response to TRH provided any additional information.

It has now been established that very small doses of thyroxine may inhibit TSH secretion after TRH without inducing any departure of plasma T_4 and T_3 from the normal range. Similarly, Saberi and Utiger[21] found that slight lowering of thyroid hormone secretion induced by 2 weeks of oral iodide produced a slight but significant rise in basal TSH levels and a doubling of the response to TRH. Such findings indicate how finely poised is the feedback mechanism to detect and respond to slight excess or insufficiency in thyroid hormone supply.

2.4. Gonadotropins

2.4.1. Plasma and Urine Gonadotropins

Improved methods of measuring gonadotropins have been reported in 1975. A radioreceptor assay (RRA) for follicle-stimulating hormone (FSH) was developed by Reichert et al.,[22] employing a rat testes tubular preparation, and by Cheng,[23] in which the receptor was partially purified plasma membranes from bovine testes. Both of these methods are highly specific for FSH. Reichert and co-workers report an index of discrimination (RRA/RIA) of 5.4 for postmenopausal serum. A much smaller index of discrimination, namely, 1.71, was found by Cheng for two pituitary extracts, but in serum, the index of discrimination was reported to be almost unity. The apparent greater receptor, as compared with immunoassay, activity of gonadotropins in serum is not observed with other peptide hormones; with them, radioimmunoassays detect substantially more material than does the radioreceptor assay.

More information has been acquired concerning free α- and β-glycopeptide hormone subunits in peripheral serum. It was observed by Hagen and McNeilly[24] that LRH caused an increase in α-subunit of 176–1760% over baseline, which in many cases preceded the rise in LH. The α-subunit response was proportional to the changes in plasma LH. Also, a rise occurred in LH β-subunits; peak values occurred 1–4 min after the peak values of LH. The magnitude of β-subunit response correlated with that of α-subunit, LH, and FSH responses. The rise in α-subunit concentration following TRH was considerably less than that following LH–RH. Edmonds et al.[25] have provided evidence that the α-subunits are secreted by the pituitary, not derived from circulating LH. After an infusion of LH, either over a 30-min period or as a single bolus, no change in the α-subunit concentration was observed.

The diagnostic usefulness of an isolated measurement of serum LH or FSH is limited because of the frequent pulsatile pattern of secretion of the hormones. For this reason, an integrated measurement of serum gonadotropins would be superior to single baseline values, although practical difficulties of repeated sampling over a period of time are considerable. To overcome this problem, investigators have correlated urinary measurements with plasma measurements. Hansen and Ross[26] measured gonadotropins in the first morning voiding of urine, and expressed this measurement as the ratio of gonadotropins to creatinine. In adult normal women, the estimated 24-hr secretion calculated in this way correlated well with the total 24-hr urine collection and with serum gonadotropin measurements. Kulin and his co-workers[27] approached the problem differently. They collected a timed 3-hr urine specimen during the day, and correlated this result with results obtained from repeated blood specimens obtained every 20 min. The 3-hr timed urine specimen provided an excellent index of the integrated blood level of LH and FSH. These two studies suggest that urinary measurements of gonadotropin, somewhat neglected in the early flush of accomplishments of radioimmunoassay of plasma hormone, may have a very practical usefulness in clinical research and in diagnosis.

Methods of measurement of the production rate of FSH have come under scrutiny by Raiti et al.[28] FSH, carefully iodinated to minimize damage, was administered to men in a priming dose, followed by constant intravenous infusion for a period of 3 hr. Blood samples were taken at intervals for the next 5–10 hr. The specific activity of FSH in plasma after equilibrium and in a pooled urine specimen was measured. The production rate of FSH of normal men, as calculated by urine excretion, was 20–45 IU/24 hr, whereas, by the constant-infusion method, the production rate was 69–108 IU/24 hr. The authors attribute the discrepancy to the uncertain immunological nature of serum and urinary FSH. It is likely that alterations in the immunological properties of this hormone occur after pituitary secretion.

2.4.2. Gonadotropins in Mother and Fetus

A detailed study of the concentrations of FSH, leutinizing hormone (LH), and chorionic gonadotropin in fetal serum and amniotic fluid has been reported by Clements et al.[29] Specific radioimmunoassays for LH and chorionic gonadotropin were developed using β-subunits for the induction of specific antisera. Little or no LH or FSH could be detected in fetal pituitary, serum, or amniotic fluid prior to 12 weeks of gestation, but chorionic gonadotropin was easily measured. Chorionic gonadotropin peaked at 11–14 weeks, with fetal serum values as high as 550 ng/ml. At the same time, amniotic fluid concentrations of 7400 ng/ml were encountered. LH became detectable after 12 weeks of gestation, and increased progressively. Fetal serum LH was still generally lower than chorionic gonadotropin during this critical period up to 20 weeks in gestation. These measurements suggest that chorionic gonadotropin is predominant in the stimulation of the fetal Leydig's cells required for masculine differentiation of the genital tract. It is noteworthy that concentrations of FSH and LH in the pituitary, serum, and amniotic fluid between 12 and 20 weeks were lower in male than in female fetuses. The authors attributed this difference to feedback inhibition by testosterone.

2.4.3. Gonadotropins in Children

The changes of gonadotropin levels in postnatal life have been described by Winter et al.[30] Chorionic gonadotropin disappears within the first 5 days. FSH is less than 5.5 μg LER-907/100 ml in both newborn male and female infants. However, between 1 week and 3 months, FSH levels rose in male infants to a value of 55 μg/100 ml. By 4 months, plasma FSH had fallen to the very low levels characteristic of the prepubertal boy. In infant girls, the postnatal rise of FSH was greater than in infant boys, reaching values of 160 μg/100 ml. Elevated levels of FSH persisted longer than in boys, and did not reach prepubertal baseline levels until 4 years of age. The situation was different with respect to LH. Peak values were reached in boys at 1 month and then declined to very low levels, but in girls, the LH value was lower. These general findings were largely confirmed in an independent study carried out by Ryle and co-workers[31] in England.

The alterations of gonadotropin secretion that occur at the time of puberty have been further studied by Parker *et al.*[32] in a series of 5 pairs of twin boys. They confirmed the earlier observations by Boyar and co-workers[33] that in early puberty, there are episodic pulses of LH release during the night, with relatively little activity during the day. This pattern was observed in 16 of the 18 nights of the twin pairs in stages of puberty 1–4; minimal daytime secretion of LH was observed during pubertal stages 1–3. Daytime activity increased during stage 4, and was equal nighttime secretion in stage 5. Measurements of serum testosterone indicated that nocturnal increases in testosterone are also occasioned by early puberty. In the earliest stages of puberty, the rises in testosterone are relatively small, but increase as puberty progresses. In the later stages of puberty, testosterone levels are equally elevated during the daytime hours. In the 5 pairs of twins, there was a striking similarity in the hormone patterns during the sleeping-waking cycles, these patterns correlating well with the stage of sexual development.

The establishment of monthly cycles of gonadotropin secretion prior to the onset of menarche was investigated by Hansen and co-workers.[34] They measured gonadotropins in overnight urine specimens from premenarchal girls for 60 consecutive days. Monthly peaks of FSH secretion were observed, with smaller changes in LH. These cycles qualitatively resembled the monthly periodicity established after menarche.

2.4.4. Gonadotropin Responses to Luteinizing Hormone–Releasing Hormone

The gonadotropin response to LH–RH has received intensive investigation during 1975. Snyder and co-workers[35] have characterized the response in men of different ages. After preliminary studies of the response to different doses, the authors injected 250 μg LH–RH intravenously for comparative studies. Despite the slight increase in basal LH that occurred with increasing age, the response to LH–RH decreased with age, almost 50% when age groups of 20–39 years and 60–79 years were compared. A similar decrease in FSH response also occurred. Treatment of normal males with clomiphene citrate, 100 mg/day for 5 days, elevated basal LH, FSH, estradiol, and testosterone levels, but markedly decreased the response to LH–RH.[36] The authors speculated that clomiphene blocked the positive feedback of endogenous estradiol on the pituitary, resulting in the low response to LH–RH. Essentially identical observations were made by Hashimoto et al.,[37] who interpreted their results as indicative of inhibition by testosterone of the LH–RH stimulation of LH secretion.

It is now evident that endogenous estrogens and progesterone greatly influence the functional capacity of the gonadotropins of the pituitary and their response to LH–RH. This interrelationship has been carefully studied in two somewhat similar investigations. Lasley et al.[38] administered 10 μg LH–RH every 2 hr for 10 hr to women during the early follicular phase of their cycle. The initial response to the first dose of LH–RH was considered to be an index of sensitivity of pituitary gonadotropins, while the integrated release over the total 10-hr period was a measure of total pituitary gonadotropin reserve. Under these conditions, there was a relatively stable increased secretion of both LH and FSH. Pretreatment of women with estradiol benzoate for 4 days was sufficient to raise the plasma estradiol to almost 400 pg/ml, and increased both sensitivity to LH–RH and the total gonadotropin reserve. While both gonadotropins were affected, the most definite changes occurred in LH secretion. When a similar dose of estrogen was followed by injection of 10 mg progesterone and the challenge of LH–RH injections started 4 hr later, there was a marked increase in sensitivity to LH–RH and in total gonadotropin secretory reserve. These investigations clearly show the complex interrelationship of estrogen and progesterone in establishing the high degree of sensitivity of the gonadotropins in the preovulatory period.

Keye and Jaffe[39] investigated how the duration of estrogen effect influences the subsequent response to LH–RH. After normal women were given an initial injection of estradiol benzoate, 5 μg/kg i.m., they received 2.5 μg/kg every 12 hr for various periods. Twelve hours after the last injection, they received LH–RH. Thirty-six hours after the first injection of estradiol, the response of LH and FSH was generally suppressed. An augmentation was evident after 60 hr, and was maximal after 108 hr of estrogen exposure. At this time, gonadotropin levels were up to 9 times those achieved during the control cycle. The modulating effects of estradiol on pituitary reserve are therefore dependent on the duration of exposure of the hypothalamus and pituitary to increased concentrations of estradiol. The late-follicular-phase rise in serum estradiol is probably responsible for the augmented response of gonadotropins at midcycle.

Gonadotropin response to LH–RH has been measured in a number of functional disturbances of puberty.[40] The LH response, but not the FSH response, to LH–RH administration was increased in children with precocious puberty, as compared with normal prepubertal or pubertal children. No increase in LH response could be found in patients with premature adrenarche and premature thelarche. Treatment of girls suffering from precocious puberty with medroxyprogesterone acetate led to a decrease in the LH response to LH–RH. These variable responses to LH–RH may have clinical application in differentiating functional abnormalities of puberty in their early stages.

Many studies have appeared describing gonadotropin levels in primary hypogonadal conditions. The sensitivity of this analysis is shown by the results obtained by Laron et al.[41] concerning gonadotropin response to LH–RH in boys with surgically corrected cryptorchidism. It had previously been established that hypertrophy of the uninvolved testis occurs. Basal LH and testosterone concentrations were normal, but FSH was significantly higher. When these patients were given LH–RH, plasma LH and FSH rose to much higher levels than occurred in age-matched normal boys. It is clear that even slight increases in gonadotropin secretion may reflect great increases in gonadotropin secretory reserve.

The pattern of gonadotropin secretion in girls with gonadal dysplasia (Turner's syndrome) during the prepubertal years is of interest, because it allows one to evaluate hypothalamic–pituitary function in the absence of feedback influence from gonadal steroids. FSH levels are definitely elevated until age 4, followed by a period from age 4 to 10 when much lower levels are encountered.[42] After age 10, there occurs a rapid rise in FSH levels to the greatly elevated levels that characterize adult patients with this condition. The pattern of LH secretion is similar to that of FSH, but the actual values in terms of LER960 are $\frac{1}{3}$–$\frac{1}{10}$ as high. The pattern of gonadotropin secretion in these agonadal individuals is qualitatively similar to that in normal prepubertal children, but is quantitatively greater. The easily demonstrable elevations of FSH below the age of 4 years may be helpful in diagnosing agonadal individuals. From age 4 to 10 years, gonadotropin levels fall, presumably because of increased sensitivity of the hypothalamus–pituitary to inhibition by steroids of adrenal origin. The subsequent rise to greatly elevated levels that occurs after hypothalamic–pituitary "puberty" is attributable to a decrease in the sensitivity to inhibition by adrenal sex steroids. Despite the high level of gonadotropin secretion in adult patients with gonadal insufficiency, gonadotropin secretory reserve as determined with LH–RH is unimpaired.[43]

Gonadotropin secretory reserve in patients with testicular disease has been evaluated by de Kretser et al.[44] A 4½-hour infusion of 1 μg/min LH–RH provided more reliable information than that obtained with a single intravenous bolus of LH–RH. Normal subjects exhibited a biphasic pattern of LH response, but not of FSH response, to LH–RH infusion. Exaggerated responses to LH–RH were obtained in patients with Klinefelter's syndrome and with the Sertoli-cell-only syndrome. An exaggerated response to LH–RH could not be demonstrated in prepubertal subjects by de Behar *et al.,*[45] which suggests that the gonad is normally inhibiting the hypothalamic–pituitary system during this period.

The pituitary gonadotropin secretion in a number of systemic illnesses has been investigated using modern methods. The hypogonadism of myotonic dystrophy was found not to have a uniform character.[46] Both hypogonadotropic and hypergonadotropic cases were found within a single affected family. In the Prader-Willi syndrome (neonatal hypotonia, mental retardation, hypogonadism, and obesity), 2 women were found to have low levels of gonadotropins and estrogens. An increase in LH and FSH occurred during 5 weeks of clomiphene therapy. One of the 2 women had a normal response to LH–RH; the other's response was similar to that of prepubertal girls. In patients with chronic renal or hepatic failure, basal gonadotropins may be low or slightly elevated. The response to LH–RH is delayed, but persists abnormally long.[47] It is possible, but not yet established, that the persistent elevation of gonadotropins in uremia is the result of decreased metabolic clearance of LH and FSH.

Amenorrhea is an almost universal manifestation of anorexia nervosa. The alterations of pituitary and ovarian function in this condition have been the subject of several investigations. Palmer *et al.*[48] examined 12 women between 16 and 24 years of age. Body weight and basal plasma FSH and LH were positively correlated. When challenged with 50 μg LH–RH, the LH response was deficient or absent in those patients with the most severe weight loss. In 4 women, the response of FSH to LH–RH was greater than that of LH. This pattern resembles that of prepubertal subjects. With successful dietary treatment, there was a restoration of normal responsiveness to LH–RH. This study is of interest because it also included 2 male patients—an unusual finding in anorexia nervosa. One patient was severely malnourished, and did not respond to LH–RH. The other patient was less underweight, and responded normally.

In the study of Warren *et al.,*[49] the LH–RH response in anorexia nervosa was correlated with the percentage deviation from ideal body weight. Deficient responses of LH to 50 μg LH–RH i.v. were found when the body weight was more than 25% below ideal. Some of these patients did, however, have an FSH response. When body weight was only 15 to 25% less than ideal, LH responses to LH–RH were either normal or supranormal, and the response of FSH was supranormal. After patients had regained normal weight, the response to LH–RH generally returned to normal. In patients with amenorrhea without weight loss, responses to LH–RH were generally normal.

A third study of anorexia nervosa, by Sherman *et al.,*[50] also demonstrated low LH responses to LH–RH in patients whose body weight was 36–47% below ideal; the FSH response to LH was not abnormal. Nutritional rehabilitation was followed by normal or supranormal LH responses to LH–RH. Because estradiol levels in these patients were less than 33 pg/ml, the authors asked whether absence of positive feedback may have limited response to LH–RH. However, pretreatment with 25 μg ethinyl estradiol for 3 days did not restore normal LH response to LH–RH in patients with severe weight loss.

These studies of anorexia nervosa are consistent in showing an impaired LH response to LH–RH in patients with moderate to severe anorexia nervosa. In contrast, the FSH response to LH–RH may be normal. These studies do not localize the disturbance of LH secretion to either the pituitary gonadotropic cells or the LH–RH-secreting cells of the hypothalamus. The decreased response could be due to a primary alteration in gonadotropic cell response to LH–RH due to the nutritional deficiency. The second possibility would be that the release of LH–RH was primarily affected, and that gonadotropic cells in the pituitary had involuted, accounting for their failure to respond to a single bolus of LH–RH. In favor of the latter view is the observation that stimulation of patients for 18–20 hr with LH–RH did result in a sustained increase in LH secretion.

In contrast to these studies of gonadotropin secretion in women with anorexia nervosa are the observations of Smith *et al.*[51] on pituitary gonadal function in men with protein–caloric malnutrition. Clinical signs of hypogonadism were present, and plasma testosterone levels were low. Plasma LH and FSH levels were high in untreated subjects and decreased during nutritional rehabilitation. A few patients had low plasma LH despite low plasma testosterone levels. Although it was suspected that impaired Leydig cell function was usually responsible for the hypogonadism, administration of chorionic gonadotropin, 4000 IU/day for 3 days, induced elevations of plasma testosterone. This finding suggests that the presumed defect in Leydig cell function could be overcome by large doses of gonadotropin, but the responses were less than those observed in normal American men receiving this dose of HCG. The lack of appropriate controls in this study renders interpretation difficult.

Gonadotropin response to LH–RH is affected by other hormones. Both corticosteroid administration and Cushing's disease decrease the LH response to LH–RH.[52] It is interesting that treatment with metyrapone for only 1 day increased the LH response to LH–RH, a finding that was attributed to decreased cortisol levels.[53]

Idiopathic hypogonadotropic hypogonadism in men, unassociated with other hormonal deficiencies, is generally considered to result from failure of LH–RH to stimulate pituitary gonadotropic cells. Such patients rarely respond to prolonged clomiphene administration with increases in plasma LH or FSH.[53] When such patients were given a single injection of

LH–RH, the LH response was either absent or decreased.[54,55] However, after repeated injections given for 1–2 weeks, the response of LH to a single intravenous injection of LH–RH was markedly increased. These findings support the hypothesis that this disease is the result of impaired LH–RH secretion, which is required for the maintenance of gonadotropin secretory capacity. In this respect, the gonadotropins differ from thyrotropins in that the secretory capacity of the latter is unimpaired in hypothyrotropic hypothyroidism.

Rarely, selective deficiency of only one gonadotropin is present, with normal secretion of the other pituitary gonadotropin. Bell *et al.*[56] have studied an interesting woman with isolated FSH deficiency. Following treatment with menotropin (Pergonal), this woman developed antibodies directed against FSH, suggesting that the hormone was recognized as a foreign antigen. When LH–RH was given to this woman, there was a rise in LH, but no change in FSH. An intriguing finding was the sharp rise in α-subunit after LH–RH. A possible explanation for this finding is a selective defect in FSH α-subunit synthesis, with excessive secretion of unutilized α-subunit.

Isolated LH deficiency occurs in the "fertile eunuch" syndrome, in which men who appear to be hypogonadal maintain spermatogenesis and have normal FSH secretion. When such a patient was given LH–RH, a normal rise in LH was observed.[57] This finding suggests a defect in LH–RH stimulation of LH secretion, but this hypothesis does not explain the maintenance of FSH secretion without invoking a separate releasing factor for FSH.

Administration of LH–RH fails to stimulate secretion of FSH and LH when hypogonadotropic hypogonadism is due to a pituitary tumor,[54] even though hypogonadotropism may be related to prolactin suppression of gonadotropins, rather than to destruction of gonadotropins by the tumor. Prolonged LH–RH secretion will stimulate LH secretion in patients with suprasellar tumors.

2.5. Prolactin

Interest in the normal and abnormal regulation of prolactin secretion remains high. The high level of prolactin that has been observed in amniotic fluid during midpregnancy has led to detailed studies of prolactin in mother and fetus. Winters *et al.*[58] measured prolactin in fetal plasma at ages of 16–19 weeks, 20–34 weeks, and 35–42 weeks, and found that the mean levels were 53, 233, and 371 ng/ml, respectively. These workers speculated that the increase in serum prolactin was temporally correlated with the increase in the adrenal weight and duration of gestation. The possibility that prolactin may increase adrenal weight was raised. It should be pointed out, however, that the relative increase in fetal adrenal size occurs in certain species in which increase in fetal and maternal prolactin does not occur.

Fang and Kim[59] compared the circulating prolactin in maternal and fetal plasma and in amniotic fluid at term. They confirm the high level of prolactin in amniotic fluid and plasma. Gel filtration of maternal and fetal plasma revealed a higher fraction of "big" prolactin in maternal plasma. On the other hand, amniotic fluid prolactin resembled fetal plasma prolactin in having less "big" prolactin. Almost all the prolactin in amniotic fluid was shown to be in the small prolactin fraction. The differences in molecular species of prolactin between maternal plasma and amniotic fluid suggested that the latter was not derived from the mother, but was derived from fetal plasma by filtration, with poor tubular reabsorption by immature kidneys. The concentration of the prolactin in the amniotic sac during midpregnancy was accounted for by the dynamic turnover of fluid involving fetal swallowing.

The high levels of prolactin in the late stages of pregnancy prompted Boyar and colleagues[60] to investigate the 24-hr secretory patterns to see whether they differed from those of nonpregnant women. Prolactin was measured at 20-min intervals for 24 hr in women during their 12th, 20th, and 32nd weeks of pregnancy. In each subject, the episodic spiking of prolactin secretion was augmented during nocturnal sleep, similar to the pattern seen in normal women. The number of spikes was not increased, but the absolute concentration of prolactin was. This finding could indicate increased secretion per secretory episode.

The role of prolactin in pregnancy and lactation was investigated by Tyson and co-workers.[61] They confirmed the secretory response to nursing present in lactating women, and observed that the increment of plasma prolactin decreased as the period of lactation continued. During the period of lactation, intravenous TRH provoked a large secretion of prolactin. Following administration of TRH, the mean percentage protein concentration in the milk did not change, but milk fat concentration did increase from 2.45% to a mean value of 3.81%. At this time, significant breast engorgement and discomfort were noted. Experimental induction of lactation in normal women was attempted by treating them with 2.5 mg Premarin twice daily for 14 days. During this period, there was an increase in response of plasma prolactin to TRH. Nipple stimulation during the last week of estrogen therapy did not increase plasma prolactin, but a definite prolactin response to breast stimulation occurred during the first 3 days after estrogen withdrawal. Breast engorgement and milk letdown was noted, and milk of normal fat and protein content was obtained from both women. One of the women adopted a baby at this time, and successfully nursed the child for 60 days.

An unusual opportunity presented itself to study an 18-year-old woman who suffered pituitary necrosis secondary to acute postpartum hemorrhage. One hour after delivery, plasma prolactin levels were between 150 and 200 ng/ml, which is normal, but after 48 hr, they were undetectable. Breast engorgement did not occur. One month later, challenge with TRH and chlorpromazine induced no rise in plasma prolactin.

It is known that estrogens will increase basal plasma prolactin in women. This led Vekemans and Robyn[62] to determine the effect of estrogens on the circadian periodicity of prolactin in women, in which the normal rise of plasma prolactin occurs in the mid or late hours of sleep. Following the administration of 400 μg ethinyl estradiol/day for 10 days, plasma prolactin began to rise before sleep, and lasted for a longer period of time than in the normal control cycles.

The effect of altered thyroid function on prolactin secretion has also received attention. Fossati and co-workers[63] measured plasma prolactin in 14 patients with myxedema, 3 of whom had galactorrhea. No elevations of serum prolactin were encountered, and the circadian rhythm of prolactin secretion during the night was not affected. As previously reported by others, the response to TRH was frequently exaggerated in hypothyroidism. It should be noted that earlier investigators had reported modest to moderate increases in basal plasma prolactin in hypothyroidism with galactorrhea. The effects of increased levels of thyroid hormone on prolactin secretion were investigated by Malarkey and Beck.[64] A single large dose of thyroxine was given to 4 normal women. No alteration in the 24-hr pattern of prolactin secretion was observed. Also, the rise in prolactin following chlorpromazine administration was normal, and the fall of serum prolactin after L-DOPA was not altered. In 3 patients with pathological lactation, similar results were obtained. These observations provide further evidence that the secretion of prolactin is not linked to that of TSH, and make it unlikely that TRH functions as a physiologically significant regulator of prolactin secretion.

The effects of glucocorticoids on the secretion of prolactin, as well as of other hormones, was reported by Copinschi et al.[65] A dose of 1 mg dexamethasone on the preceding night was sufficient to blunt the rise in prolactin, but not that of GH, following induction of hypoglycemia on the next day. When a larger dose of dexamethasone, 1 mg every 6 hr for 2 days, was administered, adrenal response to hypoglycemia was entirely abolished, and both basal and posthypoglycemic rises of prolactin were blocked. GH secretion remained only partly suppressed.

Interest in pharmacological and hormonal agents that modify prolactin secretion remains high. One of the more surprising results is the observation of Smythe and collaborators[66] that 3-iodo-L-tyrosine is an important secretagogue for prolactin in man. Ingestion of 1 g monoiodo-tyrosine in normal subjects led to a peak prolactin level of 36.3 ng/ml after about 90 min. This agent did not stimulate secretion of GH, TSH, or LH, and there were no significant changes of T_3, T_4, or cortisol. The absence of any untoward effects suggested that this agent might be a useful provocative test for prolactin secretion.

The effects on prolactin secretion of morphine administered intravenously in connection with gynecological surgery were studied by Tollis and co-workers.[67] Increased prolactin secretion occurred without alteration in plasma GH, TSH, or cortisol. The effect of morphine was blocked by apomorphine. The authors speculated that the increase was not a nonspecific stress response, but occurred via suppression of the prolactin-inhibiting factor or activation of a specific prolactin-releasing factor.

The effect of pharmacological agents is greatly influenced by the physiological conditions in which they are studied. Serotonin has been invoked as a regulator of both GH and prolactin secretion. The importance of serotonin-mediated mechanisms in the secretion of these hormones during sleep was studied by Mendelson and co-workers.[68] In normal male volunteers pretreated for 48 hr with methylsergide, a serotonin antagonist, the sleep-related peak of GH secretion was increased, and prolactin secretion was decreased by 70%. The authors confirmed earlier reports that methylsergide inhibited the GH response to hypoglycemia. These observations suggested that serotonin may be a significant modulating agent of GH secretion, inhibiting the sleep-related release of GH and stimulating the response to metabolic stimuli in the waking subject. Serotonin seems to have a greater role in increasing the nocturnal secretion of prolactin. This action is not surprising, considering the long-suspected role of serotonergic mechanisms in sleep.

One of the most important symptoms of excessive prolactin secretion in women is amenorrhea. The actual frequency of elevated prolactin levels in women with amenorrhea was studied in a busy clinic in England by Franks and co-workers.[69] They found normal levels of serum prolactin in patients whose amenorrhea appeared to be due to excessive obesity or pathological thinness and in patients with primary ovarian failure. Among 40 patients without obvious explanation for the secondary amenorrhea, prolactin levels were elevated in 8. All but 1 of 13 patients subsequently shown to have pituitary tumor had moderate to greatly elevated serum prolactin levels. Only 3 of this latter group suffered from galactorrhea. These studies underline the importance of excessive prolactin secretion as a cause of secondary amenorrhea, even in the absence of galactorrhea. It is important to recognize these cases, because therapy with prolactin-suppressing drugs may result in resumption of normal menstrual periods and fertility.

It is now recognized that prolactin is probably the most common hormone secreted in excess in patients with pituitary tumors. Child *et al.*[70] described a group of patients who presented with hypogonadism and enlarged sella turcica. All 17 women had increased prolactin levels, and 1 of 6 men had similar elevations. This series is notable because of the association of galactorrhea with hyperprolactemia in 14 of 17 women. Other authors have found a lower percentage. There was a fairly good correlation between the prolactin level and the size of the pituitary tumor, as judged by the cross-sectional area of the pituitary fossa. These patients were characterized by a low level of plasma LH. When patients were challenged with 100μg LH–RH intravenously, subnormal responses were observed in 8.

Zarate and co-workers[71] studied 7 similar women with amenorrhea, hyperprolactemia, and sellar enlargement. Only minimal responses of LH and FSH followed the administration of 50 μg LH–RH. None of these women had galactorrhea.

In a further study of the relationship between galactorrhea and prolactin, Malarkey[72] observed that most women who maintained normal menstrual periods had normal serum prolactin; the actual cause of the galactorrhea in these cases is obscure. Most of the women with amenorrhea as well as galactorrhea had elevated serum prolactin levels. In many cases, a diagnosis of pituitary tumor associated with excessive prolactin secretion remains difficult. It had been reported by Buckman and co-workers[73] that an oral water load resulted in a 50% suppression of plasma prolactin levels in normal subjects, but was without effect in patients with pituitary tumors. Adler and his co-workers[74] failed to confirm this observation. In 10 normal men, there was actually a small rise in mean prolactin, occurring within a half hour of ingestion of a water load. Also, it was noted that neither hypotonic nor hypertonic saline infusions produced significant alterations of serum prolactin. These authors did note, however, a negative correlation between plasma osmolality and plasma prolactin during water-loading.

Ergot derivatives provide a promising therapeutic approach to the treatment of galactorrhea. Many European investigators have described the favorable effects of bromocryptine administration. Five women with galactorrhea were treated with an investigational drug, Lergotril, by Cleary *et al.*,[75] and all had cessation of breast secretion within 72 hr after initiation of the drug. These patients were of interest because only 1 of the 5 had elevated serum prolactin, but the drug produced lowering of the normal level of prolactin in the other 4 patients. It would appear from the reported experiences of various authors that the ergot drugs are very effective in lowering serum prolactin and inducing ovulation in many of these patients. The length of therapy in most cases has been too short to assure that this type of drug therapy will be without serious side effects.

2.6. Somatotropin

2.6.1. Chemistry

It is now recognized that GH and prolactin do not exist as single molecular species in the pituitary or in plasma. Hummel *el al.*[76] extracted individual monkey and human pituitaries, and subjected the extracts to isoelectric focusing. This technique is a powerful method for separating closely related proteins on the basis of their isoelectric points. Single human pituitaries contained four separate bands of GH and the same number of prolactin bands. Clinical-grade human GH had five such bands. It is not known to what extent these differences in isoelectric point represent simple deamidation or more extensive changes in the molecule.

Clinical-grade preparations of GH were gel-filtered by Holmstrom and Fholenhag.[77] Those preparations derived from acetone-treated glands contained aggregated GH as a major constituent; those prepared from frozen pituitaries and subjected to gel filtration had little or no large molecular components. Aggregates of GH may be a prime determinant of antigenicity.

Another type of heterogeneity of GH and prolactin is the presence of larger-molecular-weight species that have been called "big" and "big big," depending on their elution pattern in gel filtration. Guyda[78] found that the normal or adenomatous human pituitary *in vitro* released the same patterns of these larger GH and prolactin components as was present in the patient's serum, but frequently in lower relative amounts. There was no interconversion of peaks in refiltration. The larger species of GH had lower radioreceptor activity as compared with radioimmunological reactivity, but this was not the case with prolactin. These studies provide no evidence for the preferential secretion of a larger-molecular-weight form of GH and prolactin by the pituitary. Intermolecular disulfide bonds may be responsible for "big" GH.[79] Treatment of human pituitary extracts with mercaptoethanol led to a 60% conversion of "big" to "small" GH. Further conversion was obtained when urea was added. The significance of "big" GH remains obscure, and as yet there is little evidence that it represents a true prohormone. It may be simply a by-product of monomer synthesis.

It is now known that not all circulating GH reacts equally with radioreceptors on biological membranes. Sneid *et al.*[80] compared the apparent GH measured by the receptor on pregnant rabbit liver membrane (RRA) and levels of GH measured by radioimmunoassay (RIA). Under basal conditions, the results of both assays were in good agreement. After administration of GH secretagogues, the RIA/RRA activity ratio was 1.77, suggesting an excess of nonreceptor-bound hormone.

The biological activity of GH is unaffected by treatment with some proteolytic enzymes, and is increased by treatment with others. Activation of GH by plasmin is inconstant, but Lewis *et al.*[81] studied a bacterial fibrinolysin that produces a modified hormone with a 4- to 5-fold enhancement of the biological potency when tested by the rat tibial line assay. The prolactin activity of GH was similarly increased. Three products of enzyme treatment that lacked amino acids 138–147 were isolated. Other molecular changes were not characterized. The authors speculate that the loss of the amino acids 138–147 also occurs *in vivo* during or after secretion, and results in a two-chain active molecule analogous to the conversion of proinsulin to insulin. Irrespective of this hypothesis, enzyme activation of GH may be of practical importance in extending the limited supply of biologically active human hormone.

2.6.2. Regulation of Secretion

The episodic secretion of GH in human beings is influenced by physical activity, sleep patterns, diet, emotion, and other factors. Because of the ease with which secretion of GH is modified by environmental influences, it has been very difficult to determine accurately the GH secretory pattern of normal ambulatory subjects. Plotnick *et al.*[82] aspirated small amounts of blood continuously for 24 hr with a portable withdrawal pump that did not restrict ambulatory physical activity. Hourly samples were pooled to permit recognition of secretory episodes. Unlike the findings in earlier investigations of subjects whose activities were restricted, secretory episodes were observed during the day in prepubertal, as well as in pubertal and adult, subjects. A general trend existed toward low levels of secretion in the forenoon, increasing toward evening. Despite the spike of secretion early in sleep, the general nighttime trend was downward. In this small series of subjects, who were largely male, the mean integrated 24-hr GH level in prepubertal subjects was 5.10 ng/ml; in pubertal subjects, 7.37 ng/ml; and in young adult men, 3.47 ng/ml. Analysis of their data indicated that GH secretion was not restricted to the recognized secretory episodes.

Hypoglycemia provokes GH and cortisol secretion in most normal subjects, but it is not known to what extent these hormonal insulin antagonists modify the recovery from hypoglycemia. Feldman *et al.*[83] investigated this question by inhibiting GH and cortisol secretion with the serotonin antagonist cyprohepatidine. After 2 days of administration of this drug, the cortisol response to hypoglycemia was inhibited 81% and the GH secretion 73%. Despite this modification in the secretion of insulin antagonists, no alteration in the induction of and recovery from hypoglycemia was observed. It was concluded that although these hormones must be present for normal recovery from hypoglycemia, an acute increase in their secretion is not required.

The importance of calcium in modifying a number of secretory processes *in vitro* led Ajlouni and Hagen[84] to investigate whether acute hypercalcemia modifies GH secretion. Infusions of calcium led to a rise in serum GH by 60 min, the rise increasing during a subsequent 180 min of observations. Hypercalcemia, however, was without effect on the rise of serum GH that followed L-DOPA administration.

The effects of L-DOPA and TRH on GH secretion are of interest. Normally, TRH has no effect on GH secretion, while it is a potent prolactin secretagogue. In the acromegalic patient, however, TRH is often a potent releaser of GH. L-DOPA, on the other hand, is a recognized stimulus for GH secretion in normal individuals, but usually suppresses GH secretion in acromegalic patients. These observations led Maeda and co-workers[85] to investigate the interaction of TRH and L-DOPA in the secretion of GH and prolactin in normal subjects. They found that TRH, 1 mg i.v., significantly suppressed the GH rise that followed ingestion of L-DOPA. L-DOPA, as previously reported, blocked the prolactin secretion induced by TRH. L-DOPA had unmasked the suppressive effect of TRH on GH secretion in normal subjects. The paradoxical effects in acromegaly remain unexplained. Such paradoxical reactions to TRH were previously reported in anorexia nervosa and in patients with mental depression by Maeda *et al.*[86] It is not yet known whether both the stimulatory and the inhibitory effects of TRH and L-DOPA occur at the pituitary or hypothalamic level.

The ability of somatostatin to inhibit GH secretion acutely has permitted the measurement of endogenous GH clearance in patients with disease states characterized by increased GH secretion. Pimstone *et al.*[87] found that the half-time of GH disappearance in acromegaly was 28–34 min, while in protein–calorie malnutrition, the $T_{1/2}$ ranged from 22 to 23 min. Surprisingly, when these same methods were applied to patients with severe renal and hepatic disease, half-times of disappearance were not prolonged.[88] These observations, which conflict with earlier findings, suggest that increased secretion, rather than reduced plasma clearance, is responsible for the elevations of plasma GH in these conditions.

The GH response to L-DOPA in normal subjects can be inhibited by large doses of pyridoxine given intravenously.[89] This inhibition was attributed to a stimulation of the conversion of L-DOPA to dopamine outside the CNS, thereby reducing the amount available for conversion to dopamine within the hypothalamus. That pyridoxine had no effect on the GH response to hypoglycemia suggests that pyridoxine was not acting directly on the GH secretory mechanism. Chlorpromazine, on the other hand, also decreased the response to L-DOPA, possibly by competing for dopaminergic receptors in the hypothalamus.

There is uncertainty as to whether L-DOPA stimulates GH secretion by conversion to dopamine or whether the secretion is promoted by further conversion to norepinephrine. Some insight into this question is provided by studies with clonidine. This antihypertensive drug selectively stimulates central norepinephrine receptors, and is believed to be without effect on dopaminergic receptors in the hypothalamus. Lal *et al.*[90] found that an intravenous dose of clonidine in normal men increased GH levels without altering serum levels of prolactin, FSH, LH, or TSH. On the other hand, apomorphine, which is a selective central dopaminergic agonist, caused an even greater rise in serum GH levels. This agent is also known to inhibit prolactin secretion. Lal and co-workers interpreted these observations to mean that GH secretion is increased by both dopaminergic and noradrenergic pathways.

2.6.3. Effects on Carbohydrate Metabolism

An illuminating reexamination of the effects of GH on glucose tolerance and insulin secretion was conducted by Adamson and Cerasi.[91] In their studies, GH, in doses of 5–40 μg/kg body weight, was infused for a 30-min period. After a delay of 0–24 hr, an intravenous glucose tolerance (GIT) test was performed. An impairment in glucose tolerance was present immediately after completion of the GH infusion, and increased in severity up to 5 hr. After 24 hr, a slight reduction of glucose tolerance was still evident. Of interest was the lack of any clear dose-response relationship over the range of doses of GH tested. The effects of GH administration on the insulin response to the GIT are of interest. With 10 μg/kg GH, an inhibition of insulin release, calculated as an insulinogenic index, was present at 300 min. With a higher dose of GH, 40 μg/kg, this inhibition was present at 60 min. Considerable variability of individual responses occurred at lower GH doses. The conclusion to be drawn from these studies is that GH has both an initial inhibitory action on insulin secretion and an action to promote hyperinsulinism after chronic exposure. This acute inhibition of insulin secretion, like the acute inhibition of glucose tolerance, may be of homeostatic importance.

2.6.4. New Therapeutic Applications

Investigations of the possible therapeutic usefulness of HGH in conditions other than pituitary dwarfism, and possibly in certain cases of juvenile hypoglycemia, have been limited by the availability of sufficient hormone for exploratory study. A condition that might possibly be benefited by GH treatment is acute gastric stress ulcers. This disorder occurs in association with a number of serious illnesses, and may lead to death by exsanguination. Winawer et al.[92] reasoned that a defect in normal gastric regenerative cell proliferation was responsible. Eight cancer patients with acute stress ulcer were treated with HGH, 10 mg/day. Two patients died within 3½ days, while 6 survivers received HGH for 4–18 days. While this study was not randomized, the authors considered the response suggestive considering that experience in their hospital indicates that this condition is nearly always fatal. The experimental design makes this interpretation tenuous at best, but certainly a proper examination of this question is warranted.

2.6.5. Acromegaly

Plasma lipids were measured in a large group of acromegalic patients by Nikkilä and Pelkonen.[93] Cholesterol was not elevated, but plasma triglyceride was elevated, and a Type IV pattern existed in many of the patients. The serum triglyceride did not correlate with the various hormonal measurements, except that it was more common in patients with the highest plasma insulin response. Patients with initial elevations of triglycerides had chemical improvement following successful surgical treatment of the acromegaly.

The neuromuscular complications in 17 consecutive acromegalic patients were characterized by Pickett et al.[94] Of these patients, 8 had the carpal tunnel syndrome by electrodiagnostic methods, and, in them, the mean duration of acromegaly was 14 years. Although 5 of 6 patients showed prompt symptomatic improvement after hypophysectomy, electrical conduction defects persisted for a year or more. In addition to median nerve disorders, ulnar nerve irritability was present in 2. Parasthesias of the feet occurred in 2.

Of the 17 acromegalic patients, 9 had myopathy evidenced by proximal muscle weakness and, in some cases, by myopathic EMG changes. The patients with myopathy had had their acromegaly longer than those without myopathy. Most cases complained only of decreased exercise tolerance. Difficulty was encountered in rising from chairs and elevating the arms. True atrophy of muscles was recognized in only 1 patient, but the muscles often had a flabby character. Plasma enzyme elevations were minimal. Light-microscopic findings in muscle biopsies were normal in 3 patients biopsied, but electron microscopy showed focal loss of muscle fibrils and whole sarcomeres. These findings are to be contrasted with those observed in a Chinese man with acromegaly by Cheah et al.[95]

Electron microscopy of this patient's muscle showed pleomorphic, elongated mitochondria, frequently with loss of mitochondrial cristae and contents. Increased cytoplasmic glycogen granules, inclusion bodies, and vacuoles were also present. Nine months after hypophysectomy, there was a return toward normal of these abnormal changes.

Because an abnormality in hypothalamic function in acromegaly has been widely suspected, the degree of normality or abnormality of GH secretion after selective removal of a small pituitary adenoma is of critical interest. Unfortunately, the number of adequately studied patients remains small. A patient reported by Hoyte and Martin[96] was noted to have a paradoxical suppression of serum GH levels by L-DOPA and apomorphine preoperatively. These drugs are dopamine agonists that probably act directly on the hypothalamus to influence secretion of GH-inhibiting factor (somatostatin). After elective adenomectomy, the administration of these drugs provoked GH secretion. The patient was also observed to secrete GH in response to TRH and LH–RH preoperatively, but not postoperatively. The authors conclude that the paradoxical response to dopamine agonists may have been due to a short-loop feedback inhibition of the hypothalamus by the high serum GH. How this would change the response from stimulation to suppression was not clarified. The preoperative response to TRH and LH–RH was believed to be a direct effect on the neoplastic somatotropin that had acquired receptors for these hypophysiotropic hormones. While the apparent postoperative normality of this patient argues against an underlying primary hypothalamic disorder in acromegaly, many more patients will have to be studied to determine whether other patterns of hypothalamic–pituitary function are encountered after surgical removal of pituitary somatotropic cell adenomas.

Even though hypothalamic noradrenergic and dopaminergic mechanisms may be altered during acromegaly, the peripheral secretion of norepinephrine and epinephrine appears to be normal, both in the supine position and after the upright position is assumed, according to Cryer.[97] This study does not confirm earlier studies with less elegant analytical methods.

A subtle change in the control of ACTH secretion has been reported to occur in acromegaly by Hofeldt et al.[98] They report that the cortisol response to hypoglycemia was intact in acromegaly. However, while the normal subject who receives 1 mg dexamethasone at 23:00 will have an essentially normal cortisol response to hypoglycemia the next morning, this dose of dexamethasone was effective in blocking cortisol secretion in acromegaly.

The response of 11 acromegalic patients to TRH, LH–RH, and somatostatin was described by Gomez-Pan and co-workers.[99] In response to TRH, 8 patients had a rise in serum GH, not necessarily coupled with a rise in TSH. As previously reported, the GH rise to TRH was abolished by somatostatin. In this series of patients, only 1 exhibited a major GH response to LH–RH; less definite rises in serum GH occurred in 2 other patients.

Despite the prospect of controlling acromegaly by administering somatostatin, this hope has not been realized because the brief duration of GH suppression would require repeated parenteral injection; moreover, as yet, doses that are effective in suppressing GH secretion in acromegaly also suppress secretion of insulin[100] as well as glucagon. Intensive pharmaceutical research to solve these problems is now under way.

Another possible mode of medical therapy of acromegaly has attracted interest. Camanni et al.[101] reported that 2-Br-α-ergocryptine (CB-154) acutely lowered serum GH to normal or near-normal levels in 4 of 8 acromegalic patients. Chiodini and co-workers[102] then reported that GH levels of patients who were acutely suppressed by CB-154 could be maintained at low levels for a month or more. Thorner et al.[103] were also able to maintain prolonged suppression of GH in 9 of 11 patients treated for 7–11 weeks. In addition to clinical improvement, the authors reported increased glucose tolerance and reduced hydroxyproline secretion in certain patients. Careful adjustment of dosage prevented troublesome side effects of nausea and vomiting. They concluded that CB-154 "holds promise as a safe and orally effective medical treatment."

A less favorable experience with CB-154 treatment of 8 acromegalic patients was reported by Summers et al.[104] In only 1 patient was the GH level lowered to normal. Troublesome vomiting occurred in 3 patients.

A frustrating experience is to find that apparently complete surgical emptying of the sella turcica has failed to cure an acromegalic patient. It has long been recognized that rapidly growing and invasive adenomas can invade the nasal sinuses and the middle and posterior fossae, and occasionally invade the cavernous sinuses, carotid artery, and cranial nerves. Shaffi and Wrightson[105] demonstrated that the extension of tumor cells into surrounding structures is much more frequent than hitherto suspected. They examined the dura mater of the sella turcica or diaphragma sellae in 9 operative and 4 autopsied patients with pituitary tumors of varied function, including 4 patients with acromegaly. In 9 cases, tumor cells were identified deep within the substance of the dura in an area inaccessible to usual surgical treatment. Such cells were never recognized in similar specimens obtained from patients without pituitary tumors. In addition, sinusoidal invasion was observed in 8 cases without evidence of distant metastases, and invasion of cavernous sinuses was detected in 3 patients.

It is remarkable that dural invasion was not restricted to clinically invasive tumors, but also occurred with otherwise benign tumors. This study provides an explanation for the difficulty encountered in eradicating hormone-secreting pituitary tumor cells in some patients. Operative intervention at an early stage of the disease may decrease the likelihood of dural extension.

There is continued enthusiasm for selective transsphenoidal hypophysectomy in acromegaly. This form of therapy was selected for 59 of 100 cases of acromegaly seen at Middlesex Hospital in London.[106] Only 8 of these patients were previously untreated. Serum GH levels less than 5 ng/ml were achieved in 46 of the patients. Of these, 20 did not have clinically significant deficits of other pituitary hormones postoperatively. Radiation therapy was employed for those patients whose GH levels had not fallen to a normal range and who had not previously been irradiated. Essentially similar results of transsphenoidal hypophysectomy were reported by Atkinson *et al.*[107] in a smaller series of 17 acromegalic patients. Pelkonen and Grahne[108] added cryoapplication to suspicious areas of dura observed during transsphenoidal operation. They suggest, without convincing evidence, that this addition improved the results of the operation.

2.6.6. Hypopituitarism

In most cases, idiopathic hypopituitarism in children appears to be the result of hypothalamic disease. Direct evidence that the hyposomatotropism is due to a defect in GH-releasing factor cannot be obtained until this hypophysiotropic hormone is identified, synthesized, and administered to these patients. However, an autopsy of a woman with familial isolated hyposomatotropism has provided ultrastructural and radioimmunoassay evidence of the presence of GH in the patient's pituitary.[109] Although the number of somatotropic cells was reduced to 20% of normal, these cells contained characteristic granules 210–380 nm in diameter. Extraction of the fixed pituitary demonstrated radioimmunoassayable GH, but comparison with normal pituitaries was rendered difficult by the prior fixation. This case and a similar case reported by Rimoin and Schecter[110] suggest that in this disorder, somatotropic cells are present, but are not stimulated to secrete GH.

The recognition of GH deficiency in neonatal infants is seldom achieved. Most hypopituitary dwarfs are of near-normal size at birth, and attract attention only when growth achievement falls below normal standards some time after the first year of life. Lovinger *et al.*[111] described 4 infants who were noted to have neonatal hypoglycemia and microphallus. Subsequent studies established hyposomatotropism. TSH and prolactin responses to TRH suggested an underlying hypothalamic, rather than pituitary, disorder. The microphallus was improved by early testosterone treatment. Pediatricians should be alerted to these clinical findings of hypopituitarism that are evident soon after birth.

The hypoglycemia of older hypopituitary children was reinvestigated by Hopwood et al.[112] Of 52 pituitary dwarfs, 9 had symptomatic and 14 had asymptomatic hypoglycemia. This latter observation indicates the need for studies of fasting blood sugar in pituitary dwarfs. Hypoglycemia was most frequent below age 4 in relatively lean patients. A defect in mobilization of alanine and other gluconeogenic substrates was the presumed cause of hypoglycemia.

Confirmatory studies continue to appear that TSH and prolactin responses to TRH are normal in patients with "idiopathic" pituitary dwarfism.[113] While the acute LH and FSH responses to LH–RH are frequently subnormal, these patients improved markedly after LH–RH administration for 1 month.

In a provocative report, Bernasconi et al.[114] found that α-MSH administration caused a small but significant increase in GH secretion in 3 of 5 hypopituitary children with craniopharyngiomas. Other provocative tests for GH secretion were ineffective. The authors speculated that the α-MSH was acting directly as a secretagogue on the somatotropic cells—a hypothesis that fails to explain why 5 other patients with idiopathic hypopituitarism failed to respond in a similar fashion.

The great number of provocative tests of GH secretory capacity that have appeared suggest that none is really completely satisfactory. This state of affairs has led most workers to require more than one test before making the diagnosis of hypopituitarism. A number of tests utilizing combinations of secretagogues are now appearing. Weldon et al.[115] administered L-DOPA, 125–500 mg on the basis of weight, and arginine, 0.5 g/kg body weight. The combination of agents induced a higher response than the individual agents, and allowed the authors to recognize children with partial GH secretion. The question might well be asked whether such potent GH secretagogues might exclude children who would benefit from GH treatment.

The pituitary–adrenal axis of idiopathic pituitary dwarfs was studied by Lombardi et al.[116] While baseline levels of cortisol and ACTH were low normal, the rise in plasma ACTH after insulin-induced hypoglycemia was markedly impaired (91 ± 17.5 pg/ml, vs 312 ± 50 pg/ml for controls). Likewise, the pituitary–thyroid axis is also frequently abnormal. In 8 patients, the mean T_3 concentration was 36.2 ng/dl, vs. a mean for normals in this laboratory of 107 ng/dl. Also, the plasma T_3 after TRH rose only to 62 ng/dl.

Patients with idiopathic GH deficiency who initially appear to be euthyroid may become hypothyroid during GH treatment, exhibiting a decreasing growth rate, symptoms of hypothyroidism, and low levels of T_4 and T_3 in their plasma. Lippe *et al.*[117] described their experiences with 6 such children. During GH treatment, TSH response to TRH was either absent or diminished in 4 of 6 patients. Discontinuation of GH treatment was followed by a return to euthyroidism in 3 children, and reinstitution of GH treatment was followed by a return of hypothyroidism. This study emphasizes the frequency of GH-induced hypothyroidism. The mechanism of GH inhibition of TSH secretion is obscure.

It has generally been considered that the normal pituitary is peculiarly resistant to radiation damage, and that postradiation hypopituitarism seldom results. Samaan *et al.*,[118] however, found evidence of endocrine deficiency in 14 of 15 patients subjected to intensive radiation treatment for nasopharyngeal cancer. Most commonly observed was a high basal serum prolactin level, which did not rise further after chlorpromazine. This finding suggests hypothalamic rather than pituitary damage. In 11 cases, the GH response to hypoglycemia was deficient, and 6 of these patients also failed to have the expected rise in cortisol during this test. In 3 cases, the TSH response to TRH was absent. These studies indicate that both hypothalamic and pituitary deficiency can occur secondary to therapeutic radiation.

References

1. Liotta, A. and Krieger, D. T., 1975, A sensitive bioassay for the determination of human plasma ACTH levels, *J. Clin. Endocrinol. Metab.* **40:**268–277.
2. Krieger, D. T., and Allen, W., 1975, Relationship of bioassayable and immunoassayable plasma ACTH and cortisol concentrations in normal subjects and in patients with Cushing's disease, *J. Clin. Endocrinol. Metab.* **40:**675–687.
3. Gilkes, J. J. H., Bloomfield, G. A., Scott, A. P., Lowery, P. J., Ratcliffe, J. G., Landon, J., and Rees, L. H., 1975, Development and validation of a radioimmunoassay for peptides related to β-melanocyte stimulation hormone in human plasma: The lipotropins, *J. Clin. Endocrinol. Metab.* **40:**450–457.
4. Hirata, Y., Sakamoto, N., Matsukura, S. and Imura, H., 1975, Plasma levels of β-MSH and ACTH during acute stresses and metyrapone administration in man, *J. Clin. Endocrinol. Metab.* **41:**1092–1097.
5. Genazzani, A. R., Fraioli, F., Hurlimann, J., Fioretti, P., and Felber, J. P., 1975, Immunoreactive ACTH and cortisol plasma levels during pregnancy. Detection and partial purification of corticotrophin-like placental hormone: The human chorionic corticotrophin (HCC), *Clin. Endocrinol.* **4:**1–14.
6. Pekary, A. E., Hershman, J. M., and Parlow, A. F., 1975, A sensitive and precise radioimmunoassay for human thyroid-stimulating hormone, *J. Clin. Endocrinol. Metab.* **41:**676–684.
7. Golstein-Golaire, J., and Vanhaelst, L., 1975, Gel filtration profile of circulating immunoreactive thyrotropin and subunits of myxedematous sera, *J. Clin. Endocrinol. Metab.* **41:**575–580.

8. Kourides, I. A., Weintraub, B. D., Ridgway, E. C., and Maloof, F., 1975, Pituitary secretion of free alpha and beta subunit of human thyrotropin in patients with thyroid disorders, *J. Clin. Endocrinol. Metab.* **40:**872–885.

9. Edmonds, M., Molitch, M., Pierce, J., and Odell, W. D., 1975, Secretion of alpha and beta subunits of TSH by the anterior pituitary, *Clin. Endocrinol.* **4:**525–530.

10. Petersen, V., Smith, B. R., and Hall, R., 1975, A study of thyroid stimulating activity in human serum with the highly sensitive cytochemical bioassay, *J. Clin. Endocrinol. Metab.* **41:**199–202.

11. Vanhaelst, L., Bonnyns, M., and Golstein-Golaire, J., 1975, Pituitary TSH in normal subjects and in patients with asymptomatic atrophic thyroiditis: Evidence for its immunological heterogeneity, *J. Clin. Endocrinol. Metab.* **41:**115–119.

12. Illig, R., Krawczyńska, H., Torresani, T., and Prader, A., 1975, Elevated plasma TSH and hypothyroidism in children with hypothalamic hypopituitarism, *J. Clin. Endocrinol. Metab.* **41:**722–728.

13. Kuku, S. F., Harsoulis, P., Kjeld, M., and Fraser, T. R., 1975, Human thyrotrophic hormone kinetics and effects in euthyroid males, *Horm. Metab. Res.* **7:**54–59.

14. Weeke, J., Hansen, A. P., and Lundaek, K., 1975, Inhibition by somatostatin of basal levels of serum thyrotropin (TSH) in normal men, *J. Clin. Endocrinol. Metab.* **41:**168–171.

15. Lucke, C., Höffken, B., and von zur Mühlen. A., 1975, The effect of somatostatin on TSH levels in patients with primary hypothyroidism, *J. Clin. Endocrinol. Metab.* **41:**1082–1084.

16. Guansing, A. R., Leung, Y., Ajlouni, K., and Hagen, T. C., 1975, The effect of hypoglycemia on TSH release in man, *J. Clin. Endocrinol. Metab.* **40:**755–758.

17. Vinik, A. J., Kalk, W. J., McLaren, H., Hendricks, S., and Pimstone, B. L., 1975, Fasting blunts the TSH response to synthetic thyrotropin-releasing hormone (TRH), *J. Clin. Endocrinol. Metab.* **40:**509–515.

18. Ramey, J. N., Burrow, G. N., Polackwich, R. J., and Donabedian, R. K., 1975, The effect of oral contraceptive steroids on the response of thyroid-stimulating hormone to thyrotropin-releasing hormone, *J. Clin. Endocrinol. Metab.* **40:**712–714.

19. Harada, A., Kojima, A., Tsukui, T., Onaya, T., Yamada, T., Ikejiri, K., and Yukimura, Y., 1975, Pituitary unresponsiveness to thyrotropin-releasing hormone in thyrotoxic patients during chronic anti-thyroid drug therapy and in rats previously treated with excess thyroid hormone, *J. Clin. Endocrinol. Metab.* **40:**942–948.

20. Krugman, L. G., Hershman, J. M., Chopra, I. J., Levine, G. A., Pekary, A. E., Geffner, D. L., and Chua Teco, G. N., 1975, Patterns of recovery of the hypothalamic–pituitary–thyroid axis in patients taken off chronic thyroid therapy, *J. Clin. Endocrinol. Metab.* **41:**70–80.

21. Saberi, M., and Utiger, R. D., 1975, Augmentation of thyrotropin responses to thyrotropin-releasing hormone following small decreases in serum thyroid hormone concentrations, *J. Clin. Endocrinol. Metab.* **40:**435–441.

22. Reichert, L. E., Jr., Ramsey, R. B., and Carter, E. B., 1975, Application of a tissue receptor assay to measurement of serum follitropin (FSH), *J. Clin. Endocrinol. Metab.* **41:**634–637.

23. Cheng, K.-W., 1975, A radioreceptor assay for follicle-stimulating hormone, *J. Clin. Endocrinol. Metab.* **41:**581–589.

24. Hagen, C., and McNeilly, A. S., 1975, Changes in circulating levels of LH, FSH, LHβ- and α-subunit after gonadotropin-releasing hormone, and of TSH, LHβ- and α-subunit after thyrotropin-releasing hormone, *J. Clin. Endocrinol. Metab.* **41**:466–470.
25. Edmonds, M., Molitch, M., Pierce, J. G., and Odell, W. D., 1975, Secretion of alpha subunits of luteinizing hormone (LH) by the anterior pituitary, *J. Clin. Endocrinol. Metab.* **41**:551–555.
26. Hansen, J. W., and Ross, G. T., 1975, A new method simplifying collection of serial specimens for gonadotropin determinations, *J. Clin. Endocrinol. Metab.* **41**:241–244.
27. Kulin, H. E., Bell, P. M., Santen, R. J., and Ferber, A. J., 1975, Integration of pulsatile gonadotropin secretion by timed urinary measurements: An accurate and sensitive 3-hour test, *J. Clin. Endocrinol. Metab.* **40**:783–789.
28. Raiti, S., Blizzard, R. M., Penny, R., and Migeon, C. J., 1975, Critical analysis of methods for estimating production rates of FSH, *Acta Endocrinol.* **80**:275–283.
29. Clements, J. A., Reyes, F. I., Winter, J. S. D., and Faiman, C., 1976, Studies on human sexual development. III. Fetal pituitary and serum, and amniotic fluid concentrations of LH, CG and FSH, *J. Clin. Endocrinol. Metab.* **42**:9–19.
30. Winter, J. S. D., Faiman, C., Hobson, W. C., Prasad, A. V., and Reyes, F. I., 1975, Pituitary–gonadal relations in infancy. I. Patterns of serum gonadotropin concentrations from birth to four years of age in man and chimpanzee, *J. Clin. Endocrinol. Metab.* **40**:545–551.
31. Ryle, M., Stephenson, J., Williams, J., and Stuart, J., 1975, Serum gonadotrophins in young children, *Clin. Endocrinol.* **4**:413–419.
32. Parker, D. C., Judd, H. L., Rossman, L. G., and Yen, S. S. C., 1975, Pubertal sleep–wake patterns of episodic LH, FSH and testosterone release in twin boys, *J. Clin. Endocrinol. Metab.* **40**:1099–1109.
33. Boyar, R. M., Finkelstein, J., Roffwarg, H., Kapen, S., Weitzman, E., and Hellman, L., 1972, Synchronization of augmented luteinizing hormone secretion with sleep during puberty, *N. Engl. J. Med.* **287**:582–586.
34. Hansen, J. W., Hoffman, H. J., and Ross, G. T., 1975, Monthly gonadotropin cycles in premenarcheal girls, *Science* **190**:161–163.
35. Snyder, P. J., Reitano, J. F., and Utiger, R. D., 1975, Serum LH and FSH responses to synthetic gonadotropin-releasing hormone in normal men, *J. Clin. Endocrinol. Metab.* **41**:938–945.
36. Wang, C. F., Lasley, B. L., and Yen, S. S. C., 1975, The role of estrogen in the modulation of pituitary sensitivity to LRF (luteinizing hormone–releasing factor) in men, *J. Clin. Endocrinol. Metab.* **41**:41–43.
37. Hashimoto, T., Miyai, K., Matsumoto, K., Izumi, K., and Kumahara, Y., 1975, LH and FSH response to synthetic LHRH after consecutive administration of clomiphene citrate in normal males, *J. Clin. Endocrinol. Metab.* **41**:1110–1112.
38. Lasley, B. L., Wang, C. F., and Yen, S. S. C., 1975, The effects of estrogen and progesterone on the functional capacity of the gonadotrophs, *J. Clin. Endocrinol. Metab.* **41**:820–826.
39. Keye, W. R., Jr., and Jaffe, R. B., 1975, Strength–duration characteristics of estrogen effects on gonadotropin response to gonadotropin-releasing hormone in women. I. Effects of varying duration of estradiol administration, *J. Clin. Endocrinol. Metab.* **41**:1003–1008.
40. Reiter, E. O., Kaplan, S. L., Conte, F. A., and Grumbach, M. M., 1975,

Responsivity of pituitary gonadotropes to luteinizing hormone–releasing factor in idiopathic precocious puberty, precocious thelarche, precocious adrenarche, and in patients treated with medroxyprogesterone acetate, *Pediatr. Res.* **9:**111–116.

41. Laron, Z., Dickerman, Z., Prager-Lewin, R., Keret, R., and Halabe, E., 1975, Plasma LH and FSH response to LRH in boys with compensatory testicular hypertrophy, *J. Clin. Endocrinol. Metab.* **40:**977–981.

42. Conte, F. A., Grumbach, M. M., and Kaplan, S. L., 1975, A diphasic pattern of gonadotropin secretion in patients with the syndrome of gonadal dysgenesis, *J. Clin. Endocrinol. Metab.* **40:**670–674.

43. Huang, K.-E., 1975, Pituitary response to synthetic luteinizing hormone–releasing hormone in patients with Turner's syndrome, *J. Clin. Endocrinol. Metab.* **41:**771–776.

44. de Kretser, D. M., Burger, H. G., and Dumpys, R., 1975, Serum LH and FSH response in four-hour infusions of luteinizing hormone–releasing hormone in normal men, Sertoli cell only syndrome, and Klinefelter's syndrome, *J. Clin. Endocrinol. Metab.* **41:**876–886.

45. de Behar, B. R., Mendilaharzu, H., Rivarola, M. A., and Bergadá, C., 1975, Gonadotropin secretion in prepubertal and pubertal primary hypogonadism: Response to LHRH, *J. Clin. Endocrinol. Metab.* **41:**1070–1075.

46. Febres, F., Scaglia, H., Lisker, R., Espinosa, J., Morato, T., Shkurovich, M., and Pérez-Palacios, G., 1975, Hypothalamic–pituitary–gonadal function in patients with myotonic dystrophy, *J. Clin. Endocrinol. Metab.* **41:**833–840.

47. Schalch, D. S., Gonzalez-Barcena, D., Kastin, A. J., Landa, L., Lee, L. A., Zamora, M. T., and Schally, A. V., 1975, Plasma gonadotropins after administration of LH-releasing hormone in patients with renal or hepatic failure, *J. Clin. Endocrinol. Metab.* **41:**921–925.

48. Palmer, R. L., Crisp, A. H., Mackinnon, P. C. B., Franklin, M., Bonnar, J., and Wheeler, M., 1975, Pituitary sensitivity to 50 μg LH/FSH-RH in subjects with anorexia nervosa in acute and recovery stages, *Br. Med. J.* **I:**179–182.

49. Warren, M. P., Jewelewicz, R., Dyrenfurth, I., Ans, R., Khalaf, S., and Vande Wiele, R. L., 1975, The significance of weight loss in the evaluation of pituitary response to LH–RH in women with secondary amenorrhea, *J. Clin. Endocrinol. Metab.* **40:**601–611.

50. Sherman, B. M., Halmi, K. A., and Zamudio, R., 1975, LH and FSH response to gonadotropin-releasing hormone in anorexia nervosa: Effect of nutritional rehabilitation, *J. Clin. Endocrinol. Metab.* **41:**135–142.

51. Smith, S. R., Chhetri, M. K., Johanson, A. J., Radfar, N., and Migeon, C. J., 1975, The pituitary–gonadal axis in men with protein–calorie malnutrition, *J. Clin. Endocrinol. Metab.* **41:**60–69.

52. Boccuzzi, G., Angeli, A., Bisbocci, D., Fonzo, D., Gaidano, G. P., and Ceresa, F., 1975, Effect of synthetic luteinizing hormone releasing hormone (LH–RH) on the release of gonadotropins in Cushing's disease, *J. Clin. Endocrinol. Metab.* **40:**892–895.

53. Sakakura, M., Takebe, K., and Nakagawa, S., 1975, Inhibition of luteinizing hormone secretion induced by synthetic LRH by long-term treatment with glucocorticoids in human subjects, *J. Clin. Endocrinol. Metab.* **40:**774–779.

54. Hashimoto, T., Miyai, K., Uozumi, T., Mori, S., Watanabe, M., and Kumahara, Y., 1975, Effect of prolonged LH-releasing hormone administration on gonadotropin response in patients with hypothalamic and pituitary tumors, *J. Clin. Endocrinol. Metab.* **41:**712–716.

55. Reitano, J. F., Caminos-Torres, R., and Snyder, P. J., 1975, Serum LH and

FSH responses to the repetitive administration of gonadotropin-releasing hormone in patients with idiopathic hypogonadotropic hypogonadism, *J. Clin. Endocrinol. Metab.* **41**:1035–1042.

56. Bell, J., Benveniste, R., Spitz, I., and Rabinowitz, D., 1975, Isolated deficiency of follicle-stimulating hormone: Further studies, *J. Clin. Endocrinol. Metab.* **40**:790–794.

57. Williams, C., Wieland, R. G., Zorn, E. M., and Hallberg, M. C., 1975, Effect of synthetic gonadotropin-releasing hormone (GnRH) in a patient with the "fertile eunuch" syndrome, *J. Clin. Endocrinol. Metab.* **41**:176–179.

58. Winters, A. J., Colston, C., MacDonald, P. C., and Porter, J. C., 1975, Fetal plasma prolactin levels, *J. Clin. Endocrinol. Metab.* **41**:626–629.

59. Fang, V. S., and Kim, M. H., 1975, Study on maternal, fetal, and amniotic human prolactin at term, *J. Clin. Endocrinol. Metab.* **41**:1030–1034.

60. Boyar, R. M., Finkelstein, J. W., Kapen, S., and Hellman, L., 1975, Twenty-four hour prolactin (Prl) secretory patterns during pregnancy, *J. Clin. Endocrinol. Metab.* **40**:1117–1120.

61. Tyson, J. E., Khojandi, M., Huth, J., and Andreassen, B., 1975, The influence of prolactin secretion on human lactation, *J. Clin. Endocrinol. Metab.* **40**:764–773.

62. Vekemans, M., and Robyn, C., 1975, The influence of exogenous estrogen on the circadian periodicity of circulating prolactin in women, *J. Clin. Endocrinol. Metab.* **40**:886–889.

63. Fossati, P., L'Hermite, M., Derrien, G., Golstein, J., VanHaelst, L., Robyn, C., and Linguette, M., La prolactinémie chez les myxoedémateuses, *Ann. Endocrinol.* **36**:145–151.

64. Malarkey, W. B., and Beck, P., 1975, Twenty-four hour prolactin profiles in normal and disease states: Failure of thyroxine to modify prolactin secretion, *J. Clin. Endocrinol. Metab.* **40**:708–712.

65. Copinschi, G., L'Hermite, M., LeClercq, R., Golstein, J., Vanhaelst, L., Virasoro, E., and Robyn, C., 1975, Effects of glucocorticoids on pituitary hormonal responses to hypoglycemia. Inhibition of prolactin release, *J. Clin. Endocrinol. Metab.* **40**:442–449.

66. Smythe, G. A., Compton, P. J., and Lazarus, L., 1975, The stimulation of human prolactin secretion by 3-iodo-L-tyrosine, *J. Clin. Endocrinol. Metab.* **40**:714–716.

67. Tolis, G., Hickey, J., and Guyda, H., 1975, Effects of morphine on serum growth hormone, cortisol, prolactin, and thyroid stimulating hormone in man, *J. Clin. Endocrinol. Metab.* **41**:797–800.

68. Mendelson, W. B., Jacobs, L. S., Reichman, J. D., Othmer, E., Cryer, P. E., Trivedi, B., and Daughaday, W. H., 1975, Methylsergide: Suppression of sleep-related prolactin secretion and enhancement of sleep-related growth hormone secretion, *J. Clin. Invest.* **56**:690–697.

69. Franks, S., Murray, M. A. F., Jequier, A. M., Steele, S. J., Nabarro, J. D. N., and Jacobs, H. S., 1975, Incidence and significance of hyperprolactinaemia in women with amenorrhoea, *Clin. Endocrinol.* **4**:597–607.

70. Child, D. F., Nader, S., Mashiter, K., Kjeld, M., Banks, L., and Russell Fraser, T., 1975, Prolactin studies in "functionless" pituitary tumours, *Br. Med. J.* **1**:604–606.

71. Zárate, A., Canales, E. S., Villalobos, H., Soria, J., Jacobs, L. S., Kastin, A. J., and Schally, A. V., 1975, Pituitary hormonal reserve in patients presenting hyperprolactinemia, intrasellar masses, and amenorrhea without galactorrhea, *J. Clin. Endocrinol. Metab.* **40**:1034–1037.

72. Malarkey, W. B., 1975, Nonpuerperal lactation and normal prolactin regulation, *J. Clin. Endocrinol. Metab.* **40**:198–204.
73. Buckman, M. T., Kaminsky, N., Conway, M., and Peake, G. T., 1973, Utility of L-Dopa and water loading in evaluation of hyperprolactinemia, *J. Clin. Endocrinol. Metab.* **36**:911–919.
74. Adler, R. A., Noel, G. L., Wartofsky, L., and Frantz, A. G., 1975, Failure of oral water loading and intravenous hypotonic saline to suppress plasma prolactin in man, *J. Clin. Endocrinol. Metab.* **41**:383–389.
75. Cleary, R. E., Crabtree, R., and Lemberger, L., 1975, The effect of Lergotrile on galactorrhea and gonadotropin secretion, *J. Clin. Endocrinol. Metab.* **40**:830–833.
76. Hummel, B. C. W., Brown, G. M., Hwang, P., and Friesen, H. G., 1975, Human and monkey prolactin and growth hormone: Separation of polymorphic forms by isoelectric focusing, *Endocrinology* **97**:855–867.
77. Holmström, B., and Fhölenhag, K., 1975, Characterization of human growth hormone preparations used for the treatment of pituitary dwarfism: A comparison of concurrently used batches, *J. Clin. Endocrinol. Metab.* **40**:856–862.
78. Guyda, H. J., 1975, Heterogeneity of human growth hormone and prolactin secreted *in vitro:* Immunoassay and radioreceptor assay correlations, *J. Clin. Endocrinol. Metab.* **41**:953–967.
79. Benveniste, R., Stachura, M. E., Szabo, M., and Frohman, L. A., 1975, Big growth hormone (GH): Conversion to small GH without peptide bond cleavage, *J. Clin. Endocrinol. Metab.* **41**:422–425.
80. Sneid, D. S., Jacobs, L. S., Weldon, V. V., Trivedi, B. L., and Daughaday, W. H., 1975, Radioreceptor-inactive growth hormone associated with stimulated secretion in normal subjects, *J. Clin. Endocrinol. Metab.* **41**:471–474.
81. Lewis, U. J., Pence, S. J., Singh, R. N. P., and VanderLaan, W. P., 1975, Enhancement of the growth promoting activity of human growth hormone, *Biochem. Biophys. Res. Commun.* **67**:617–624.
82. Plotnick, L. P., Thompson, R. G., Kowarski, A., De Lacerda, L., Migeon, C. J., and Blizzard, R. M., 1975, Circadian variation of integrated concentration of growth hormone in children and adults, *J. Clin. Endocrinol. Metab.* **40**:240–247.
83. Feldman, J. M., Plonk, J. W., and Bivens, C. H., 1975, The role of cortisol and growth hormone in the counter-regulation of insulin-induced hypoglycemia, *Horm. Metab. Res.* **7**:378–381.
84. Ajlouni, K., and Hagen, T. C., 1975, The effect of acute hypercalcemia on growth hormone release in man, *J. Clin. Endocrinol. Metab.* **40**:780–782.
85. Maeda, K., Kato, Y., Chihara, K., Ohgo, S., Iwasaki, Y., and Imura, H., 1975, Suppression by thyrotropin-releasing hormone (TRH) of human growth hormone release induced by L-Dopa, *J. Clin. Endocrinol. Metab.* **41**:408–411.
86. Maeda, K., Kato, Y., Ohgo, S., Chihara, K., Yoshimoto, Y., Yamaguchi, N., Kuromaru, S., and Imura, H., 1975, Growth hormone and prolactin release after injection of thyrotropin-releasing hormone in patients with depression, *J. Clin. Endocrinol. Metab.* **40**:501–505.
87. Pimstone, B. L., Becker, D., and Kronheim, S., 1975, Disappearance of plasma growth hormone in acromegaly and protein–calorie malnutrition after somatostatin, *J. Clin. Endocrinol. Metab.* **40**:168–171.
88. Pimstone, B. L., Le Roith, D., Epstein, S., and Kronheim, S., 1975, Disappearance rates of plasma growth hormone after intravenous somatostatin in renal and liver disease, *J. Clin. Endocrinol. Metab.* **41**:392–395.

89. Mims, R. B., Scott, C. L., Modebe, O. M., and Bethune, J. E., 1975, Inhibition of L-Dopa-induced growth hormone stimulation by pyridoxine and chlorpromazine, *J. Clin. Endocrinol. Metab.* **40:**256–259.
90. Lal, S., Tolis, G., Martin, J. B., Brown, G. M., and Guyda, H., 1975, Effect of clonidine on growth hormone, prolactin, luteinizing hormone, follicle-stimulating hormone and thyroid-stimulating hormone in the serum of normal men, *J. Clin. Endocrinol. Metab.* **41:**827–832.
91. Adamson, U., and Cerasi, E., 1975, Acute effects of exogenous growth hormone in man: Time- and dose-bound modification of glucose tolerance and glucose-induced insulin release, *Acta Endocrinol.* **80:**247–261.
92. Winawer, S. J., Sherlock, P., Sonenberg, M., and Vanamee, P., 1975, Beneficial effect of human growth hormone on stress ulcers, *Arch. Intern. Med.* **135:**569–572.
93. Nikkilä, A. E. A., and Pelkonen, R., 1975, Serum lipids in acromegaly, *Metabolism* **24:**829–838.
94. Pickett, J. B. E., III, Layzer, R. B., Levin, S. R., Schneider, V., Campbell, M. J., and Sumner, A. J., 1975, Neuromuscular complications of acromegaly, *Neurology* **25:**638–645.
95. Cheah, J. S., Chua, S. P., and Ho, C. L., 1975, Ultrastructure of the skeletal muscles in acromegaly—before and after hypophysectomy, *Amer. J. Med. Sci.* **269:**183–187.
96. Hoyte, K. M., and Martin, J. B., 1975, Recovery from paradoxical growth hormone responses in acromegaly after transsphenoidal selective adenomectomy, *J. Clin. Endocrinol. Metab.* **41:**656–659.
97. Cryer, P. E., 1975, Plasma norepinephrine and epinephrine in acromegaly, *J. Clin. Endocrinol. Metab.* **41:**542–545.
98. Hofeldt, F. D., Levin, S. R., Von Werder, K., Becker, N., Schneider, V., Hane, S., Seymour, R., Adams, J. E., and Forsham, P. H., 1975, Altered hypothalamic–pituitary–adrenal responsiveness to dexamethasone–insulin tolerance test in active acromegaly, *J. Clin. Endocrinol. Metab.* **41:**399–401.
99. Gomez-Pan, A., Tunbridge, W. M. G., Duns, A., Hall, R., Besser, G. M., Coy, D. H., Schally, A. V., and Kastin, A. J., 1975, Hypothalamic hormone interaction in acromegaly, *Clin. Endocrinol.* **4:**455–460.
100. Giustina, G., Peracchi, M., Reschini, E., Panerai, E., and Pinto, M., 1975, Dose-response study of the inhibiting effect of somatostatin on growth hormone and insulin secretion in normal subjects and acromegalic patients, *Metabolism* **24:**807–815.
101. Camanni, F., Massara, F., Belforte, L., and Molinatti, G. M., 1975, Changes in plasma growth hormone levels in normal and acromegalic subjects following administration of 2-bromo-α-ergocryptine, *J. Clin. Endocrinol. Metab.* **40:**363–366.
102. Chiodini, P. G., Liuzzi, A., Botalla, L., Oppizzi, G., Müller, E. E., and Silvestrini, F., 1975, Stable reduction of plasma growth hormone (hGH) levels during chronic administration of 2-Br-α-ergocryptine (CB-154) in acromegalic patients, *J. Clin. Endocrinol. Metab.* **40:**705–708.
103. Thorner, M. O., Chait, A., Aitken, M., Benker, G., Bloom, S. R., Mortimer, C. H., Sanders, P., Stuart Mason, A., and Besser, G. M., 1975, Bromocriptine treatment of acromegaly, *Br. Med. J.* **1:**299–303.
104. Summers, V. K., Hipkin, L. J., Diver, M. J., and Davis, J. C., 1975, Treatment of acromegaly with bromocryptine, *J. Clin. Endocrinol. Metab.* **40:**904–906.

105. Shaffi, O. M., and Wrightson, P., 1975, Dural invasion by pituitary tumours, *N. Z. Med. J.* **81:**386–390.
106. Williams, R. A., Jacobs, H. S., Kurtz, A. B., Millar, J. G. B., Oakley, N. W., Spathis, G. S., Sulway, M. J., and Nabarro, J. D. N., 1975, The treatment of acromegaly with special reference to trans-sphenoidal hypophysectomy, *Q. J. Med.* **44:**79–98.
107. Atkinson, R. L., Becker, D. P., Martins, A. N., Schaaf, M., Dimond, R. C., Wartofsky, L., and Earll, J. M., 1975, Acromegaly. Treatment by transsphenoidal microsurgery, *J. Amer. Med. Assoc.* **233:**1279–1283.
108. Pelkonen, R., and Grahne, B., 1975, Treatment of acromegaly by transsphenoidal hypophysectomy with cryoapplication, *Clin. Endocrinol.* **4:**53–64.
109. Merimee, T. J., Ostrow, P., and Aisner, S. C., 1975, Clinical and pathological studies in a growth hormone–deficient dwarf, *Johns Hopkins Med. J.* **136:**150–154.
110. Rimoin, D. L., and Schechter, J. E., 1973, Histological and ultrastructural studies in isolated growth hormone deficiency, *J. Clin. Endocrinol. Metab.* **37:**725–735.
111. Lovinger, R. D., Kaplan, S. L., and Grumbach, M. M., 1975, Congenital hypopituitarism associated with neonatal hypoglycemia and microphallus: Four cases secondary to hypothalamic hormone deficiencies, *J. Pediatr.* **87:**1171–1181.
112. Hopwood, N. J., Forsman, P. J., Kenny, F. M., and Drash, A. L., 1975, Hypoglycemia in hypopituitary children, *Amer. J. Dis. Child.* **129:**918–926.
113. Demura, R., Jujo, K., Takano, K., Odagiri, E., Maeda, T., Suda, T., Demura, H., and Shizume, K., 1975, Hypothalamic–pituitary functions in patients with idiopathic pituitary dwarfism, *Endocrinol. Jpn.* **22:**97–103.
114. Bernasconi, S., Torresani, T., and Illig, R., 1975, The effect of α-MSH on plasma growth hormone, cortisol and TSH in children, *J. Clin. Endocrinol. Metab.* **40:**759–763.
115. Weldon, V. V., Gupta, S. K., Klingensmith, G., Clarke, W. L., Duck, S. C., Haymond, M. W., and Pagliara, A. S., 1975, Evaluation of growth hormone release in children using arginine and L-DOPA in combination, *J. Pediatr.* **87:**540–544.
116. Lombardi, G., Minozzi, M., Faggiano, M., Carella, C., Jaquet, P., Carayon, P., and Oliver, C., 1975, Plasma immunoreactive T_3, TSH and ACTH before and after provocative tests in idiopathic hypopituitary dwarfism, *J. Clin. Endocrinol. Metab.* **40:**143–151.
117. Lippe, B. M., Van Herle, A. J., La Franchi, S. H., Uller, R. P., Lavin, N., and Kaplan, S. A., 1975, Reversible hypothyroidism in growth hormone–deficient children treated with human growth hormone, *J. Clin. Endocrinol. Metab.* **40:**612–618.
118. Samaan, N. A., Bakdash, M. M., Caderao, J. B., Cangir, A., Jesse, R. H., Jr., and Ballantyne, A. J., 1975, Hypopituitarism after external irradiation, evidence for both hypothalamic and pituitary origin, *Ann. Intern. Med.* **83:**771–777.

3

The Thyroid

Kenneth A. Woeber and Lewis E. Braverman

3.1. Introduction

This chapter will cover those new aspects relating to the physiology and pathophysiology of the thyroid that have appeared in critically reviewed journals during 1975; it will not be an exhaustive compilation of the literature during this period. Since advances have occurred in virtually all the major areas relating to thyroid hormone economy, we deemed it advisable to organize the chapter along classic lines. The organization has been done in this way not only for reasons of expediency, but also because each major area, in effect, is a discipline in its own right.

KENNETH A. WOEBER • Department of Medicine, Mt. Zion Hospital and Medical Center; and University of California, San Francisco, California. LEWIS E. BRAVERMAN • Department of Medicine, University of Massachusetts Medical School, Worcester, Massachusetts.

3.2. Neuroendocrine Regulation of Thyroid Function

The availability of synthetic thyrotropin-releasing hormone (TRH) has led to a continued exploration of the potential factors that may influence the pituitary tropic hormone responses to this hypothalamic tripeptide. Furthermore, the recent development of a radioimmunoassay for TRH is beginning to provide some information concerning the factors that might affect the synthesis and release of endogenous TRH.

Earlier observations had suggested that TRH might have a salutary effect in depressive states in man. These observations appeared to be consonant with the more recent finding that TRH is also found in extrahypothalamic areas of the CNS, leading to the suggestion that TRH may function as a neurotransmitter as well as a releasing hormone. Accordingly, several controlled studies were undertaken to evaluate the role of TRH as an antidepressant; most have failed to confirm such an effect of TRH, however.[1] In addition, pituitary responsiveness to TRH in depressive states has been evaluated. In the most extensive study, the thyrotropin-stimulating hormone (TSH) response to TRH was depressed, whereas that of prolactin was enhanced. This latter observation is of interest in light of the behavioral role that prolactin appears to play in some animals. Also of interest was the observation that in some depressed patients, a response of growth hormone to TRH was found, a finding not seen in normal man.[2]

A variety of pharmacological agents have been shown to influence the responsiveness of the pituitary to TRH. The monoamine dopamine and its precursor, L-DOPA, impair the responses of both TSH and prolactin to TRH.[3] Whether dopamine exerts its effect through the mediation of prolactin-inhibiting factor (and TSH-inhibiting factor), or whether it acts directly on the pituitary, is not clear. Apomorphine, a dopaminergic agonist, impairs the prolactin, but not the TSH, response to TRH, while morphine provokes prolactin, but not TSH, release.[4,5] These observations indicate that dopaminergic mechanisms are important in the regulation of prolactin release, and suggest that they may also be important in the regulation of TSH secretion. Dopaminergic mechanisms may also be involved in the regulation of growth hormone (GH), since L-DOPA provokes GH release. TRH administration, however, inhibits this induction of GH release by L-DOPA, suggesting that TRH, in addition to its role in regulating TSH and prolactin secretion, may also play a role in the regulation of GH release.[6] Noradrenergic mechanisms appear not to be involved in the regulation of TSH secretion. For example, clonidine, a norepinephine agonist, provokes release of GH but not of TSH or prolactin.[7] On the other hand, the failure to observe an increased TSH response to this agent could be due to an increased output of somatostatin, which has been shown to inhibit TSH secretion,[8,9] and which may accompany an increase in GH release. Other pharmacological agents have been shown to influence TSH secretion and its response to TRH. Ovulatory suppressants may increase basal concentrations of TSH in serum[10] and enhance TSH responsiveness to TRH.[11]

A variety of physiological and pathological circumstances have been reported to be accompanied by alterations in the dynamics of TSH secretion. Fasting for 36 hr appears to decrease the responses of both TSH and prolactin to TRH,[12] whereas fasting for 3–4 weeks had previously been reported not to affect TSH responsiveness to TRH. In contrast to prolonged fasting, protein–calorie malnutrition and anorexia nervosa are associated with altered TSH responsiveness to TRH, the former[13] being accompanied by an increased response, the latter[14] by a delayed response. Prolactin responsiveness to TRH is normal in both states.

As suggested earlier, a relationship may exist between the mechanisms regulating GH secretion and TSH secretion. This view is supported by a recent observation that TSH release is provoked by hypoglycemia in certain clinical circumstances of GH deficiency, under conditions in which the expected increase in GH in response to hypoglycemia does not occur.[15] Moreover, reversible trophoprivic hypothyroidism may accompany GH therapy in GH-deficient children.[16] These observations could be ascribed to the known inhibitory effect of somatostatin on TSH secretion, since increases in somatostatin may accompany increases in either endogenous or exogenously administered GH.

The exquisite sensitivity of the anterior pituitary to physiological changes in the concentration of T_4 and T_3 in the plasma has been well documented in the past. Small increases in serum T_4 and T_3 concentrations, induced by the exogenous administration of a combination of T_4 and T_3, decreased basal serum TSH concentration and the TSH response to exogenous TRH, whereas small decreases in serum T_4 and T_3 concentrations, during the short-term administration of pharmacological quantities of iodide, increased basal serum TSH concentrations and the TSH response to TRH. Further studies on the influence of thyroid hormones on the secretion of TSH and its responsiveness to TRH were carried out during 1975. The time course of the inhibitory effect of essentially physiological amounts of 3,5,3'-L-triiodothyronine (T_3) on the TSH response to TRH has been examined. Following the ingestion of a single dose of T_3, there is a progressively increasing inhibition of TSH responsiveness to TRH that attains a maximum at about 3 days after ingestion, well after the early elevation of plasma T_3 concentration has returned to normal.[17,18] This inhibition decreases over the ensuing 3 to 4 days, so that by the seventh day, responsiveness to TRH is near normal. A greater delay, perhaps necessitated by the conversion of L-thyroxine (T_4) to T_3, has been noted with a large oral dose of T_4.[18] Whether the delay observed with T_3 is due to a requirement for the synthesis of an inhibitory protein within the pituitary, or, as has recently been suggested,[19] is due to delayed transfer of T_3 across the blood-brain interface, is uncertain.

The development of a radioimmunoassay for measuring TRH in blood, urine, CSF, and tissue extracts had led to some preliminary observations concerning the dynamics of endogenous TRH secretion. The concentration of TRH in the blood of the rat appears to be independent of the thyroid state. Cold exposure, which is known to provoke TSH release in this species, has been reported by one group to increase plasma TRH[20] and by another group to have no effect.[21] In man, the concentrations of TRH in plasma and CSF appear to be independent of gender.[22,23] It should be emphasized, however, that methodological difficulties encountered in the TRH assay have not been completely resolved, and, accordingly, the foregoing observations should be considered preliminary.

The development of radioimmunoassays that selectively measure the α and β subunits of TSH has permitted an evaluation of the subunit concentrations in plasma in patients with various thyroid disorders.[24] Since neither subunit is increased in patients with the ophthalmopathy of Graves' disease, the exophthalmos-producing factor is probably not the α or β subunit of TSH *per se*, but may be some other fragment of TSH, as has been suggested by others.[25-27]

3.3. Thyroid Hormones

3.3.1. Synthesis and Secretion

A number of advances have taken place in this area, most noteworthy of which are the further elucidation of the mechanism of TSH action and the demonstration of a possible short feedback loop responsive to thyroid hormones.

Work with a calcium ionophore has indicated that calcium ion has effects similar to those of TSH and cyclic adenosine monosphosphate (cAMP) on thyroid iodide transport and glucose oxidation.[28] In addition, in the presence of an ionophore, calcium increased both cyclic guanidine monophosphate (cGMP) concentration and the binding of iodide to thyroid proteins in the absence of TSH.[29] These observations suggest that calcium ion may be the ultimate arbiter of some effects of TSH and perhaps of other thyroid stimulators.

It is well known that iodide inhibits some of the actions of TSH on the thyroid. A recent study[30] has served to synthesize these multifaceted effects of iodide by demonstrating that this ion inhibits the accumulation of cAMP, and the stimulation of glucose oxidation, lactate formation, and iodothyronine secretion, in the thyroid response to TSH. Similarly, iodide inhibited the accumulation of cAMP and the stimulation of iodothyronine secretion in response to prostaglandin E_1. On the other hand, iodide did not inhibit the stimulatory effects of dibutyryl cAMP, suggesting that the inhibitory effect of iodide is proximal to the generation of cAMP. As has previously been demonstrated for other effects, oxidation of iodide is a prerequisite to these inhibitory effects on the thyroid.

The property of TSH to promote thyroid growth may reside in its ability to stimulate the synthesis of polyamines. Since the enzyme ornithine decarboxylase catalyzes a rate-limiting step in polyamine synthesis, it is noteworthy that TSH enhances the activity of this enzyme, an effect that may require new protein synthesis and may be mediated by cAMP or prostaglandins.[31,32]

The identity of the oxygen species responsible for the iodination of tyrosyl residues has recently been reexamined. Superoxide dismutase, which catalyzes the transformation of the superoxide radical to hydrogen peroxide, does not interfere with iodinations, suggesting that the superoxide radical is not the oxidizing agent *per se*. On the other hand, catalase, which catalyzes the degradation of H_2O_2, inhibited iodinations.[33] Confirmation of the locus of iodination of thyroglobulin at the cell–colloid interface was provided by electron-microscopic autoradiography.[34]

The induction of goiter by large doses of iodide, which previously had been shown to occur in man, chicken, and mouse, has now been demonstrated to occur in the hog.[35] It should be pointed out that iodide-induced goiter in man almost always occurs in the presence of underlying thyroid disease, and is often accompanied by hypothyroidism. Other work has demonstrated that the stability of thyroglobulin correlates more closely with iodothyronine content than with total iodine content.[36] It has further been demonstrated that asialothyroglobulin is associated with poor thyroid hormone formation,[37] and that incomplete thyroglobulin saccharide chains result in an increase in membrane-bound thyroglobulin and impaired iodothyronine synthesis, as may be found in "cold" thyroid nodules.[38]

Several workers have provided evidence that thyroid hormones themselves inhibit the action of exogenous TSH on thyroid secretory activity in man and mouse, as judged from colloid droplet formation, release of hormone iodine, and measurement of serum T_4.[39–41] The data are conflicting, however, as to whether the inhibitory action of thyroid hormones in this short feedback loop occurs prior to or subsequent to the synthesis of cAMP.

3.3.2. Peripheral Metabolism

Since the demonstration of the quantitative importance of the peripheral monodeiodination of T_4 in the generation of T_3, a great deal of activity has been directed toward examining the factors that influence the conversion of T_4 to T_3. Although the exact quantities of T_3 that are derived from peripheral deiodination of T_4 and directly from thyroid secretion have been open to debate, it is generally agreed that almost all the circulating T_3 is generated peripherally from T_4. Another product of the monodeiodination of T_4 that has recently been identified in plasma is 3,3′,5′-triiodothyronine (reverse T_3, rT_3). Reverse T_3 arises from T_4 through monodeiodination of the inner ring, whereas T_3 is derived through monodeiodination of the outer ring. Reverse T_3 is essentially biologically inactive, while T_3 is 2–3 times more potent than T_4. Accordingly, it has been suggested that the poise between inner and outer ring monodeiodination of T_4 may represent an important peripheral regulatory mechanism for modulating the quantity of biologically active hormones at the tissue level.

A variety of physiological and pathological circumstances are accompanied by qualitative alterations in the monodeiodination of T_4. In virtually all these circumstances, the alteration is one in which the generation of T_3 (outer-ring monodeiodination) is selectively depressed, with the result that the plasma concentration of T_3 is disproportionately decreased relative to that of T_4. In those circumstances in which rT_3 has been measured, the decrease in T_3 is almost invariably accompanied by a reciprocal increase in rT_3. Circumstances in which the conversion of T_4 to T_3 is impaired include the fetal and early neonatal periods,[42] advanced age, fasting, protein–calorie malnutrition, anorexia nervosa, severe systemic illnesses including cirrhosis and chronic renal failure,[43-47] and the period following surgery.[48] The administration of propylthiouracil,[49,50] but not methimazole, and of pharmacological doses of glucocorticoids[51] also impairs the conversion of T_4 to T_3. In those clinical states of decreased conversion of T_4 to T_3, basal serum TSH and its response to TRH may be increased, indicating a compensatory response on the part of the hypothalamic–pituitary axis to the decreased serum T_3 concentration. Studies in fetal sheep have indicated that the decrease in T_3 generation is due not only to decreased T_3 production, but also to increased metabolic clearance.[52] Conversely, the increase in rT_3 in this circumstance is due both to increased production and to decreased metabolic clearance. The observation that T_3 is very low in the fetus and amniotic fluid[53] in the face of a high maternal concentration provides the most convincing evidence to date that maternal-to-fetal transfer of T_3 is at best minimal, and that the maintenance of a eumetabolic state in the fetus is accomplished primarily through the secretion of T_4 by the fetal thyroid.

Although there have been several reports of measurements of the fractional rate of conversion of T_4 to T_3 in normal subjects and in hypothyroid patients rendered eumetabolic by T_4, there is a paucity of data concerning such measurements in patients with untreated hypothyroidism or thyrotoxicosis. A recent study has suggested that the fractional rate of conversion of T_4 to T_3 is increased in untreated hypothyroidism relative to the euthyroid state, and declines with T_4 replacement.[54] Such data are not available for thyrotoxic patients.

Two important studies have appeared concerning the metabolism of thyronine-binding globulin (TBG).[55,56] In man, TBG has a metabolic clearance rate approaching 1 liter/day, and it appears that desialylation may be the rate-limiting step in its metabolism by liver.

3.3.3. Metabolic Action

The major activity in this area has continued to be concerned with the binding of thyroid hormones to subcellular constituents. The characteristics of the saturable nuclear T_3 and T_4 binding interactions appear to have been established for rat liver, and the nuclear binding component has been extracted and appears to be some component of chromatin.[57-59] Saturable binding sites for T_3 and T_4 have also been demonstrated in the mitochondrial fraction of rat liver.[60] The relative biological importance of these different subcellular sites may bear on the multiple actions of thyroid hormones. It is tempting to speculate that mitochondrial binding of thyroid hormones may be a prerequisite for their action in regulating energy metabolism, while nuclear binding may initiate and sustain the effects of thyroid hormones on growth and development.

Thyroid hormones have been shown to stimulate the uptake of certain amino acids in rat thymocytes. This stimulatory effect, unlike that of insulin or dibutyryl cAMP, resides in an inhibition of amino acid efflux, rather than a stimulation of influx.[61]

The potentiation of adrenergic responsiveness in thyrotoxicosis and its attenuation in hypothyroidism have received general acceptance. These phenomena are supported by recent studies in which it was shown that the plasma cAMP response to glucagon and the urinary cAMP response to epinephrine in man are enhanced in thyrotoxicosis and impaired in hypothyroidism.[62,63] Moreover, the administration of a large dose of T_3 to the dog has been shown to increase plasma cAMP, but not to affect plasma cGMP.[64] (See Chapter 8 for a full discussion of thyroid–catecholamine interrelationships.)

The urinary excretion of the collagen metabolites, hydroxylysyl glucosides, has been measured in patients with thyrotoxicosis and hypothyroidism. As has been shown to be the case for urinary hydroxyproline excretion, values were increased in thyrotoxicosis and decreased in hypothyroidism.[65]

3.4. Clinical Aspects of Thyroidology

Several novel aspects relating to clinical thyroidology appeared in the literature during the year of review. For purposes of convenience, these aspects will be considered according to the major disease categories.

3.4.1. Thyrotoxicosis

In view of the confusion concerning the terminology of the non-TSH immunoglobulin stimulators of Graves' disease, a new nomenclature has been proposed. It has been suggested that the long-acting thyroid stimulator (LATS) be termed mouse-thyroid stimulator (MTS), in view of its delayed stimulatory properties in mouse, but not in human thyroid tissue. LATS-protector (LATS-P) has recently been found in the sera of most patients with Graves' disease; it is an immunoglobulin that prevents the binding of LATS by human thyroid tissue and does not stimulate the mouse thyroid. Thus, in view of its stimulatory properties in human but not mouse thyroid tissue, LATS-P would then be designated human-thyroid stimulator (HTS). The generic term embracing both thyroid-stimulating immunoglobulins would be thyroid-stimulating antibodies (TSAb).[66]

The etiology of Graves' disease continues to be an enigma. The early enthusiasm for the primary role of LATS (or, preferably, MTS) in this disorder has been somewhat dampened by the failure to find a consistent correlation between the presence of MTS and abnormal thyroid suppressibility. Furthermore, remission of thyrotoxic Graves' disease may occur despite the presence of MTS in the serum. More sensitive assays for MTS and the discovery of LATS-P (or, preferably, HTS) have again stimulated a great deal of interest in this area. TSAb has now been reported to be present in all patients with untreated Graves' disease, and the titers appear to correlate in a positive manner with the values for the early thyroid uptake of radioiodine. Following treatment with antithyroid drugs or radioiodine, TSAb disappeared in approximately 50% of the patients, whereas following partial thyroidectomy, TSAb disappeared in 83%.[67] These values accord well with those previously reported for the return of normal suppressibility of thyroid function following the different treatment modalities. High titers of maternal TSAb near delivery are invariably accompanied by neonatal thyrotoxicosis.[68] Consequently, it is deemed advisable that TSAb be measured near term in all women with Graves' disease in order to be alerted to the possibility of neonatal thyrotoxicosis. Finally, TSAb has been detected in a high proportion of patients with generally enlarged thyroid glands who developed iodine-induced thyrotoxicosis following iodine supplementation in an area of endemia.[69] This observation suggests that some patients who are prone to develop the jod-Basedow phenomenon have underlying Graves' disease.

In view of the problems noted above in ascribing the etiology of Graves' disease to TSAb, a great deal of interest has been generated in defining the role of cell-mediated immunity in the pathogenesis of thyroid disease. Migration-inhibition factor is often present in patients with thyroid disease, including Graves' disease, Hashimoto's thyroiditis, and primary hypothyroidism. Lymphocyte-mediated cytoxicity, as well as migration-inhibition factor, has been found in patients with these disorders, and both were unaffected by treatment.[70] On the other hand, in contrast to earlier observations, patients with Graves' disease or primary hypothyroidism do not display quantitative or qualitative abnormalities in the circulating lymphocyte population.[71] Finally, to determine whether there exists a primary abnormality intrinsic to the thyroid gland of Graves' disease that may have pathogenetic significance, a study of the adenylate cyclase–cAMP–protein kinase system was undertaken; no abnormalities were detected, however.[72]

Some work has been reported in relation to other varieties of hyperthyroidism. The so-called molar thyrotropin that is in all likelihood the stimulator in the hyperthyroidism associated with hydatidiform mole may be chorionic gonadotropin.[73] This report confirms the work of others published earlier. A recent report described a patient with hyperthyroidism in whom the disease was accompanied by an increase in basal TSH and enhanced responsiveness to TRH, suggesting a resetting of the threshold of feedback inhibition.[74] There have been several reports of a clinical entity comprising thyrotoxicosis, painless goiter, and a very low thyroid radioiodine uptake in the absence of iodine or thyroid hormone ingestion. This entity has been interpreted as representing either painless or silent subacute thyroiditis or a functional variant of Hashimoto's thyroiditis. In the one study in which thyroid biopsy was undertaken, the histopathology was consistent with Hashimoto's, rather than subacute, thyroiditis.[75] Since the course of this disorder is self-limited, specific antithyroid therapy is not indicated. The phenomenon of iodine-induced thyrotoxicosis (jod-Basedow) in persons with no apparent underlying abnormality of thyroid function has been reported from France.[76] This report follows previous observations that iodine-induced thyrotoxicosis may occur in patients with nontoxic goiter residing in iodine-sufficient areas. Prior to these findings, jod-Basedow had been reported to occur only in endemic iodine-deficient areas following iodine supplementation. Thus, the prevalence of jod-Basedow in iodine-sufficient areas may be higher than previously suggested, and should be recognized as a definite clinical entity. The existence of "T_4 toxicosis" has been suggested on the basis of elevated serum free T_4 and normal or low total T_3 or free T_3 concentrations in patients with nonthyroidal illness.[77] It appears likely that the foregoing chemical profile is due to the underlying illness, and not to a peculiarity in the nature of the thyroid hyperfunction. A normal or augmented TSH response to TRH would effectively exclude the latter. Finally, it has been reported that the development of thyrotoxic crisis does not require a serum T_3 concentration that exceeds that found in uncomplicated thyrotoxicosis.[78]

There has been some work relating to various aspects of the treatment of thyrotoxicosis. Inorganic iodide as sole therapy in Graves' disease has been shown to lead to only a transient decrease in serum T_4 and T_3 concentrations, confirming earlier impressions.[79] Glucocorticoids have been shown to abruptly decrease serum T_4 and T_3 concentrations in Graves' disease, an effect that may be due to an inhibition of hormone secretion and to an inhibition of peripheral T_4 to T_3 conversion.[80] In keeping with the clinical experience that some patients treated with radioiodine develop a transient worsening of thyrotoxicosis, it has been shown that serum T_3 and T_4 concentrations rise during the first 1–2 days following radioiodine therapy.[81] The pharmacokinetics of propylthiouracil in man have been studied, revealing a very rapid plasma half-life of approximately 1½ hr;[82,83] no values for thyroid tissue half-life are presently available, however.

3.4.2. Hypothyroidism

There has been relatively less activity in this area. However, the development of a neonatal screening program for the detection of hypothyroidism represents a major contribution. Here, a T_4 radioimmunoassay is performed on a filter paper spot of blood obtained on the fifth day of postnatal life. With this screening, the incidence of neonatal hypothyroidism is of the order of 1/7000 births.[84] The development of a similar spot test for serum TSH has been described.[85]

Several reports have previously appeared in which apparent trophoprivic hypothyroidism was associated with increased basal TSH and enhanced TSH responsiveness to TRH. In some children with apparent hypothalamic hypothyroidism, similar findings have been reported. It has been suggested that the defect may reside in the elaboration by the pituitary of a biologically less active TSH.[86]

The pattern of recovery of the functional integrity of the hypothalamic–pituitary–thyroid complex following withdrawal of chronic thyroid suppression in euthyroid patients has been studied.[87 88] During the first week or two following withdrawal, serum TSH is undetectable and is unresponsive to TRH despite a decline in serum T_4 and T_3 concentrations to subnormal values. Thereafter, serum TSH becomes detectable in the basal state, and responsiveness to TRH is restored, followed by a progressive return to normal of serum T_4 and T_3 concentrations over the ensuing 2–3 weeks. This sequence of events, in conjunction with the observation that basal serum TSH and its response to TRH are lower than would be expected in light of the subnormal values for serum T_4 and T_3 concentrations, suggests that prolonged suppression therapy leads to depletion of pituitary TSH. A similar phenomenon has been reported to occur in treated hyperthyroid patients during the initial period following attainment of a eumetabolic state.[89] In the patient who has been receiving chronic thyroid treatment, the absolute value of serum T_4 during T_3 administration may be used to differentiate a potentially normal hypothalamic–pituitary–thyroid complex from either primary or trophoprivic hypothyroidism. In the latter, but not the former, circumstance, serum T_4 decreased to below the limits of assay detectability.[90]

The hemorrhagic tendency of patients with hypothyroidism has previously been ascribed, at least in part, to a decrease in some coagulation factors. Recent work indicates that platelet adhesiveness is also impaired. This impairment is corrected by treatment with T_4.[91] Finally, the decreased red cell mass in hypothyroidism may be due, at least in part, to decreased erythropoietin elaboration; the converse phenomenon appears to be the case in thyrotoxicosis.[92]

The recent suggestion that mild hypothyroidism, such as may occur in Hashimoto's disease, is associated with an increased incidence of breast cancer in women[93] deserves further consideration. A possible role for prolactin in this circumstance has not been examined.

3.4.3. Thyroid Cancer

The association of low-dose irradiation to the head, neck, and chest area early in life with the later development of thyroid cancer is now well recognized. This relationship has been reemphasized in recent publications.[94,95] Thyroid abnormalities are detectable by palpation or scintiscan in about one-quarter of asymptomatic irradiated individuals, and of this group, as many as one-half may harbor a carcinoma. It is noteworthy that even in the initial absence of palpable thyroid abnormalities, hypofunctioning areas detected by scintiscanning techniques may also be associated with thyroid cancer. Whether such lesions are significant from the standpoint of biological behavior remains to be determined, however. The availability of a radioimmunoassay for human thyroglobulin antigen in plasma has provided a means of detecting a potential tumor marker.[96] It should be borne in mind, however, that the presence of thyroglobulin antigen in serum is not specific for differentiated thyroid cancer, since it has been found in the serum of patients with Graves' disease and subacute thyroiditis, and is factitiously elevated in the serum of patients with Hashimoto's disease who have high titers of circulating thyroglobulin antibody.[97] It seems very likely that circulating thryoglobulin antigen will be detected in all circumstances in which the thyroid gland is subject to hyperstimulation by either TSH or TSAb.

3.5. Miscellaneous Aspects of Thyroidology

This section encompasses those aspects of thyroidology that cannot be conveniently incorporated elsewhere.

The oral administration of a single dose of monoiodotyrosine has been shown to provoke selectively the release of prolactin in man.[98] In view of its lack of toxicity, this monoamine may prove to be a useful tool for assessing prolactin reserve. A radioimmunoassay has been developed for measuring diiodotyrosine in plasma, and it has been shown that the values obtained are independent of sex and decline with age.[99]

Finally, a useful table has been published that presents the radiation-absorbed dose to various organs for different radioisotopes of iodine. For example, in a normal subject with a thyroid uptake of isotope of 25%, 50 μC of ^{131}I (half-life, 8 days) delivers 65 rads to the thyroid, whereas the same dose of ^{123}I (half-life, 13 hr) delivers only 0.7 rad.[100]

References

1. Hall, R., Hurter, P. R., Price, J. S., and Mountjoy, C. Q., 1975, Thyrotropin-releasing hormone in depression, *Lancet* 1:162.
2. Maeda, K., Kato, Y., Ohgo, S., Chihara, K., Yoshimoto, Y., Yamaguchi, N., Kuromaru, S., and Imura, H., 1975, Growth hormone and prolactin release after injection of thyrotropin-releasing hormone in patients with depression, *J. Clin. Endocrinol. Metab.* **40**:501–505.
3. Besses, G. S., Burrow, G. N. Spaulding, S. W., and Donabedian, R. K., 1975, Dopamine infusion acutely inhibits the TSH and prolactin response to TRH, *J. Clin. Endocrinol. Metab.* **41**:985–988.

4. Nilsson, K. O., Wide, L., and Hökfelt, B., 1975, The effect of apomorphine on basal and TRH stimulated release of thyrotrophin and prolactin in man, *Acta Endocrinol.* **80:**220–229.
5. Tolis, G., Hickey, J., and Guyda, H., 1975, Effects of morphine on serum growth hormone, cortisol, prolactin, and thyroid stimulating hormone in man, *J. Clin. Endocrinol. Metab.* **41:**797–800.
6. Maeda, K., Kato, Y., Chihara, K., Ohgo, S., Iwasaki, Y., and Imura, H., 1975, Suppression by thyrotropin-releasing hormone (TRH) of human growth hormone release induced by L-DOPA, *J. Clin. Endocrinol. Metab.* **41:**408–411.
7. Lal, S., Tolis, G., Martin, J. B., Brown, G. M., and Guyda, H., 1975, Effect of clonidine on growth hormone, prolactin, luteinizing hormone, follicle-stimulating hormone, and thyroid-stimulating hormone in the serum of normal men, *J. Clin. Endocrinol. Metab.* **41:**827–832.
8. Weeke, J., Hansen, A. P., and Lundaek, K., 1975, Inhibition by somatostatin of basal levels of serum thyrotropin (TSH) in normal men, *J. Clin. Endocrinol. Metab.* **41:**168–171.
9. Lucke, C., Höffken, B., and von zur Mühlen, A., 1975, The effect of somatostatin on TSH levels in patients with primary hypothyroidism, *J. Clin. Endocrinol. Metab.* **41:**1082–1084.
10. Weeke, J., and Hansen, A. P., 1975, Serum TSH and serum T₃ levels during normal menstrual cycles and during cycles on oral contraceptives, *Acta Endocrinol.* **79:**431–438.
11. Ramey, J. N., Burrow, G. N., Polackwich, R. J., and Donabedian, R. K., 1975, The effect of oral contraceptive steroids on the response of thyroid-stimulating hormone to thyrotropin-releasing hormone, *J. Clin. Endocrinol. Metab.* **40:**712–714.
12. Vinik, A. I., Kalk, W. J., McLaren, H., Hendricks, S., and Pimstone, B. L., 1975, Fasting blunts the TSH response to synthetic thyrotropin-releasing hormone (TRH), *J. Clin. Endocrinol. Metab.* **40:**509–511.
13. Becker, D. J., Vinik, A. I., Pimstone, B. L., and Paul, M., 1975, Prolactin response to thyrotropin-releasing hormone in protein–calorie malnutrition, *J. Clin. Endocrinol. Metab.* **41:**782–783.
14. Miyai, K., Yamamoto, T., Azukizawa, M., Ishibashi, K., and Kumahara, Y., 1975, Serum thyroid hormones and thyrotropin in anorexia nervosa, *J. Clin. Endocrinol. Metab.* **40:**334–338.
15. Guansing, A. R., Leung, Y., Ajlouni, K., and Hagen, T. C., 1975, The effect of hypoglycemia on TSH release in man, *J. Clin. Endocrinol. Metab.* **40:**755–758.
16. Lippe, B. M., Van Herle, A. J., LaFranchi, S. H., Uller, R. P., Lavin, N., and Kaplan, S. A., 1975, Reversible hypothyroidism in growth hormone–deficient children treated with human growth hormone, *J. Clin. Endocrinol. Metab.* **40:**612–618.
17. Azizi, F., Vagenakis, A. G., Ingbar, S. H., and Braverman, L. E., 1975, The time course of changes in TRH responsiveness in man following a single dose of liothyronine, *Metabolism* **24:**691–694.
18. Wenzel, K. W., Meinhold, H., and Schleusener, H., 1975, Different effects of oral doses of triiodothyronine or thyroxine on the inhibition of thyrotrophin releasing hormone (TRH) mediated thyrotrophin (TSH) response in man, *Acta Endocrinol.* **80:**42–48.
19. Takaishi, M., Miyachi, Y., and Shishiba, Y., 1975, Delayed equilibrium of

pituitary triiodothyronine (T_3) following an acute T_3 administration, *Endocrinol. Jpn.* **22**:461–463.

20. Montoya, E., Seibel, M. J., and Wilber, J. F., 1975, Thyrotropin-releasing hormone secretory physiology: Studies by radioimmunoassay and affinity chromatography, *Endocrinology* **96**:1413–1418.

21. Emerson, C. H., and Utiger, R. D., 1975, Plasma thyrotropin-releasing hormone concentrations in the rat. Effect of thyroid excess and deficiency and cold exposure, *J. Clin. Invest.* **56**:1564–1570.

22. Saito, S., Musa, K., Yamamoto, S., Oshima, I., and Funato, T., 1975, Radioimmunoassay of thyrotropin releasing hormone in plasma and urine, *Endocrinol. Jpn.* **22**:303–309.

23. Shambaugh, G. E., III, Wilber, J. F., Montoya, E., Ruder, H., and Blonsky, E. R., 1975, Thyrotropin-releasing hormone (TRH): Measurements in human spinal fluid, *J. Clin. Endocrinol. Metab.* **41**:131–134.

24. Kourides, I. A., Weintraub, B. D., Ridgway, E. C., and Maloof, F., 1975, Pituitary secretion of free alpha and beta subunits of human thyrotropin in patients with thyroid disorders, *J. Clin. Endocrinol. Metab.* **40**:872–885.

25. Valk, T. W., Taylor, R. E., Jr., and Barker, S. B., 1975, Production and measurement of exophthalmos-producing factor in guinea pigs, *Endocrinology* **96**:151–159.

26. Kohn, L. D., and Winand, R. J., 1975, Exophthalmogenic activity of the β^3 subunit of thyrotropin, *Endocrinology* **96**:1592–1594.

27. Kohn, L. D., Winand, R. J., and Bates, R. W., 1975, Relationship of thyrotropin to exophthalmos-producing substance: Formation of an exophthalmos-producing factor by pepsin digestion of mouse pituitary tumor and human thyrotropin preparations, *Endocrinology* **96**:1329–1332.

28. Yamashita, K., Aiyoshi, Y., Oka, H., and Ogata, 1975, Effects of calcium ionophore (A-23187) on glucose oxidation and iodide transport in dog thyroid slices, *Endocrinol. Jpn.* **22**:415–418.

29. Van Sande, J., Decoster, C., and Dumont, J. E., 1975, Control and role of cyclic 3′,5′-guanosine monophosphate in the thyroid, *Biochem. Biophys. Res. Commun.* **62**:168–175.

30. Van Sande, J., Grenier, G., Willems, C., and Dumont, J. E., 1975, Inhibition by iodide of the activation of the thyroid cyclic 3′,5′-AMP system, *Endocrinology* **96**:781–786.

31. Zusman, D. R., and Burrow, G. N., 1975, Thyroid-stimulating hormone regulation of ornithine decarboxylase activity in the thyroid, *Endocrinology* **97**:1089–1095.

32. Matsuzaki, S., and Suzuki, M., 1975, Thyroid function and polyamines II. Thyrotropin stimulation of polyamine biosynthesis in the rat thyroid, *Endocrinol. Jpn.* **22**:339–345.

33. Yamamoto, K., and DeGroot, L. J., 1975, Participation of NADPH–cytochrome C reductase in thyroid hormone biosynthesis, *Endocrinology* **96**:1022–1029.

34. Ekholm, R., and Wollman, S. H., 1975, Site of iodination in the rat thyroid gland deduced from electron microscopic autoradiographs, *Endocrinology* **97**:1432–1444.

35. Tarutani, O., Kondo, T., and Horiguchi-Sho, K., 1975, The effect of iodide administration on hog thyroid gland and the composition of thyrogrobulin and 27-S iodoprotein, *Endocrinol. Jpn.* **22**:389–397.

36. Fukuda, H., and Greer, M. A., 1975, The relative roles of iodination and

iodothyronine content on thyroglobulin stability, *Acta Endocrinol.* **78**:468–480.

37. Monaco, F., Grimaldi, S., Dominici, R., and Robbins, J., 1975, Defective thyroglobulin synthesis in an experimental rat thyroid tumor: Iodination and thyroid hormone synthesis in isolated tumor thyroglobulin, *Endocrinology* **97**:347–351.

38. Monaco, F., Monaco, G., and Andreoli, M., 1975, Thyroglobulin biosynthesis in "cold" and "hot" nodules in the human thyroid, *J. Clin. Endocrinol. Metab.* **41**:253–259.

39. Gafni, M., Sirkis, N., and Gross, J., 1975, Inhibition of the response of mouse thyroid to thyrotropin induced by chronic triiodothyronine treatment, *Endocrinology* **97**:1256–1262.

40. Vigneri, R., Squatrito, S., Pezzino, V., Filetti, S., and Polasa, P., 1975, The effect of short-term triiodothyronine administration on thyroxine response to exogenous TSH in man, *J. Clin. Endocrinol. Metab.* **41**:974–976.

41. Shishiba, Y., Takaishi, M., Miyachi, Y., and Ozawa, Y., 1975, Alteration of thyroidal responsiveness to TSH under the influence of circulating thyroid hormone: Short feed-back regulatory effect, *Endocrinol. Jpn.* **22**:367–371.

42. Chopra, I. J., Sack, J., and Fisher, D. A., 1975, Circulating 3,3′,5′-triiodothyronine (reverse T_3) in the human newborn, *J. Clin. Invest.* **55**:1137–1141.

43. Chopra, I. J., and Smith, S. R., 1975, Circulating thyroid hormones and thyrotropin in adult patients with protein–calorie malnutrition, *J. Clin. Endocrinol. Metab.* **40**:221–227.

44. Moshang, T., Parks, J. S., Baker, L., Vaidya, V., Utiger, R. D., Bongiovanni, A. M., and Snyder, P. J., 1975, Low serum triiodothyronine in patients with anorexia nervosa, *J. Clin. Endocrinol. Metab.* **40**:470–473.

45. Bermudez, F., Surks, M. I., and Oppenheimer, J. H., 1975, High incidence of decreased serum triiodothyronine concentration in patients with nonthyroidal disease, *J. Clin. Endocrinol. Metab.* **41**:27–40.

46. Chopra, I. J., Chopra, U., Smith, S. R., Reza, M., and Solomon, D. H., 1975, Reciprocal changes in serum concentrations of 3,3′,5′-triiodothyronine (reverse T_3) and 3,3′,5-triiodothyronine (T_3) in systemic illnesses, *J. Clin. Endocrinol. Metab.* **41**:1043–1049.

47. Nomura, S., Pittman, C. S., Chambers, J. B., Jr., Buck, M. W., and Shimizu, T., 1975, Reduced peripheral conversion of thyroxine to triiodothyronine in patients with hepatic cirrhosis, *J. Clin. Invest.* **56**:643–652.

48. Burr, W. A., Griffiths, R. S., Black, E. G., Hoffenberg, R., Meinhold, H., and Wenzel, K. W., 1975, Serum triiodothyronine and reverse triiodothyronine concentrations after surgical operation, *Lancet* **2**:1277–1279.

49. Saberi, M., Sterling, F. H., and Utiger, R. D., 1975, Reduction in extrathyroidal triiodothyronine production by propylthiouracil in man, *J. Clin. Invest.* **55**:218–223.

50. Geffner, D. L., Azukizawa, M., and Hershman, J. M., 1975, Propylthiouracil blocks extrathyroidal conversion of thyroxine to triiodothyronine and augments thyrotropin secretion in man, *J. Clin. Invest.* **55**:224–229.

51. Chopra, I. J., Williams, D. E., Orgiazzi, J., and Solomon, D. H., 1975, Opposite effects of dexamethasone on serum concentrations of 3,3′,5-triiodothyronine (reverse T_3) and 3,3′,5-triiodothyronine (T_3), *J. Clin. Endocrinol. Metab.* **41**:911–920.

52. Chopra. I. J., Sack, J., and Fisher, D. A., 1975, 3,3′,5′-triiodothyronine (reverse T_3) and 3,3′,5-triiodothyronine (T_3) in fetal and adult sheep:

Studies of metabolic clearance rates, production rates, serum binding, and thyroidal content relative to thyroxine, *Endocrinology* **97**:1080–1088.

53. Chopra, I. J., and Crandall, B. F., 1975, Thyroid hormones and thyrotropin in amniotic fluid, *N. Engl. J. Med.* **293**:740–743.

54. Inada, M., Kasagi, K., Kurata, S., Kazama, Y., Takayama, H., Torizuka, K., Fukase, M., and Soma, T., 1975, Estimation of thyroxine and triiodothyronine distribution and of the conversion rate of thyroxine to triiodothyronine in man, *J. Clin. Invest.* **55**:1337–1348.

55. Refetoff, S., Fang, V. S., and Marshall, J. S., 1975, Studies on human thyroxine-binding globulin (TBG) IX. Some physical, chemical, and biological properties of radioiodinated TBG and partially desialylated TBG, *J. Clin. Invest.* **56**:177–187.

56. Cavalieri, R. R., 1975, Preparation of ^{125}I-labeled human thyroxine-binding alpha globulin and its turnover in normal and hypothyroid subjects, *J. Clin. Invest.* **56**:79–87.

57. Spindler, B. J., Macleod, K. M., Ring, J., and Baxter, J. D., 1975, Thyroid hormone receptors. Binding characteristics and lack of hormonal dependency for nuclear localization, *J. Biol. Chem.* **250**:4113–4119.

58. Surks, M. I., Koerner, D. H., and Oppenheimer, J. H., 1975, *In vitro* binding of L-triiodothyronine to receptors in rat liver nuclei. Kinetics of binding, extraction properties, and lack of requirement for cytosol proteins, *J. Clin. Invest.* **55**:50–60.

59. DeGroot, L. J., and Torresani, J., 1975, Triiodothyronine binding to isolated liver cell nuclei, *Endocrinology* **96**:357–369.

60. Sterling, K., and Milch, P. O., 1975, Thyroid hormone binding by a component of mitochondrial membrane, *Proc. Nat. Acad. Sci. U.S.A.* **72**:3225–3229.

61. Goldfine, I. D., Simons, C. G., and Ingbar, S. H., 1975, Stimulation of uptake of α-aminoisobutyric acid in rat thymocytes of L-triiodothyronine: A comparison with insulin and dibutyryl cyclic AMP, *Endocrinology* **96**:802–805.

62. Elkeles, R. S., Lazarus, J. H., Siddle, K., and Campbell, A. K., 1975, Plasma adenosine 3′,5′-cyclic monophosphate response to glucagon in thyroid disease, *Clin. Sci. Mol. Med.* **48**:27–31.

63. Guttler, R. B., Shaw, J. W., Otis, C. L., and Nicoloff, J. T., 1975, Epinephrine-induced alterations in urinary cyclic AMP in hyper- and hypothyroidism, *J. Clin. Endocrinol. Metab.* **41**:707–711.

64. Fernandez-Pol, J. A., and Hays, M. T., 1975, Alterations in cyclic nucleotides in dogs after triiodothyronine, *Acta Endocrinol.* **79**:66–75.

65. Askenasi, R., and Demeester-Mirkine, N., 1975, Urinary excretion of hydroxylysyl glycosides and thyroid function, *J. Clin. Endocrinol. Metab.* **40**:342–344.

66. Adams, D. D., *et al.*, 1975, Nomenclature of thyroid-stimulating antibodies, *Lancet* **1**:1201.

67. Mukhtar, E. D., Smith, B. R., Pyle, G. A., Hall, R., and Vice, P., 1975, Relation of thyroid-stimulating immunoglobulins to thyroid function and effects of surgery, radioiodine, and antithyroid drugs, *Lancet* **1**:713–715.

68. Dirmikis, S. M., and Munro, D. S., 1975, Placental transmission of thyroid-stimulating immunoglobulins, *Br. Med. J.* **2**:665–666.

69. Adams, D. D., Kennedy, T. H., Stewart, J. C., Utiger, R. D., and Vidor, G. I., 1975, Hyperthyroidism in Tasmania following iodide supplementation:

Measurements of thyroid-stimulating autoantibodies and thyrotropin, *J. Clin. Endocrinol. Metab.* **41:**221–228.

70. Amino, N., and DeGroot, L. J., 1975, Insoluble particulate antigen(s) in cell-mediated immunity of autoimmune thyroid disease, *Metabolism* **24:**45–56.

71. Mulaisho, C., Abdou, N. I., and Utiger, R. D., 1975, Lack of T-cell immune abnormalities in peripheral blood lymphocytes in patients with Graves' disease or hypothyroidism, *J. Clin. Endocrinol. Metab.* **41:**266–270.

72. Orgiazzi, J., Chopra, I. J., Williams, D. E., and Solomon, D. H., 1975, Evidence for normal thyroidal adenyl cyclase, cyclic AMP–binding and protein-kinase activities in Graves' disease, *J. Clin. Endocrinol. Metab.* **40:**248–255.

73. Kenimer, J. G., Hershman, J. M., and Higgins, H. P., 1975, The thyrotropin in hydatidiform moles is human chorionic gonadotropin, *J. Clin. Endocrinol. Metab.* **40:**482–491.

74. Gershengorn, M. C., and Weintraub, B. D., 1975, Thyrotropin-induced hyperthyroidism caused by selective pituitary resistance to thyroid hormone. A new syndrome of "inappropriate secretion of TSH," *J. Clin. Invest.* **56:**633–642.

75. Gluck, F. B., Nusynowitz, M. L., and Plymate, S., 1975, Chronic lymphocytic thyroiditis, thyrotoxicosis, and low radioactive iodine uptake, *N. Engl. J. Med.* **293:**624–628.

76. Savoie, J. C., Massin, J. P., Thomopoulos, P., and Leger, F., 1975, Iodine-induced thyrotoxicosis in apparently normal thyroid glands, *J. Clin. Endocrinol. Metab.* **41:**685–691.

77. Britton, K. E., Quinn, V., Ellis, S. M., Cayley, A. C. D., Miralles, J. M., Brown, B. L., and Ekins, R. P., 1975, Is "T₄ toxicosis" a normal biochemical finding in elderly women?, *Lancet* **2:**141–142.

78. Brooks, M. H., Waldstein, S. S., Bronsky, D., and Sterling, K., 1975, Serum triiodothyronine concentration in thyroid storm, *J. Clin. Endocrinol. Metab.* **40:**339–341.

79. Emerson, C. H., Anderson, A. J., Howard, W. J., and Utiger, R. D., 1975, Serum thyroxine and triiodothyronine concentrations during iodide treatment of hyperthyroidism, *J. Clin. Endocrinol. Metab.* **40:**33–36.

80. Williams, D. E., Chopra, I. J., Orgiazzi, J., and Solomon, D. H., 1975, Acute effects of corticosteroids on thyroid activity in Graves' disease, *J. Clin. Endocrinol. Metab.* **41:**354–361.

81. Shafer, R. B., and Nuttall, F. Q., 1975, Acute changes in thyroid function in patients treated with radioactive iodine, *Lancet* **2:**635–637.

82. Sitar, D. S., and Hunninghake, D. B., 1975, Pharmacokinetics of propylthiouracil in man after a single oral dose, *J. Clin. Endocrinol. Metab.* **40:**26–29.

83. McMurry, J. F., Jr., Gilliland, P. F., Ratliff, C. R., and Bourland, P. D., 1975, Pharmacodynamics of propylthiouracil in normal and hyperthyroid subjects after a single oral dose, *J. Clin. Endocrinol. Metab.* **41:**362–364.

84. Dussault, J. H., Coulombe, P., Laberge, C., Letarte, J., Guyda, H., and Khoury, K., 1975, Preliminary report on a mass screening program for neonatal hypothyroidism, *J. Pediatr.* **86:**670–674.

85. Irie, M., Enomoto, K., and Naruse, H., 1975, Measurement of thyroid-stimulating hormone in dried blood spot, *Lancet* **2:**1233–1234.

86. Illig, R., Krawczyńska, H., Torresani, T., and Prader, A., 1975, Elevated

plasma TSH and hypothyroidism in children with hypothalamic hypopituitarism, *J. Clin. Endocrinol. Metab.* **41**:722–728.

87. Vagenakis, A. G., Braverman, L. E., Azizi, F., Portnay, G. I., and Ingbar, S. H., 1975, Recovery of pituitary thyrotropic function after withdrawal of prolonged thyroid-suppression therapy, *N. Engl. J. Med.* **293**:681–684.

88. Krugman, L. G., Hershman, J. M., Chopra, I. J., Levine, G. A., Pekary, A. E., Geffner, D. L., and Teco, G. N. C., 1975, Patterns of recovery of the hypothalamic–pituitary–thyroid axis in patients taken off chronic thyroid therapy, *J. Clin. Endocrinol. Metab.* **41**:70–80.

89. Harada, A., Kojima, A., Tsukui, T., Onaya, T., Yamada, T., Ikejiri, K., and Yukimura, Y., 1975, Pituitary unresponsiveness to thyrotropin-releasing hormone in thyrotoxic patients during chronic anti-thyroid drug therapy and in rats previously treated with excess thyroid hormone, *J. Clin. Endocrinol. Metab.* **40**:942–948.

90. Duick, D. S., Stein, R. B., Warren, D. W., and Nicoloff, J. T., 1975, The significance of partial suppressibility of serum thyroxine by triiodothyronine administration in euthyroid man, *J. Clin. Endocrinol. Metab.* **41**:229–234.

91. Edson, J. R., Fecher, D. R., and Doe, R. P., 1975, Low platelet adhesiveness and other hemostatic abnormalities in hypothyroidism, *Ann. Intern. Med.* **82**:342–346.

92. Das, K. C., Mukherjee, M., Sarkar, T. K., Dash, R. J., and Rastogi, G. K., 1975, Erythropoiesis and erythropoietin in hypo- and hyperthyroidism, *J. Clin. Endocrinol. Metab.* **40**:211–220.

93. Itoh, K., and Maruchi, N., 1975, Breast cancer in patients with Hashimoto's thyroiditis, *Lancet* **2**:1119–1121.

94. Refetoff, S., Harrison, J., Karanfilski, B. T., Kaplan, E. L., DeGroot, L. J., and Bekerman, C., 1975, Continuing occurrence of thyroid carcinoma after irradiation to the neck in infancy and childhood, *N. Engl. J. Med.* **292**:171–175.

95. Becker, F. O., Economou, S. G., Southwick, H. W., and Eisenstein, R., 1975, Adult thyroid cancer after head and neck irradiation in infancy and childhood, *Ann. Intern. Med.* **83**:347–351.

96. Van Herle, A. J., and Uller, R. P., 1975, Elevated serum thyroglobulin. A marker of metastases in differentiated thyroid carcinomas, *J. Clin. Invest.* **56**:272–277.

97. Ochi, Y., Hachiya, T., Yoshimura, M., Miyazaki, T., Majima, T., Kaimatsu, I., and Takahashi, H., 1975, Radioimmunoassay for estimation of thyroglobulin in human serum, *Endocrinol. Jpn.* **22**:351–356.

98. Smythe, G. A., Compton, P. J., and Lazarus, L., 1975, The stimulation of human prolactin secretion by 3-iodo-L-tyrosine, *J. Clin. Endocrinol. Metab.* **40**:714–716.

99. Nelson, J. C., Weiss, R. M., Palmer, F. J., Lewis, J. E., and Wilcox, R. B., 1975, Serum diiodotyrosine, *J. Clin. Endocrinol. Metab.* **41**:1118–1124.

100. M I R D/Dose Estimate Report No. 5, Summary of current radiation dose estimates to humans from ^{123}I, [124]I, ^{125}I, [130]I, ^{131}I, and [132]I as sodium iodide, *J. Nucl. Med.* **16**:857–860.

The Ovary

Mortimer B. Lipsett and Griff T. Ross

4.1. Introduction

We have interpreted our assignment to discuss the ovary broadly, and
have considered those areas of current interest that encompass ovarian
physiology, products of ovarian secretion, and problems related to the
female sex steroids. Many of the topics have almost exclusive relevance to
man; in others, the experiments in animals have proved decisive. Nevertheless, we have attempted to confine our survey of topics for discussion to
those areas that directly illuminate human physiology or disease.

MORTIMER B. LIPSETT and GRIFF T. ROSS • National Institutes of Health,
Bethesda, Maryland.

4.2. Estrogen Secretion Rates

4.2.1. Normal Women

Despite the immense past effort in the study of the estrogens, there still remains new ground to be broken, even in aspects of estradiol* metabolism. In a definitive study, Baird and Fraser[1] measured blood production and ovarian secretion rates of estradiol and estrone, using the now classic technique of estimating production rate from the metabolic clearance rate and the plasma concentrations, together with secretion rate by catheterization of the ovarian veins. They calculated that 95% of plasma estradiol is secreted by the preovulatory follicle of the corpus luteum. The contralateral ovary is relatively inactive. They also showed that the ovulatory fall in estradiol concentration was due to cessation of ovarian secretion at this time.

By contrast, about 50% of the estrone production rate resulted from peripheral conversion from androstenedione. This source of estrone will vary throughout the cycle, since plasma androstenedione concentrations increase with ovulation and are higher during the luteal than during the follicular phase of the cycle. The plasma concentrations of estradiol and estrone were compared to intrafollicular concentrations (see below).

4.2.2. Anovulatory Bleeding

In women with persistent ovarian follicles and dysfunctional uterine bleeding, estradiol was secreted by the ovary that contained the follicles at a rate comparable to that seen around ovulation or during the early luteal phase.[2,3] This finding offers no clue as to the reasons these follicles persist, but the combined studies indicate that a plasma estrogen concentration appropriate for the preovulatory period in anovulatory women means that large follicles persist in the ovary.

4.2.3. Hyperthyroidism

The effects of hyperthyroidism on estrogen metabolism have been examined repeatedly because of the associated menstrual abnormalities and disagreements about results. Ridgway et al.[4] noted, as had others, that the metabolic clearance rate of estradiol was decreased in hyperthyroid-

---

*The following trivial names for steroids have been used:
  androstenedione (androst-4-ene-3,17-dione)
  androstanediol (5α-androstane-3α,17β-diol)
  dihydrotestosterone (17β-hydroxy-5α-androstan-3-one)
  2-hydroxyestrone [2,3-dihydroxy-1,3,5(10)-estratriene-17-one]
  2-hydroxyestradiol [1,3,5,(10)-estratriene-2,3,17β-triol]
  2-hydroxyestriol [1,3,5,(10)-estratriene-2,3,16α,17β-tetrol]

ism, in association with the increased concentration of estrogen and testosterone-binding globulin, but that plasma estradiol levels were only slightly elevated, and production rates remained within normal limits. Since the production rate was normal, it seems probable that the plasma free E_2 was normal, because the two parameters are related directly in a responsive negative feedback system. In partial confirmation of this are the findings of Kono et al.[5] that urinary unconjugated estradiol is not increased in hyperthyroidism; this implies that the plasma free estradiol concentration is normal, since the free urinary steroid is a function of free plasma steroid.

4.2.4. Oral Estrogens

Of particular note for the clinician was the finding that micronized estradiol was effective by mouth. In a large study of postmenopausal women, Callantine et al.[6] showed that doses of 1–2 mg/day controlled symptoms. Yen et al.[7] showed that one tablet containing 2 mg micronized estradiol produced a maximal increment of plasma estradiol of 80 pg/ml at 5 hr after ingestion, with persistence of effect for as long as 24 hr. The increment in estrone was over 400 pg/ml 6 hr after ingestion. The finding that estrone showed the larger increment suggested that estradiol is converted to estrone in the gastrointestinal tract.

4.2.5. Catechol Estrogens

The metabolism of secreted hormones to other active compounds, either peripherally or intracellularly, has been of continuing interest over the past decade. The Montefiore group continues to provide evidence regarding their metabolism, and their latest studies of the origin and possible roles of the catechol estrogens are important. Fishman[8] established that 2-hydroxylation is a major pathway in the metabolism of estradiol and estrone (Fig. 1). Improvement in methods has permitted more facile analysis of these 2-hydroxylated compounds in urine. The excretion of 2-hydroxyestrone (2-OHE$_1$), measured throughout the menstrual cycle, was 20–40 μg/day, with a peak at ovulation.[9] In pregnancy, 2-OHE$_1$ was excreted at rates exceeding 2 mg/day in the second trimester, a rate higher than that of estradiol. Quantitatively, 2-OHE$_1$ was the most important of the catechol estrogens,[10] but the 2-hydroxyderivatives of estradiol and estriol were also identified. Although 2-OHE$_1$ and 2-hydroxyestradiol (2-OHE$_2$) have been shown to have no uterotropic potency, Martucci and Fishman[11] demonstrated that 2-OHE$_2$ had a binding affinity for uterine cytosol receptor 24% that of estradiol; similarly, Davies et al.[12] found that 2-hydroxylation of estrone and estradiol reduced their

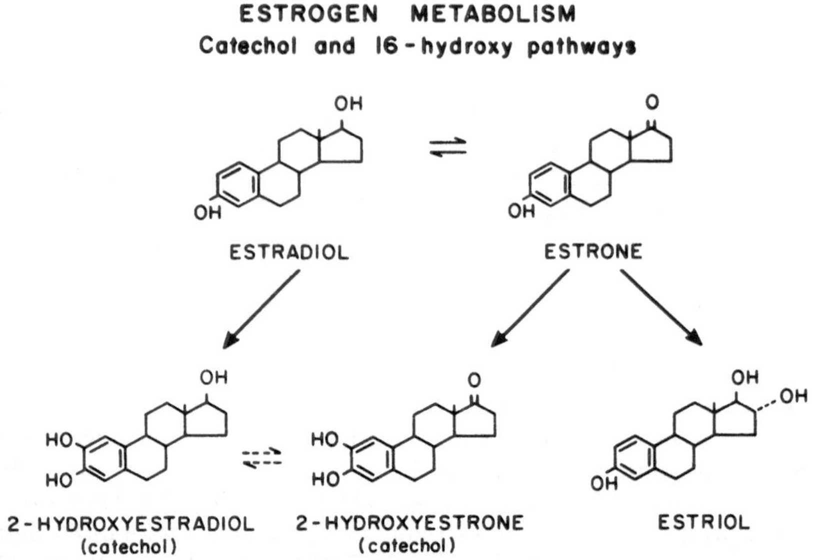

ESTROGEN   METABOLISM
Catechol and 16-hydroxy pathways

Fig. 1.   Catechol estrogens.

binding affinities for the cytosol receptors in the rat pituitary and hypo-thalamus by 40%. Because of this high-affinity binding of compounds that are not estrogenic by bioassay, a role as antiestrogens has been suggested. Naftolin et al.,[13] testing this hypothesis, reported that 2-OHE$_1$ induced a rise in plasma luteinizing hormone (LH) concentration in the rat; presumably, the compound acted as an antiestrogen, and thus behaved as clomiphene citrate.

In view of this relationship between the binding affinities of the 2-hydroxycatechol estrogens and their biological effect, modulation of estrogen action at the cellular level seems possible. These actions cannot be considered in isolation, and the recent studies of estriol metabolism have direct relevance, particularly since estriol and 2-hydroxyestrone are the major metabolites of estradiol.

4.2.5.1. Estriol

Estriol is produced in significant amounts in normal women, and circulates as the unconjugated steroid. Flood et al.[14] analyzed the clear-ance rates and production rates of estriol in cycling and in postmenopau-sal women. The metabolic clearance rates were the same as those of estrone, indicating that estriol had no specific plasma binding protein.

Estriol production rates were 14 μg/day in the follicular phase and 23 μg/ day during the early luteal phase. In 4 postmenopausal women, production rates varied from 5 to 22 μg/day. Thus, although the biological contribution of estriol in the menstruating woman is small, it may be of importance in the postmenopausal woman whose estradiol production is low. Since estriol is not bound to testosterone-binding globulin and estradiol is, the relative biological effectiveness of the apparently low blood levels of estriol will be magnified. Estriol has been shown to act as an antiestrogen or as a weak estrogen, depending on the experimental protocol. These conflicting results have now been resolved by the finding that estriol binds to rat uterine cytosol receptor with an affinity some 10% that of estradiol.[11,15] However, the dissociation of the estriol–receptor complex is rapid,[16] accounting for its low biological potency when given as a single dose. When estriol is given at short intervals, its biological potency is about equal to that of estrone.[16]

Since the two principal metabolites of estradiol act as an estrogen and an antiestrogen, factors altering the routes of metabolism could be expected to alter the total estrogenic biological effect. The hypothesis that estriol inhibits the development of breast cancer because of its antiestrogenic potency[17] cannot be correct in view of the more recent findings. The 2-hydroxyestrogens could conceivably play this role. The factors influencing the metabolism of estradiol have not been investigated extensively, but some data are available. Thyroid status profoundly alters the routes of metabolism of estradiol, hyperthyroidism favoring 2-hydroxylation.[18] Obese women excreted more estriol than did a control population,[19] and a recent study showed that inanition favored 2-hydroxylation, while obesity promoted 16-hydroxylation.[20] The conditions that favor 2- vs. 16-hydroxylation need further exploration because the resultant net estrogenic effect of estradiol secretion will depend on them. The possibility has been raised that the excess estriol in obesity contributes to a higher total estrogen production rate, and is therefore a factor in the production of the menstrual disturbances of obesity.

4.3. Regulation of Follicular Growth

4.3.1. Intrafollicular Steroid Concentrations

The definition of the factors regulating follicular growth has proceeded rapidly, and the correlations of intrafollicular hormones and receptors with follicular activity are being made. Manipulation of intraovarian steroid hormone levels with immunological and chemical antagonists of estrogens and androgens has been shown to affect gonadotropic stimulation of both follicular growth and atresia in an animal model system.[21-25] Estrogens enhanced follicular growth and reduced atresia, whereas androgens inhibited granulosa cell proliferation and increased atresia in ovaries of hypophysectomized immature female rats given gonadotropins.[23-25] Cytosol of granulosa cells from preantral follicles was shown to contain receptors specific for androgens and for estrogens, providing one of the components required for nuclear translocation of sex steroid hormones in these cells, as in other cells that respond to steroid hormones.[26-28] These studies have led to the hypothesis that the local steroid hormone milieu is one determinant of the route followed by a maturing follicle to atresia or ovulation. Mechanisms for regulating intra-follicular hormone levels are implicit in this hypothesis.[29]

Extensive studies of cyclic changes in the human intraovarian hormone milieu over the past year suggest that mechanisms exist for regulating both steroid and gonadotropin levels within follicles in the human ovary. Baird and Fraser[1] measured estradiol and estrone concentrations in specimens of ovarian follicular fluid and venous effluent collected during laparotomy performed at varying times during the menstrual cycle for diseases unrelated to the ovaries. During the early follicular phase of the cycle, mean estradiol concentrations were of the order of 3–4 nmole/liter in plasma from both ovaries, and remained at these levels throughout the cycle in the ovary without a large preovulatory follicle or corpus luteum. However, in the mid- to late follicular phase, mean estradiol concentrations of 49 nmole/liter were 20-fold higher in plasma from the ovary containing the dominant follicle than from the contralateral ovary. Similarly, mean estradiol concentrations ranged from 16 nmole/liter during the early luteal phase to 28 nmole/liter during the mid- to late luteal phase in plasma from the ovary containing a corpus luteum. These levels were 4–8-fold higher than mean estrogen concentrations in plasma collected during the luteal phase from the contralateral ovary. In general, changes in estrone concentrations paralleled changes in estradiol concentrations, being higher in plasma specimens containing higher concentrations of estradiol.

In follicular fluid, concentrations of both estrogens were 1–2 orders of magnitude higher than those in peripheral blood. Though wide variations were seen, estradiol concentrations ranged from 70 to 1050 nmole/liter at all stages of the cycle except during the mid- and late proliferative phases, when a mean estradiol concentration of 5390 nmole/liter was detected in specimens collected from follicles greater than 1 cm in diameter. These results are consistent with those obtained in earlier studies showing that steroid hormone concentrations in antral fluid increase with increasing diameter of human ovarian follicles throughout the follicular phase of the cycle.[30] Since ovarian secretion is the principal source of estradiol in the peripheral blood of women during the reproductive years, rising concentrations of the steroid in peripheral blood reflect biosynthesis of the hormone by the ovary containing the dominant follicle.

McNatty and co-workers[31,32] studied cyclic changes in the gonadotropic and sex steroid hormones of antral fluid, and suggested that the order of these changes is important for both the growth and the secretory activity of granulosa cells prior to and following ovulation. At laparotomy, specimens of antral fluid were collected from ovaries either *in situ* during surgery or from follicles dissected out of ovarian tissue excised up to 2 hr earlier. Concentrations of follicle-stimulating hormone (FSH), LH, prolactin, and steroid hormones, including estradiol and progesterone, were measured by radioimmunoassay. In specimens obtained from 97 women, concentrations of hormones in antral fluid from follicles less than 8 mm in diameter were compared to those in antral fluid from follicles equal to or greater than 8 mm in diameter recovered in early, middle, and late follicular, and early, middle, and late luteal phases of the cycle. Intrafollicular concentrations, in turn, were compared with concentrations of the same hormones in peripheral blood. Antral fluid estradiol and progesterone concentrations rose during the middle and later follicular phases, and were higher in fluid from larger than from smaller follicles, consistent with earlier observations.[30,33] Kemeter *et al.*[34] measured antral fluid testosterone, estradiol, and progesterone concentrations, and found lower testosterone levels, but higher estradiol and progesterone levels, in control fluid from larger follicles. It has become evident, then, that the process of follicular growth leading to ovulation is accompanied by progressive increases in follicular steroid synthesis and accumulation of steroids in the follicular fluid. Whether this latter phenomenon is a passive accompaniment of follicular growth, or whether it is a necessary step for ovulation, is unknown.

4.3.2. Protein Hormones in the Follicles

Although profiles of serum prolactin concentrations were similar to those seen in normal women, McNatty *et al.*[32] found that prolactin concentrations were higher in serum specimens collected intraoperatively from women stressed by surgery and anesthesia. Nonetheless, mean antral fluid prolactin concentrations fell from mean early follicular phase levels of 60 ng/ml to mean late follicular phase levels of 10 ng/ml in fluid from follicles less than 8 mm in diameter, with a secondary rise during the midluteal phase to 30 ng/ml. Though concentrations were lower in antral fluid from follicles greater than 8 mm in diameter, patterns of change were similar. While these data suggest that a mechanism exists for regulating antral fluid prolactin concentrations in the human ovary, the physiological significance of these changes remains to be shown.

FSH concentrations in follicles less than 8 mm in diameter were maximal either during or just after maximal plasma concentrations that occur during early follicular midcycle, or during late luteal phases of the cycle. In contrast, FSH concentrations in antral fluid from follicles greater than 8 mm in diameter rose despite declining serum FSH levels in the mid- and late follicular phases. Since the follicle destined to ovulate is one of these maturing larger follicles, increasing concentrations of FSH may be important in regulating this phase of follicular maturation. In this regard, it is noteworthy that in specimens collected during the follicular phase of the cycle, detectable levels of FSH were associated with higher concentrations of estradiol in antral fluid.

In contrast to the discrepancies between FSH concentrations in blood and antral fluid during the follicular phase, LH concentrations in blood and antral fluid were consonant. However, during the luteal phase of the cycle, antral fluid LH concentrations in both large and smaller follicles rose despite declining serum concentrations. Antral fluid from follicles in which LH was measurable contained more progesterone, and all follicles that contained measurable LH and higher concentrations of progesterone also contained FSH. These data were interpreted to indicate that estradiol and FSH in antral fluid conditions granulosa cells to secrete progesterone in response to LH, an interpretation consistent with the observation that FSH induces LH receptors in rat granulosa cells.[35] More recently, McNatty and Sawers[31] studied the effects of *in vivo* antral fluid hormone concentration on the mitotic and secretory activity of granulosa cells *in vitro*. Mitotic activity was highest in cells recovered from antral follicles that contained FSH and estradiol. Furthermore, addition of FSH and high concentrations of estradiol stimulated mitotic activity in cells harvested from follicles in which LH was undetectable or at low levels. Mitotic rates were lower in cells isolated from follicles containing LH, irrespective of other hormones. Cells recovered from antral follicles containing LH, FSH, and estradiol secreted more progesterone *in vitro* than cells from follicles that did not contain all three hormones. Moreover, addition of all three hormones to the tissue culture media stimulated progesterone secretion by cells isolated from follicles in which none of the three hormones was detected. Follicular fluid or estrogen-free follicular fluid inhibited differentiation of rat granulosa cells in culture.[36] The factors in follicular fluid that modulate granulosa cell growth and function remain incompletely defined.

McNatty and Sawers suggest that an 8–10-day exposure to a mixture of FSH and estradiol is a prerequisite for normal progesterone secretion by granulosa cells, and presumably is therefore a prerequisite for normal corpus luteum function.[31] In this regard, it is interesting to recall that Ross et al.[37] reported that serum FSH levels and serum estradiol levels were lower during the follicular phase of cycles with short or inadequate luteal phases, and suggested this as an etiological factor. Sherman and Korenman[38,39] supported and amplified this suggestion.

4.3.3. Prostaglandins

Plunkett et al.[40] showed that addition of gonadotropins to the incubation medium stimulated PGF synthesis by human ovarian follicles maintained in organ culture for 72 hr, as had been shown previously by Moon et al.[41] for rabbit ovarian follicles. Evidence consistent with a role for PGF_2 at the level of the follicles in mediating LH-induced ovulation in rabbits has been adduced.[42] In part, this effect results from LH stimulation of follicular PGF_2 synthesis, since intrafollicular injection of indomethacin inhibits not only PGF_2 synthesis, but also LH-induced ovulation. Whether prostaglandins mediate the ovulatory role of LH in humans remains to be established.

4.4. The Postmenopausal Ovary

4.4.1. Follicle-Stimulating Hormone Regulation

The postmenopausal ovary has been the subject of increasing inquiry. Yen and Tsai[43] examined the plasma LH and FSH concentrations following ovariectomy. They reported reversal of the FSH:LH ratio due to a 10-fold increase in FSH and only a 3- to 4-fold increase in LH. Sherman and Korenman,[44] in studies of the characteristics of the menstrual cycle throughout reproductive life, noted that FSH concentrations were increased, although LH remained within the normal range in perimenopausal women. Goldenberg et al.[45] had shown previously that FSH increased whenever there was an absence of ovarian follicles. Sherman and Korenman[44] suggested that there is, then, an additional regulatory mechanism for FSH other than the estrogen feedback, and that by analogy with the male, the follicle might be secreting an "inhibin." Sherman et al.[46] provided additional evidence for this mechanism by detailed analysis of the plasma concentrations of LH, FSH, estradiol, and progesterone in older women. The hypothesis is attractive, since it provides for information exchange between the follicular components of the ovary and the hypothalamus–pituitary. As suggested by Sherman and Korenman, this could be one way of regulating the number of follicles that mature during each cycle.

4.4.2. Androgen Secretion

The postmenopausal ovary does not secrete significant estrogen, as shown by several lines of evidence, which now include direct catheterization of the ovarian effluent vein.[47] Androgen secretion does continue, and Judd et al.[48] noted that plasma testosterone and androstenedione concentrations fell following ovariectomy of the postmenopausal woman. In other studies, Judd et al.[47] found that testosterone secretion into the ovarian vein remained close to that of premenopausal women, and that the ovary was the source of much of the testosterone present in the blood. Vermeulen,[49] using similar techniques, reported that about 50% of the testosterone was derived from the ovary, and showed that human chorionic gonadotropin (HCG) could increase ovarian testosterone secretion. These studies raise the question of the cells of origin of testosterone in the ovary. There are many studies demonstrating that the ovarian stroma has the capacity to synthesize androgens *de novo*. Savard et al.[50] emphasized the uniquely greater capacity of the stromal compartment for androgen synthesis. Morris and Scully[51] reviewed the evidence that stromal thecal cells were concerned with androgen synthesis, and Guraya[52] considered the histology of these cells extensively. The reports of virilization associated with hyperthecosis[53-55] show that the luteinized stromal thecal cell can be a source of excessive testosterone secretion. From these data, it is now fair to conclude that the stromal thecal cell and the interstitial cell are the sources of the ovarian secretion of testosterone, and that this ovarian function continues after the menopause.

4.5. Idiopathic Hirsutism

4.5.1. The Ovary

The role of the ovary in idiopathic hirsutism has received extensive attention. Kirschner and his colleagues have studied the origin of the androgens in women with idiopathic hirsutism by catheterization of ovarian and adrenal veins. In their most recent paper,[56] they summarize their data showing that the excess androgens, testosterone, and androstenedione almost always originate from the ovary. This experience has not been shared by others, and Oake et al.[57] and Northrup et al.[58] reported significant adrenal cortical secretion of androgens in some hirsute women, although the ovary was more frequently the important source, and only rarely was the adrenal cortex the sole source of the androgens. Parker et al.[59] explored the dynamics of adrenal and ovarian catheterization in detail, and commented on the problems involved in sampling and in obtaining estimates of secretion over a sufficient period of time to ensure that the effect of episodic fluctuations would be minimal. They reported that ACTH induced secretion of androgens only by the adrenal cortex, and the HCG was effective only in stimulating the ovary. However, in reaffirmation of their earlier findings, Kirschner et al.[56] showed that dexamethasone suppressed plasma testosterone in 20 of 44 hirsute women even though the ovary was shown to be the major source of testosterone and androstenedione. These data are important because they demonstrate that glucocorticoid suppression of testosterone in hirsutism cannot be equated with an adrenal origin of the disease, and that the phrase "adult adrenogenital syndrome," which is often loosely applied to these women, should be abandoned. Not in the nature of dissent, but as a complementary finding, is the heightened sensitivity of the adrenal cortex to small doses of ACTH in hirsutism.[60] The increase in plasma androstenedione concentration was clearly greater than in normal women. No explanation of this phenomenon is at hand.

4.5.2. Therapy

Although the reasons for excessive androgen production by the ovary remain obscure, the identification of the offending gland has made endocrine therapy more rational. Givens et al.[60] found that it was necessary to give oral contraceptives for at least 3 weeks to observe the maximal decrease in plasma LH and androgens. Since suppression of LH is the goal of this regimen, the contraceptives should contain higher amounts of the progestational agents. Casey[61] examined the effects of chronic treatment, and attempted to correlate them with changes in testosterone plasma levels and production rates. Adrenal suppression alone was rarely successful, although there were significant decreases in the testosterone production rate. An oral contraceptive, ethinylestradiol, 50 μg, and medroxyprogesterone, 10 mg, produced good clinical results in 5 of 9 subjects, and addition of 0.5 mg β-methasone at midnight to this regimen yielded 6 good results in 10 trials. When good results were achieved, there was a marked decrease in the androgen indexes; however, there were occasional poor clinical results obtained even when this occurred. Further study will be necessary to prove that the chronic use of glucocorticoids in addition to the oral contraceptives will be necessary.

4.5.3. Antiandrogens

Attention should be called to the use of antiandrogens in idiopathic hirsutism. Cyproterone acetate is an orally active progestational agent that shares with other progestins the capacity to inhibit LH release and to antagonize androgens at the end-organ. There is now extensive experience in Germany with this compound for the treatment of acne and hirsutism. Hammerstein *et al.*[62] summarized their experience in the treatment of more than 600 women with hirsutism, acne, or seborrhea. Acne and seborrhea responded quickly, and with a high success rate. The success rate in hirsutism varied from 60 to 80% among different clinics, and 6–9 months being necessary to observe improvement. Since cyproterone acetate is progestational, it was necessary to devise a reverse sequential regimen that included the use of ethinylestradiol to induce withdrawal bleeding. Despite the good results that have been reported, there is no evidence that the compound induced these effects because of its antiandrogenic potency. Whether comparatively high doses of other, similar progestins with equal LH suppression would achieve the same effects remains to be tested.

4.5.4. Skin Androgen Metabolism

Our knowledge of the pathogenetic events in hirsutism has advanced markedly over the past several years. The skin has been known to have the capacity to metabolize such preandrogens* as dehydroepiandrosterone and its sulfate to testosterone,[63,64] and this capacity has been shown to exist in the hair follicle.[65] There is good reason to believe that dihydrotestosterone is the active proximate androgen at the hair follicle, and Thomas and Oake[66] reported that the skin of hirsute women transformed a greater proportion of testosterone to dihydrotestosterone than did the skin of normal women. Using the adhering follicle cells of the plucked beard hair and testosterone and androstenedione as precursors, Schweikert and Wilson[67,68] could find no differences between men and women in the rate of dihydrotestosterone formation. In considering these apparently opposite findings, it should be remembered that the sebaceous glands of the skin are also testosterone-responsive, and that Schweikert and Wilson measured only the activity of hair follicle cells.

The work of Mauvais-Jarvis and his collaborators, extending over seven years, offers the possibility of analyzing these events *in vivo*. Mauvais-Jarvis *et al.*[69] showed that the skin was the most active tissue for reducing dihydrotestosterone to androstanediol. In 1973, Mauvais-Jarvis *et al.*[70] found that the excretion of androstanediol was much higher in hirsute women than in normal women, and intermediate in women with acne. They attributed these results to the role of the skin appendages in synthesizing dihydrotestosterone and then metabolizing it, primarily to androstanediol. Kuttenn and Mauvais-Jarvis[71] then examined the 5α-

---

*A preandrogen is a steroid without androgenic activity that is converted into an active androgen in peripheral tissues.

reduction of testosterone to dihydrotestosterone and to the diols in pubic skin from patients with abnormal sex differentiation. There was a good correlation between 5α-reductase activity and hair growth in sexual-area skin. Thus, the *in vitro* data confirm the *in vivo* data, and the measurement of androstanediol is likely to prove a useful index of the extent of the skin's synthesis of dihydrotestosterone.

If 5α-reduction is a necessary step for androgen action in the skin, then inhibitors of this enzyme could prove useful. Mauvais-Jarvis *et al.*[72] administered progesterone, a 5α-reductase inhibitor, by inunction on pubic skin, and found that 5α-reduction of testosterone by this skin *in vitro* was severely inhibited, while plasma testosterone levels remained unchanged. The development of 5α-reductase inhibitors, effective locally, will undoubtedly be an efficient means for preventing excessive hair growth. It might even be the locally effective depilatory for men that would obviate the need to shave.

4.6. Side Effects of Estrogen

4.6.1. Liver Tumors

Each year witnesses the reporting of new side effects of estrogens in the postmenopausal woman and of the oral contraceptives in younger women. The case control method has proved to be a powerful tool for the epidemiologist to document the association of rare events with other factors. In general, data obtained in this way have survived critical review and have been confirmed in subsequent studies, although several notable instances that received wide publicity, such as the association of coffee with myocardial infarction and the increased incidence of breast cancer in reserpine users, have not been confirmed.

Since estrogenic compounds are now used so widely and for prolonged periods of time, the increasing risk of serious complication requires a continuing reanalysis of the detriment–benefit ratio of these compounds. Some of these complications have been recognized only recently because of their rarity. In 1973, Baum *et al.*[73] suggested that oral contraceptive use was associated with benign hepatomas. Subsequently, several small series of such cases have been reported. Christopherson *et al.*[74] described four types of hepatic tumors among 13 women: focal nodular hyperplasia, adenoma, hamartoma, and carcinoma. Sherlock[75] summarized the English experience. The tumors reported were adenomatous, and often not sharply demarcated from normal liver. Occasionally, there was associated sinusoidal dilation (peliosis hepatica) that often led to bleeding. The patients had usually been taking the "pill" for more than 2 years. The presenting complaints were due to an enlarging mass, pain, or hemorrhage. Edmondson et al.[76] found that over 90% of women with liver adenomas had been taking oral contraceptives, and the mean duration of use was 6½ years.

These and other reports suggest that the frequency of hepatic tumors will increase as the duration of exposure to the contraceptives becomes longer. Thus, the extent of the problem may be considerably greater than was suspected 2 years ago.

4.6.2. Gall Bladder Disease

In 1973, the Boston Collaborative Drug Survey Program reported that the use of oral contraceptives increased the risks for gall bladder disease.[77] The same group[78] noted that estrogens had the same sequelae in postmenopausal women. Now, Bennion et al.[79] have shown that gall bladder bile is more saturated with cholesterol in women taking oral contraceptives than in normally cycling women. This finding in women has ample precedent in the experimental animal. Thus, the observed epidemiological finding is supported by laboratory study and clinical investigation.

4.6.3. Uterine Cancer

There are many data associating either increased, or more probably uninterrupted, estrogenic stimulation of the uterine endometrium with a higher frequency of endometrial cancer. MacMahon[80] summarized these and other risk factors for endometrial cancer. Two recent studies, both using the case control method, emphasize the role of estrogens. Smith et al.[81] concluded that menopausal and postmenopausal women who used estrogens had 4–5 times the risk of matched controls with respect to developing endometrial cancer. Ziel and Finkle,[82] who examined specifically the use of conjugated estrogens after the menopause, derived slightly higher risk factors. They also noted that the risk increased with duration of exposure. They were unable to tell how many of these women used the steroids intermittently or had withdrawal bleeding. Nevertheless, these two studies unfortunately confirm the many clinical reports linking estrogens with endometrial cancer.

4.6.4. Stroke

Another serious side effect that has been associated with oral contraceptives is stroke. The Collaborative Group for the Study of Stroke in Young Women[83] studied 598 women 15–44 years of age with various types of cerebrovascular disease. Again, using the case control method, they estimated that the relative risk of cerebral ischemia or thrombosis is 9 times greater in oral contraceptive users. They affirmed these results in 1975,[84] and showed that the increased risk was independent of hypertension, migraine, and smoking. To place these results in perspective, it should be noted that the absolute risk of stroke per year was still only 1 in 10,000. Bickerstaff[85] observed a recent marked increase in rarer types of cerebrovascular thrombosis in young women, and attributed it to oral contraceptive use. A dissenting voice is that of Comer *et al.*,[86] who compared the frequency of strokes in two 5-year periods in Rochester, Minnesota, and Bakersfield, California. They observed no increase that could be associated with increasing contraceptive usage, and their calculated incidence was the same as that reported in the rest of the country. Although this apparent disagreement cannot be resolved, the evidence for venous thrombosis attributable to oral contraceptive use is so strong that it is difficult to see how the cerebral vessels could be spared.

None of these reports of serious side effects taken in isolation is sufficient reason to ban the use of the most effective contraceptive available. The reports do suggest that the risk of some serious side effect imposed by oral contraceptive use is many times that of the normal population. Thus, there can be little complacency about the status of contraceptive methods, and there is every reason for supporting efforts to develop safer and equally effective techniques.

References

1. Baird, D. T., and Fraser, I. S., 1974, Blood production and ovarian secretion rates of estradiol-17β and estrone in women throughout the menstrual cycle, *J. Clin. Endocrinol. Metab.* **38:**1009–1017.
2. Fraser, I. S., and Baird, D. T., 1974, Blood production and ovarian secretion rates of estradiol-17β and estrone in women with dysfunctional uterine bleeding, *J. Clin. Endocrinol. Metab.* **39:**564–570.
3. deJong, F. H., Baird, D. T., and van der Molen, H. J., 1974, Ovarian secretion rates of oestrogens, androgens, and progesterone in normal women and in women with persistent ovarian follicles, *Acta Endocrinol.* **77:**575–587.
4. Ridgway, E. C., Longcope, C., and Maloof, F., 1975, Metabolic clearance and blood production rates of estradiol in hyperthyroidism, *J. Clin. Endocrinol. Metab.* **41:**491–497.
5. Kono, S., Loriaux, D. L., and Lipsett, M. B., 1974, A radioimmunoassay of unconjugated oestradiol in urine, *Acta Endocrinol.* **76:**741–746.
6. Callantine, M. R., Martin, P. L., Bolding, O. T., Warner, P. O., and Greaney, M. O., Jr., 1975, Micronized 17β-estradiol for oral estrogen therapy in menopausal women, *Obstet. Gynecol.* **46:**37–41.
7. Yen, S. S. C., Martin, P. L., Burnier, A. M., Czekala, N. M., Greaney, M. O., Jr., and Callantine, M. R., 1975, Circulatory estradiol, estrone, and gonado-

tropin levels following the administration of orally active 17β-estradiol in postmenopausal women, *J. Clin. Endocrinol. Metab.* **40**:518–521.

8. Fishman, J., 1963, Role of 2-hydroxyestrone in estrogen metabolism, *J. Clin. Endocrinol. Metab.* **23**:207–210.

9. Ball, P., Gelbke, H. P., and Knuppen, R., 1975, The excretion of 2-hydroxyestrone during the menstrual cycle, *J. Clin. Endocrinol. Metab.* **40**:406–408.

10. Gelbke, H. P., Böttger, M., and Knuppen, R., 1975, Excretion of 2-hydroxyestrone in urine throughout human pregnancies, *J. Clin. Endocrinol. Metab.* **41**:744–750.

11. Martucci, C., and Fishman, J., 1976, Uterine estrogen receptor binding of catecholestrogens and of estetrol [1,3,5(10)-estratriene-3,15α,16α,17β-tetrol], *Steroids* **27**:325–333.

12. Davies, I. J., Naftolin, F., Ryan, K. J., Fishman, J. and Siu, J., 1975, The affinity of catechol estrogens for estrogen receptors in the pituitary and anterior hypothalamus of the rat, *Endocrinology* **97**:554–557.

13. Naftolin, F., Morishita, H., Davies, I. J., Todd, R., Ryan, K. J., and Fishman, J., 1975, 2-Hydroxyestrone induced rise in serum luteinizing hormone in the immature male rat, *Biochem. Biophys. Res. Commun.* **64**:905–910.

14. Flood, C., Pratt, J. H., and Longcope, C., 1976, The metabolic clearance and blood production rates of estriol in normal, non-pregnant women, *J. Clin. Endocrinol. Metab.* **42**:1–8.

15. Tseng, L., and Gurpide, E., 1974, Nuclear concentration of estriol in superfused human endometrium; competition with estradiol, *J. Steroid Biochem.* **5**:273–278.

16. Anderson, J. N., Peck, E. J., Jr., and Clark, J. H., 1975, Estrogen-induced uterine responses and growth: Relationships to receptor estrogen binding by uterine nuclei, *Endocrinology* **96**:160–167.

17. Lemon, H. M., Wotiz, H. H., Parsons, L., and Mozden, P. J., 1966, Reduced estriol excretion in patients with breast cancer prior to endocrine therapy, *J. Amer. Med. Assoc.* **196**:1128–1136.

18. Fishman, J., Hellman, L., Zumoff, B., and Gallagher, T. F., 1965, Effect of thyroid on hydroxylation of estrogen in man, *J. Clin. Endocrinol. Metab.* **25**:365–368.

19. Brown, J. B., and Strong, J. A., 1965, The effect of nutritional status and thyroid function on the metabolism of oestradiol, *J. Endocrinol.* **32**:107–115.

20. Fishman, J., Boyar, R. M., and Hellman, L., 1975, Influence of body weight on estradiol metabolism in young women, *J. Clin. Endocrinol. Metab.* **41**:989–991.

21. Goldenberg, R. L., Vaitukaitis, J. L., and Ross, G. T., 1972, Estrogen and follicle-stimulating hormone interactions on follicle growth in rats, *Endocrinology* **90**:1492–1498.

22. Reiter, E. O., Goldenberg, R. L., Vaitukaitis, J. L., and Ross, G. T., 1972, Evidence for a role of estrogen in the ovarian augmentation reaction, *Endocrinology* **91**:1518–1522.

23. Harman, S. M., Louvet, J.-P., and Ross, G. T., 1975, Interaction of estrogen and gonadotropins in follicular atresia, *Endocrinology* **96**:1145–1152.

24. Louvet, J.-P., Harman, S. M., and Ross, G. T., 1975, Effects of human chorionic gonadotropin, human interstitial cell stimulating hormone and human follicle stimulating hormone on ovarian weights in estrogen-primed hypophysectomized immature female rats, *Endocrinology* **96**:1179–1186.

25. Louvet, J.-P., Harman, S. M., Schreiber, J. R., and Ross, G. T., 1975,

Evidence for a role of androgens in follicular maturation, *Endocrinology* **97**:366–372.

26. Schreiber, J. R., Reid, R., and Ross, G. T., 1976, A receptor-like testosterone binding protein in ovaries from estrogen-stimulated hypophysectomized immature female rats, *Endocrinology* **98**:1206–1213.

27. Schreiber, J. R., and Ross, G. T., 1976, Further characterization of a rat ovarian testosterone receptor with evidence of nuclear translocation, *Endocrinology* **99**:590–596.

28. Richards, J. S., 1975, Estradiol receptor content in rat granulosa cells during follicular development: Modification by estradiol and gonadotropins, *Endocrinology* **97**:1174–1184.

29. Ross, G. T., 1976, On intraovarian control of oogenesis in the human, *in: Ovulation in the Human* (P. G. Crosignani and D. R. Mishell, eds.), pp. 127–140, Academic Press, London.

30. Sanyal, M. K., Berger, M. J., Thompson, I. E., Taymor, M. L., and Horne, H. W., Jr., 1974, Development of graafian follicles in adult human ovary. I. Correlation of estrogen and progesterone concentration in antral fluid with growth of follicles, *J. Clin. Endocrinol. Metab.* **38**:828–835.

31. McNatty, K. P., and Sawers, R. S., 1975, Relationship between the endocrine environment within the graafian follicle and the subsequent rate of progesterone secretion by human granulosa cells *in vitro, J. Endocrinol.* **66**:391–400.

32. McNatty, K. P., Hunter, W. M., McNeilly, A. S., and Sawers, R. S., 1975, Changes in the concentration of pituitary and steroid hormones in the follicular fluid of human graafian follicles throughout the menstrual cycle, *J. Endocrinol.* **64**:555–571.

33. Edwards, R. G., Steptoe, P. C., Abraham, G. E., Walters, E., Purdy, J. M., and Fotherby, K., 1972, Steroid assays and preovulatory follicular development in human ovaries primed with gonadotrophins, *Lancet* **2**:611–615.

34. Kemeter, P., Salzer, H., Breitenecker, G., and Friedrich, F., 1975, Progesterone, testosterone, and estradiol-17β levels in the follicular fluid of tertiary follicles and graafian follicles of human ovaries, *Acta Endocrinol.* **80**:686–704.

35. Zeleznik, A. J., Midgley, A. R., Jr., and Reichert, L. E., Jr., 1974, Granulosa cell maturation in the rat: Increased binding of human chorionic gonadotropin following treatment with follicle-stimulating hormone *in vivo, Endocrinology* **95**:818–825.

36. Bernard, J., 1975, Effect of follicular fluid and oestradiol on the luteinization of rat granulosa cells *in vitro, J. Reprod. Fertil.* **43**:453–460.

37. Ross, G. T., Cargille, C. M., Lipsett, M. B., Rayford, P. L., Marshall, J. R., Strott, C. A., and Rodbard, D., 1970, Pituitary and gonadal hormones in women during spontaneous and induced ovulatory cycles, *Recent Prog. Horm. Res.* **26**:1–62.

38. Sherman, B. M., and Korenman, S. G., 1974, Measurement of plasma LH, FSH, estradiol, and progesterone in disorders of the human menstrual cycle: The short luteal phase, *J. Clin. Endocrinol. Metab.* **38**:89–93.

39. Sherman, B. M., and Korenman, S. G., 1974, Measurement of serum LH, FSH, estradiol, and progesterone in disorders of the human menstrual cycle: The inadequate luteal phase, *J. Clin. Endocrinol. Metab.* **39**:145–149.

40. Plunkett, E. R., Moon, Y. S., Zamecnik, J., and Armstrong, D. T., 1975, Preliminary evidence of a role of prostaglandin F in human follicular function, *Amer. J. Obstet. Gynecol.* **123**:391–397.

41. Moon, Y. S., Zamecnik, J., and Armstrong, D. T., 1974, Stimulation of prostaglandin F synthesis by luteinizing hormone in rabbit ovarian follicles grown in organ culture, *Life Sci.* **15:**1731–1738.
42. Armstrong, D. T., Grinwich, D. L., Moon, Y. S., and Zamecnik, J., 1974, Inhibition of ovulation in rabbits by intrafollicular injection of indomethacin and prostaglandin F antiserum, *Life Sci.* **14:**129–140.
43. Yen, S. S. C., and Tsai, C. C., 1971, The effect of ovariectomy on gonadotropin release, *J. Clin. Invest.* **50:**1149–1153.
44. Sherman, B. M., and Korenman, S. G., 1975, Hormonal characteristics of the human menstrual cycle throughout reproductive life, *J. Clin. Invest.* **55:**699–706.
45. Goldenberg, R. L., Grodin, J. M., Rodbard, D., and Ross, G. T., 1973, Gonadotropins in women with amenorrhea. The use of plasma follicle-stimulating hormone to differentiate women with and without ovarian follicles, *Amer. J. Obstet. Gynecol.* **116:**1003–1012.
46. Sherman, B. M., West, J. H., and Korenman, S. G., 1976, The menopausal transition: Analysis of LH, FSH, estradiol, and progesterone concentrations during menstrual cycles of older women, *J. Clin. Endocrinol. Metab.* **42:**629–636.
47. Judd, H. L., Judd, G. E., Lucas, W. E., and Yen, S. S. C., 1974, Endocrine function of the postmenopausal ovary: Concentration of androgens and estrogens in ovarian and peripheral vein blood, *J. Clin. Endocrinol. Metab.* **39:**1020–1024.
48. Judd, H. L., Lucas, W. E., and Yen, S. S. C., 1974, Effect of oophorectomy on circulating testosterone and androstenedione levels in patients with endometrial cancer, *Amer. J. Obstet. Gynecol.* **118:**793–798.
49. Vermeulen, A., 1976, The hormonal activity of the postmenopausal ovary, *J. Clin. Endocrinol. Metab.* **42:**247–253.
50. Savard, K., Marsh, J. M., and Rice, B. F., 1965, Gonadotropins and ovarian steroidogenesis, *Recent Prog. Horm. Res.* **21:**285–365.
51. Morris, J. M., and Scully, R. E., 1958, *Endocrine Pathology of the Ovary*, Mosby Co., St. Louis.
52. Guraya, S. S., 1973, Interstitial gland tissue of mammalian ovary, *Acta Endocrinol. Suppl.* **171:**5–27.
53. Bardin, C. W., Lipsett, M. B., Edgcomb, J. H., and Marshall, J. R., 1967, Studies of testosterone metabolism in a patient with masculinization due to stromal hyperthecosis, *N. Engl. J. Med.* **277:**399–402.
54. Givens, J. R. Wiser, W. L., Coleman, S. A., Wilroy, R. S., Andersen, R. N., and Fish, S. A., 1971, Familial ovarian hyperthecosis: A study of two families, *Amer. J. Obstet. Gynecol.* **110:**959–972.
55. Judd, H. L., Scully, R. E., Herbst, A. L., Yen, S. S. C., Ingersol, F. M., and Kliman, B., 1973, Familial hyperthecosis: Comparison of endocrinologic and histologic findings with polycystic ovarian disease, *Amer. J. Obstet. Gynecol.* **117:**976–982.
56. Kirschner, M. A., Zucker, I. R., and Jespersen, D., 1976, Idiopathic hirsutism—An ovarian abnormality, *N. Engl. J. Med.* **294:**637–640.
57. Oake, R. J., Davies, S. J., McLachlan, M. S. F., and Thomas, J. P., 1974, Plasma testosterone in adrenal and ovarian vein blood of hirsute women, *Q. J. Med.* **43:**603–613.
58. Northrop, G., Archie, J. T., Patel, S. K., and Wilbanks, G. D., 1975, Adrenal and ovarian vein androgen levels and laparoscopic findings in hirsute women, *Amer. J. Obstet. Gynecol.* **122:**192–198.

59. Parker, C. R., Jr., Bruneteau, D. W., Greenblatt, R. B., and Mahesh, V. B., 1975, Peripheral, ovarian, and adrenal vein steroids in hirsute women: Acute effects of human chorionic gonadotropin and adrenocorticotrophic hormone, *Fertil. Steril.* **26:**877–888.

60. Givens, J. R., Andersen, R. N., Wiser, W. L., and Fish, S. A., 1974, Dynamics of suppression and recovery of plasma FSH, LH, androstenedione and testosterone in polycystic ovarian disease using an oral contraceptive, *J. Clin. Endocrinol. Metab.* **38:**727–735.

61. Casey, J. H., 1975, Chronic treatment regimens for hirsutism in women: Effect on blood production rate of testosterone and on hair growth, *Clin. Endocrinol.* **4:**313–325.

62. Hammerstein, J., Meckies, J., Leo-Rossberg, I., Moltz, L., and Zielske, F., 1975, Use of cyproterone-acetate (CPA) in the treatment of acne, hirsutism, and virilism, *J. Steroid Biochem.* **6:**827–836.

63. Cameron, E. H. D., Baillie, A. H., Grant, J. K., Milnes, J. A., and Thomson, J., 1966, Transformation *in vitro* of (7α-³H)dehydroepiandrosterone to (³H)testosterone by skin from men, *J. Endocrinol.* **35:**19–28.

64. Hodgins, M. B., 1971, *In vitro* metabolism of dehydroepiandrosterone and dehydroepiandrosterone sulphate in breast skin of women, *Steroids* **18:**11–23.

65. Fazekas, A. G., and Lanthier, A., 1971, Metabolism of androgens by isolated beard hair follicles, *Steroids* **18:**367–379.

66. Thomas, J. P., and Oake, R. J., 1974, Androgen metabolism in the skin of hirsute women, *J. Clin. Endocrinol. Metab.* **38:**19–22.

67. Schweikert, H. U., and Wilson, J. D., 1974, Regulation of human hair growth by steroid hormones. I. Testosterone metabolism in isolated hairs, *J. Clin. Endocrinol. Metab.* **38:**811–819.

68. Schweikert, H. U., and Wilson, J. D., 1974, Regulation of human hair growth by steroid hormones. II. Androstenedione metabolism in isolated hairs, *J. Clin. Endocrinol. Metab.* **39:**1012–1019.

69. Mauvais-Jarvis, P., Bercovici, J. P., and Gauthier, F., 1969, *In vivo* studies on testosterone metabolism by skin of normal males and patients with the syndrome of testicular feminization, *J. Clin. Endocrinol. Metab.* **29:**417–421.

70. Mauvais-Jarvis, P., Charransol, G., and Bobas-Masson, F., 1973, Simultaneous determination of urinary androstanediol and testosterone as an evaluation of human androgenicity, *J. Clin. Endocrinol. Metab.* **36:**452–459.

71. Kuttenn, F., and Mauvais-Jarvis, P., 1975, Testosterone 5α-reduction in the skin of normal subjects and of patients with abnormal sexual development, *Acta Endocrinol.* **79:**164–176.

72. Mauvais-Jarvis, P., Kuttenn, F., and Wright, F., 1975, La progéstérone administrée par voie percutanée, *Ann. Endocrinol.* **36:**55–62.

73. Baum, J. K., Holtz, F., Bookstein, J. J., and Klein, E. W., 1973, Possible association between benign hepatomas and oral contraceptives, *Lancet* **2:**926–929.

74. Christopherson, W. M., Mays, E. T., and Barrows, G. H., 1975, Liver tumors in women on contraceptive steroids, *Obstet. Gynecol.* **46:**221–223.

75. Sherlock, S., 1975, Hepatic adenomas and oral contraceptives, *Gut* **16:**753–756.

76. Edmondson, H. A., Henderson, B., and Benton, B., 1976, Liver-cell adenomas associated with the use of oral contraceptives, *N. Engl. J. Med.* **294:**470–472.

77. Boston Collaborative Drug Surveillance Programme, 1973, Oral contraceptives and venous thromboembolic disease, surgically confirmed gall-bladder disease, and breast tumours, *Lancet* **1**:1399–1404.
78. Boston Collaborative Drug Surveillance Program, 1974, Surgically confirmed gall-bladder disease, venous thromboembolism, and breast tumors in relation to postmenopausal estrogen therapy, *N. Engl. J. Med.* **290**:15–18.
79. Bennion, L. J., Ginsberg, R. L., Garnick, M. B., and Bennett, P. H., 1976, Effects of oral contraceptives on the gallbladder bile of normal women, *N. Engl. J. Med.* **294**:189–192.
80. MacMahon, B., 1974, Risk factors for endometrial cancer, *Gynecol. Oncol.* **2**:122–129.
81. Smith, D. C., Prentice, R., Thompson, D. J., and Herrmann, W. L., 1975, Association of exogenous estrogen and endometrial carcinoma, *N. Engl. J. Med.* **293**:1164–1167.
82. Ziel, H. K., and Finkle, W. D., 1975, Increased risk of endometrial carcinoma among users of conjugated estrogens, *N. Engl. J. Med.* **293**:1167–1170.
83. Collaborative Group for the Study of Stroke in Young Women, 1973, Oral contraception and increased risk of cerebral ischemia or thrombosis, *N. Engl. J. Med.* **288**:871–878.
84. Collaborative Group for the Study of Stroke in Young Women, 1975, Oral contraceptives and stroke in young women: Associated risk factors, *J. Amer. Med. Assoc.* **231**:718–722.
85. Bickerstaff, E. R., 1975, *Neurological Complications of Oral Contraceptives*, Clarendon Press, New York.
86. Comer, T. P., Tuerck, D. G., Bilas, R. A., and Clow, S. F., Falero, F., and Raskind, R. R., 1975, Comparison of strokes in women of childbearing age in Rochester, Minnesota and Bakersfield, California, *Angiology* **26**:351–355.

5

The Testis
Daniel D. Federman

5.1. Introduction

The testis is critical in three phases of life. *In utero,* it controls male differentiation of the genitalia, the breast, and, to an extent unknown in man, the brain and liver. At puberty, it produces the hormones responsible for secondary sexual development. In adulthood, it is the source of gametes for sexual reproduction. This chapter reviews recent advances in testicular physiology and pathophysiology in each of these areas. In this first volume of *The Year in Endocrinology,* an attempt has been made to integrate recent advances with established knowledge in the field.

DANIEL D. FEDERMAN • Stanford University Medical School, Stanford, California.

5.2. Intrauterine and Neonatal Function

5.2.1. Embryonic Sex Differentiation

5.2.1.1. Normal Controls

The indifferent tendency of the mammalian embryo, including man, is to differentiate along female lines. A fine summary of the knowledge of these processes has been published by Goldstein and Wilson.[1] In brief, male genital differentiation requires the influence of two substances from the testis. The first is a protein of mol. wt. approximately 30,000 that is known as *Mullerian regression factor* (MRF). This substance acts locally to inhibit the Mullerian duct primordia, which would otherwise develop into a uterus and fallopian tubes. Using monolayer cultures of calf testis, Blanchard and Josso[2] demonstrated MRF production by Sertoli cells, and not by the interstitial cells. Josso[3] showed that the content of MRF in irradiated human testicular explants did not decline as the number of germ cells did; since MRF is produced by cultured tubular tissue, but not by Leydig cells, he infers that it is produced in the Sertoli cells.

The second substance required for male genital differentiation is the steroid hormone testosterone (T) and its 5α-reduced metabolite, dihydrotestosterone (DHT). Alone or in concert with MRF, T stimulates development of the Wolffian ducts into the seminal vesicle, epididymis, and vas deferens. DHT, produced from T in target tissues by the action of a 5α-reductase, is responsible for external virilization. This effect of DHT was predicted by Wilson and Lasnitzki,[4] who showed that fetal duct primordia lack the reductase at the critical stage of their differentiation, whereas the enzyme is present in the external genital anlage at that time. It was confirmed by Walsh *et al.*,[5] and by Imperato-McGinley *et al.*,[6] who have independently described a syndrome in which absence of the 5α-reductase is associated with male internal but ambiguous external differentiation. By inference, then, T is adequate for Wolffian duct development, but DHT is needed for normal external masculinization.

The mechanisms of steroidogenesis in the fetal testis are being clarified (see Fig. 1). It was at least theoretically possible that androstenedione and testosterone synthesis could have proceeded by enzymatic conversion of C-21 steroids derived from the placenta, i.e., that the early steps of steroid synthesis from acetate would occur in the placenta, and thus would not require a gonadotropin effect on the fetal testis. For this sequence, the last steps would require only maturation in the testis of the relevant enzymes for conversion of C-21 to C-19 steroids. Important evidence on this point has been acquired in the rabbit, in which Catt *et al.*[8] showed that the onset of fetal testosterone synthesis at the 19th gestational day was precisely correlated with the appearance of receptors specific for luteiniz-

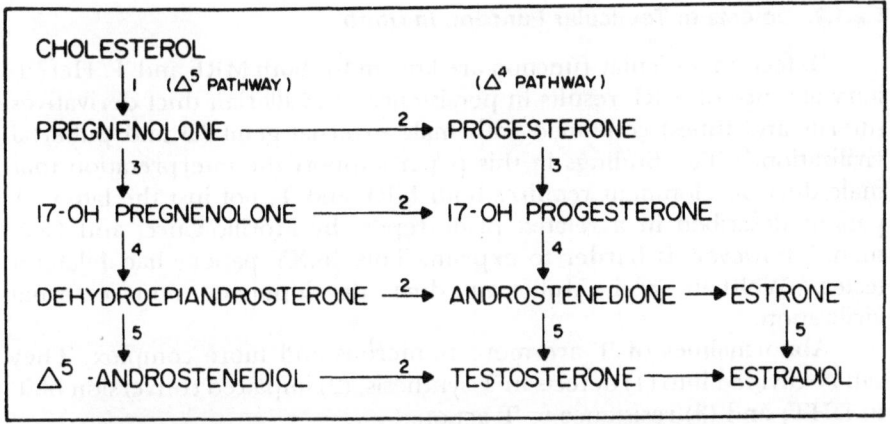

Fig. 1. Pathways of biosynthesis of testosterone. The defects are noted. (Reproduced from Givens *et al.*[7] with permission.)

ing hormone (LH) and human chorionic gonadotropin (HCG). This finding indicates that testosterone synthesis proceeds from acetate via cholesterol and pregnenolone, the latter step requiring gonadotropin. This interpretation was confirmed when Payne and Jaffe[9] showed that testicular homogenates from a 107-day human fetus were able to form androgens from pregnenolone sulfate. Similarly, Ahluwalia *et al.*[10] studied steroid biosynthesis in human testicular minces incubated with labeled acetate, cholesterol, or progesterone. These workers found that testes from 12–16 week fetuses synthesized testosterone from each of the precursors, that HCG stimulated formation of testosterone from acetate and cholesterol (but not from progesterone), and that cAMP served as a second messenger for the gonadotropin effect. Since the fetal pituitary does not appear to produce significant LH early in pregnancy, Leydig cell function at that time is almost certainly under HCG control. At least one clinical observation, however, suggests that the fetal pituitary plays a significant role in the last trimester. Patients with hypogonadotropic hypogonadism have a significant frequency of nondescent of the testis and even occasional hypospadias. These findings suggest that there has been partial androgen deficiency in the last trimester; since the lesion in this syndrome is absence of the hypothalamic LH-releasing factor, and since there is thus deficiency of fetal LH, one may infer that in the normal fetus, pituitary LH is functionally significant.

5.2.1.2. Defects in Testicular Function *in Utero*

Defects in testicular function are known for both MRF and T. Hereditary absence of MRF results in persistence of Mullerian duct derivatives (uterus and tubes) combined with male external genitalia and pubertal virilization.[11] The findings in this paper support the interpretation that male duct development requires both MRF and T, not just the latter. A patient described in a related prior report by Morillo-Cucci and German,[12] however, is harder to explain. This 46,XY patient had bilateral testes, Wolffian and Mullerian duct development, and external virilization.

Abnormalities of T are more numerous and more complex. They can be divided into (1) defects in T synthesis; (2) impaired conversion of T to DHT; and (3) resistance to T action.

5.2.1.2a. Defects in Synthesis. There are five enzymatic steps specific for the synthesis of testosterone from cholesterol, and hereditary defects of each have been identified (Fig. 1). Three of the enzymes are required for adrenal synthesis of cortisol: the 20α-hydroxylase, the 3β-hydroxysteroid dehydrogenase, and the 17-hydroxylase. Deficiency of either of the first two produces a life-threatening form of congenital adrenal hyperplasia that presents in infancy. 17-Hydroxylase deficiency may not present early because the patients form adequate amounts of mineralocorticoid, which protects against cortisol deficiency. In the genetic male, all three disorders produce pseudohermaphroditism with absent Mullerian structures (i.e., MRF is intact), usually normal male internal ducts, and variable external hermaphroditism. The other defects in testosterone biosynthesis are of significance only in the testis; they thus produce male pseudohermaphroditism, but not adrenal insufficiency. The 17,20-desmolase (or lyase) deficiency originally reported by Zachman *et al.*[13] was found in two first cousins and possibly in an "aunt." The adrenal metabolites 17-hydroxy and 17-ketosteroids were normal. Testosterone was low, and did not increase after HCG; pregnenetriol was high; and testis homogenates could not convert progesterone or pregnenolone to testosterone. Finally, the 17-ketosteroid reductase deficiency originally reported by Saez *et al.*[14] has so far produced male pseudohermaphrodites who have looked like normal females except for clitoromegaly. At puberty, they have had primary amenorrhea as the chief complaint, owing to the absence of the uterus.

5.2.1.2b. Impaired Conversion of Testosterone to Dihydrotestosterone. Two groups have reported male pseudohermaphroditism associated with impaired conversion of T to DHT. Imperato-McGinley *et al.*[6] identified an autosomal recessive trait among a strongly inbreeding group in Santa Domingo, and Walsh *et al.*[5] found similar patients in this country. In both, the genetic males have male internal genitalia and ambiguous external development. In both, *in vitro* conversion of T to DHT by usual target tissues is deficient, but in the patients of Imperato-McGinley and co-workers, plasma DHT was low, whereas in the patients of Walsh and co-workers, it was normal. Whether this difference is significant is unknown. The implications of this disorder for embryogensis were summarized in Section 5.2.1.2a, in which the significance for pubertal development is outlined.

5.2.1.2c. Resistance to Testosterone Action. The syndrome of testicular feminization is characterized by complete resistance to the action of testosterone. This resistance is apparently due to a defect in the protein receptor for the hormone such that the receptor–steroid–chromatin complex required for the stimulation of genomic transcription does not form. Several syndromes of incomplete male pseudohermaphroditism, seemingly due to partial defects in hormone action, have been described.[15-18] Genetic males show male internal ducts and varying degrees of external virilization. Since the evidence for these defects comes largely from studies done at or after puberty, these syndromes will be discussed in detail in Section 5.3.

5.2.2. Testicular Function in Childhood

The neonatal male's peripheral blood level of testosterone is higher than that in cord blood; in the first week of life, values in both male and female fall to almost undetectable levels. In the female, the level stays down, but in the normal male, the plasma testosterone rises within a month of birth to levels about half that of the adult.[19] LH values show the same evolution, and are presumably responsible for the stimulation of the Leydig cell. Between 4 and 6 or 7 months, both LH and testosterone gradually decline to values similar to those in the female, and remain there until the rise associated with puberty.[20] The function of this infantile testosterone surge is unknown. Although it is tempting to speculate that these levels have a role in male differentiation of the CNS and liver, akin to similar phenomena in lower animals, there is scant support for this view from experimental observations. Major evidence that the human phenomena are not parallel is provided by the female pseudohermaphrodite with congenital adrenal hyperplasia. Although exposed as a newborn to pathological levels of testosterone, the genetic female with this disorder shows normal menstrual function at puberty if suitably treated with cortisol.

5.3. Puberty

Major collections of information on the regulation of the onset of puberty were published in 1974 by Grumbach and colleagues,[21] and in 1975 by Bierich.[22] These collections should be consulted for a comprehensive review of information available before this year.

A major cross-sectional study, although it antedates the year 1975, is cited here because of its significance. Faiman and Winter[23] studied 253 healthy males from 0.2 to 25 years of age. The principal observations were:

1. LH and follicle-stimulating hormone (FSH) values were usually measurable in normal males from age 1 on; until age 6, there was no significant rise.
2. Between ages 6 and 10, there was a slight but significant increase in mean LH and FSH levels.
3. This rise was paralleled by an increase in mean testis size that was the first clinically detectable sign of puberty, reliably antedating hormonal changes or secondary sex characteristics.
4. Plasma testosterone did not show any significant change during this time.
5. From ages 10 to 17, FSH continued to rise at the same rate as before, reaching mean adult values by age 15; LH rose, with an increasing slope, reaching the adult mean by age 17; testosterone showed a 20-fold rise to the adult level between ages 10 and 17.

Similar observations were made in a longitudinal study of 56 healthy males: FSH and testicular size changed first, and LH and testosterone showed significant increases in Tanner stage 2.[23] A similar longitudinal study of 46 boys was done by Lee *et al.*,[24] who found testicular enlargement to antedate FSH rise, and LH to rise before testosterone. Adult levels of testosterone were reached before completion of pubertal changes, the whole period of rise being about 2 years. The findings in any one patient may be misleading, however, since Grumbach *et al.*[25] and others have found occasional patients with slight increases in testosterone by the time testicular enlargement could be detected. Whether the radioimmunoassayable hormones being measured in childhood are biologically active is not yet clear.

The onset of puberty is a central event mediated by the hypothalamus. In the prepubertal period, the CNS sites appear to be exquisitely sensitive to negative feedback inhibition by the extremely low levels of gonadal steroids produced in childhood. According to this view, puberty begins when this threshold to negative restraint rises slightly. The consequent release of gonadotropin-releasing hormone, or luteinizing hor-

mone–releasing hormone (LH–RH), in turn stimulates pituitary production of gonadotropins, and hence gonadal steroid synthesis. The train of
events, accompanied by further elevation of the threshold to negative
feedback, ultimately results in completion of puberty and establishment of
the tropic–feedback interrelations typical of adulthood. Supporting this
view, Grumbach et al.[25] showed that the prepubertal levels of FSH could
be suppressed to immeasurable levels by doses of estrogen that were
ineffective in pubertal or adult patients, and that doses of clomiphene that
would stimulate gonadrotropin release in adults would inhibit gonadotropin and testosterone secretion in prepubertal males, presumably via weak
estrogenic effects.

Adrenal secretion of low levels of sex steroids has been suggested as
playing a role in both the childhood phase, via negative feedback, and the
onset of puberty, perhaps by a positive effect on resetting the threshold.
Sizonenko and Paunier[26] found dihydroepiandrosterone rising between
ages 7 and 10, and suggested that this component of the "adrenarche"
could contribute to resetting hypothalamic sensitivity to feedback by
testosterone or estradiol or both. Hopper and Yen[27] had found that
dihydroepiandrosterone sulfate, but not dihydroepiandrosterone, rose
before other hormonal changes of puberty were apparent, and also felt
that it could be important in initiating the events of puberty. Similar data
and interpretations were reported by Lee and Migeon.[28] Evidence supporting this hypothesis came from studies by Reiter et al.,[29] who found
that children whose bone ages were advanced because of incomplete
treatment of congenital adrenal hyperplasia showed LH–RH tests (i.e.,
gonadotropin responses to LH–RH) appropriate to their bone ages
(maturation), rather than to their chronological ages. This finding correlates with the prior knowledge that children with congenital adrenal
hyperplasia whose bone ages are sufficiently advanced will undergo precocious puberty when put on cortisol therapy.

If puberty is initiated by decreased CNS sensitivity to negative feedback, and thus enhanced release of LH–RH, the next step appears to be
stimulation of development of the pituitary gonadotropes by the releasing hormone. Evidence of this view comes from a variety of sources.[25] The
response to LH–RH is quantitatively proportional to the stage of puberty.
Little LH is released in response to LH–RH in prepubertal children,
significantly more by enpubertal subjects, and a still higher amount by
adult males (Fig. 2). There is much less change in the FSH response, and
this response is paradoxically greater in the prepubertal female.

In addition to the enhanced responsiveness to LH–RH, a nocturnal
pulse of LH release is a characteristic of puberty. Parker et al.[31] studied
the dynamics of this in 5 pairs of monozygotic twins, and found concordance for a nocturnal rise in LH and, later, T. The pattern became evident

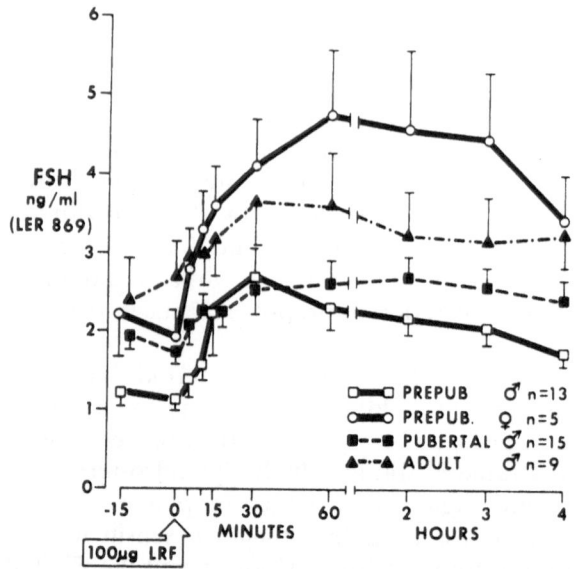

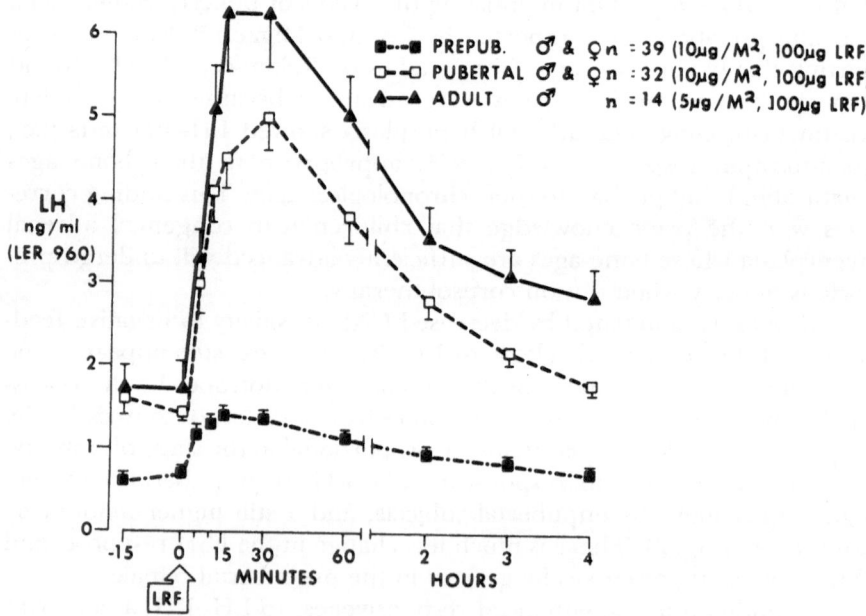

Fig. 2. Changes in plasma LH (top) and FSH (bottom) in response to LH–RH in prepubertal, pubertal, and adult subjects. (Reproduced from Grumbach et al.[30] with permission.)

in stages 2 and 3 of puberty, and reached adult pattern by stage 5. Parker and his colleagues concluded that the CNS plays a fundamental role in the sleep-entrained rise in LH and T. On this same point, it may be noted that the mid- and late-adolescent male shows a nocturnal rise in testosterone, plus several pulses of testosterone.[32] Both the rise and the pulses appear to follow prior LH pulses, and are presumably due to the effect of the LH pulses on the testis. Rowe *et al.*[33] studied the dynamics of the LH–T relationship, and showed that T responds sluggishly but consistently. Thus, although other factors may play a significant role in the release of T, LH is the predominant control.

Further evidence that LH and FSH production by the pituitary gonadotropins is dependent on initial and then sustained production of LH–RH is provided by study of patients with both congenital and acquired hypogonadotropic hypogonadism. These patients, who will be discussed in detail in Section 5.5.1, show low levels of gonadotropin and impaired responses to LH–RH.[34] After pretreatment with LH–RH for periods of several days to weeks, basal levels of LH and FSH may not rise, but the response to LH–RH reliably does.

5.4. Adult Physiology

5.4.1. The Hypothalamus and Pituitary

The initial event of puberty, as described in Section 5.3, is presumed to be a rise in the threshold of negative feedback inhibition of the release of LH–RH. Although it is not yet entirely certain, release of LH–RH appears to be mediated by α-adrenergic control, with relay via the neurosecretory neurons of the hypothalamus. Since these neurons have rich connections with the hippocampus and limbic systems, the detailed control and its change at the onset of puberty may be quite complex. Once secreted, LH–RH attaches to high-affinity receptors in the anterior pituitary, and thence activates adenyl cyclase. Levels of cAMP are elevated, calcium transport into the gland is enhanced, and gonadotropin stored in secretory granules is discharged.[35] As noted earlier, LH–RH appears to have a significant effect in developing the gonadotropes; thus, the actions described above may require an interval of earlier stimulus to cellular proliferation or growth before they are manifest.

Uncertainly persists as to whether there is one or more releasing hormones, but the evidence for one seems persuasive. LH–RH has a greater effect on LH than on FSH, but, especially at higher doses, it releases some FSH as well as the free α-subunits common to the glycoprotein hormones.[36,37] The pituitary gonadotropins are covered in Chapter 2. Their actions on the testis remain controversial. FSH stimulates adenyl cyclase and cAMP production in testicular tubules, but not in the Leydig cells. Its effect on promotion of spermatogenesis appears to require testosterone and, presumably, the synthesis of the androgen-binding protein of the testis. LH stimulates cAMP in the Leydig cells, and thus promotes testosterone synthesis; whether LH has a direct effect on the tubules is still moot.

Similar controversy surrounds the negative feedback control of gonadotropin release. It is agreed that T inhibits the release of LH, but there is controversy over whether it does so directly or via a metabolite such as estradiol (E_2) or DHT. Stewart-Bentley et al.[38] infused a dose of T calculated to mimic the normal secretion rate, and found definite inhibition of LH, but not of FSH. E_2 in an amount approximately equal to that which would be produced from the T also produced LH suppression, as did DHT. Although DHT was less effective, it allowed for the conclusion that testosterone, acting either as an androgen or via conversion to estrogen, provides the major negative feedback regulation of LH.

Santen[39] investigated this problem in a series of well-designed experiments. He infused T and E_2 at rates slightly above their physiological secretion. Although both suppressed LH, their effects on the amplitude and frequency of LH pulses were different. In addition, E_2 blunted the LH response to LH–RH, whereas T did not; this finding was taken as evidence for an effect of E_2 at the pituitary level that is not produced by T. Finally, DHT, which cannot be aromatized to an estrogen, nevertheless suppressed LH. Santen concluded that since T and E_2 have different effects on LH secretory patterns, and since DHT can suppress LH, the inhibitory effect of T on LH release does not require aromatization of the T.

Even greater argument surrounds the feedback regulation of FSH. Physiological doses of androgen do not suppress FSH as they do LH, but much larger doses may.[35] The significance of this latter finding is unclear, however, since large amounts of infused T could be partially converted to small but physiologically effective amounts of E_2, with consequent effects on sex steroid binding to sex hormone–binding globulin (SHBG) and on the hypothalamus or pituitary. The hypothalamus contains receptors for T, DHT, and E_2, and has enzymes capable of aromatizing T to E_2. Although it has been postulated that the testicular tubule secretes a substance called *inhibin* that mediates the FSH suppression, the substance has never been well characterized. Many papers have attempted to correlate diminished spermatogenesis with elevations of FSH (see Section 5.4.2.3); severe restrictions in sperm production are often accompanied by elevated FSH, but lesser degrees do not seem to correlate well. The existence of inhibin, then, remains a matter of faith, rather than of demonstration. Assuming it to exist, an interesting approach to its possible site of action was provided by Bramble *et al.,*[40] who did LH–RH tests in patients with monotropic elevation of FSH, and found a selective exaggeration of the FSH response to LH–RH. From this response in the presumed absence of inhibin, these investigators inferred that inhibin usually operates to modulate the secretion of FSH at the pituitary, rather than higher. Similar observations and conclusions were reported by Zárate *et al.,*[41] but since LH–RH is thought to promote development and secretion of the gonadotropins, hyperresponse of FSH to LH–RH may reflect increased prior stimulation by LH–RH, rather than absence of a modulating effect of inhibin. Figure 3 is an effort by Jeffcoate[42] to portray current understanding of the integration of the hypothalamic–pituitary–testicular axis. It also serves to point up the areas of uncertainty.

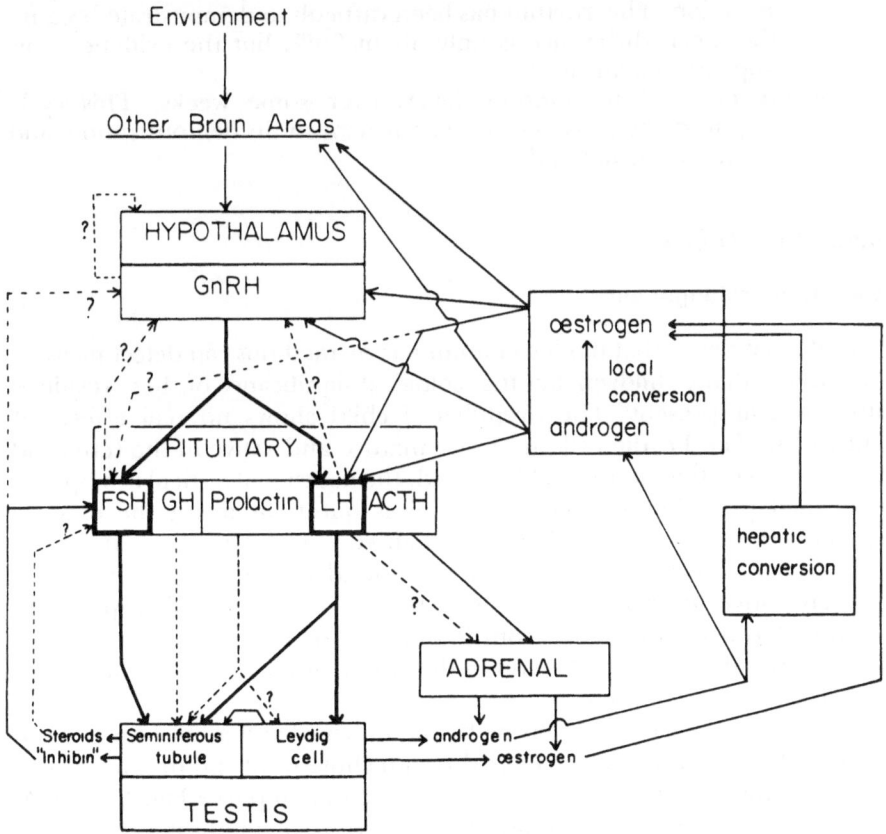

Fig. 3. Scheme proposed by Jeffcoate to illustrate hypothalamic–pituitary–testis interrelationships. (Reproduced from Jeffcoate[42] with permission.)

Physiological variations in the secretion of gonadotropin are now known in several circumstances. As increasingly sensitive methods for hormone assay have become available, it has become clear that the tonic secretion generally found in the male masks fluctuations that are small in time scale and of unknown importance. Among the known variations are the following:

1. A sleep-induced release of LH characteristic of midpuberty, and absent from prepubertal and mature males.[32]
2. A slowly rising sequence of LH pulses during the night, mostly followed by testosterone rises, resulting in a gradual nighttime rise in the level of testosterone. This sequence is not suppressed by administration of dexamethasone and consequent suppression of ACTH.[43]
3. A circadian rhythm in testosterone and, presumably, in LH secretion. This rhythm has been difficult to demonstrate because the mean difference is only about 20%, but the evidence now appears convincing.[44]
4. A cycle of testosterone levels over some weeks. This cycle required extensive statistical treatment for its demonstration, and awaits confirmation.[45]

5.4.2. The Testis

5.4.2.1. Steroidogenesis

We have seen that modern immunoassay methods can detect measurable LH in many children, but the biological significance of these results is unknown at present. The prepubertal child shows no real effects of androgen. The Leydig cells are more mature and active in the fetus and newborn male than in the child. Indeed, the occasional testicular biopsy in a normal prepubertal child always raises questions about the existing status of the Leydig cells. Their virtual absence at that time is reflected in the studies of Payne and Jaffe,[9] who showed that although fetal testes actively converted pregnenolone sulfate to testosterone, this capacity diminished during the span from 2 months to 9 years of age. It then reappeared during puberty, and in the young adult, again reached levels equal to those of the fetus.

The synthesis of testosterone by the pubertal and adult human testis follows the pathways from acetate through cholesterol and pregnenolone, with a significant stimulation by LH at the latter step (see Fig. 1). The Δ^4 pathway is favored in the rat, but evidence from man indicates that the Δ^5 pathway via 17-OH pregnenolone and dehydroepiandrosterone is used preferentially.[46] The ultrastructural location of these reactions is of interest. Cholesterol synthesis takes place in the microsomes; its cleavage to pregnenolone is carried out in the mitochondria; pregnenolone is then returned to the microsomes for synthesis of the intermediates and then of testosterone itself.

Adult levels of androgens and related estrogens are established gradually. Scholler et al.[47] measured plasma T, estrone (E_1), and E_2 in the basal state, and after HCG administration in prepubertal, enpubertal, and mature boys. He found that prepubertal boys had measurable levels of T, with some diurnal variation; that the response to HCG is less than in the adult; that an adult level of response appeared in puberty stage 2, and did not increase further; and, finally, that the response of E_1 and E_2 to HCG did increase with advancing puberty, and was thus a better index of the completion of puberty than was the T response.

The biosynthesis of testosterone in the testis is stimulated by pituitary LH, following on its combination with specific receptors on the Leydig cell membrane. The stimulation of a membrane-bound adenyl cyclase and mediation via cAMP are similar to the effects of tropic hormones on other steroid-secreting tissues. The central effect appears to be on the cholesterol-to-pregnenolone step, which requires the side-chain cleavage; as noted, this cleavage occurs in the mitochondria. In addition to this early effect, however, continued administration of LH ultimately leads to increased concentrations of many of the intermediate enzymes. Conversely, particular steps in testosterone synthesis can be inhibited by specific metabolites. Pregnenolone, progesterone, and testosterone inhibit the 20 α-hydroxylation of cholesterol[48]; 17-OH progesterone, testosterone, and androstenedione each inhibit the conversion of pregnenolone to progesterone.[49] The significance of these effects is not known, but they provide models for intratesticular control of testosterone synthesis not mediated by feedback effects on gonadotropin.

Testosterone secreted from the testis is transported in the peripheral blood in several forms. About 60% is bound to SHBG, which also binds E_2; about 38% is bound to albumin; the remaining 2% is free and presumably biologically active.[46] SHBG is remarkable in that it binds two hormones that compete with each other for certain of their biological effects; further, both hormones affect the amount of the binding protein. Testosterone lowers the level of SHBG, and results in an increased percentage of free testosterone; conversely, E_2 raises the concentration of SHBG, decreases the percentage of free testosterone, and raises the percentage of free and the total E_2. It should also be recalled that E_2 circulates in picogram, and testosterone in microgram, amounts. Thus, trivial changes in the fractional binding of E_2 may have highly significant biological effects.

Some 6–7 mg testosterone is synthesized per day. A small fraction (approximately 0.25%) of this testosterone is aromatized in the testis to E_2; in the author's view, this step is a major point of expression of genetic control by the X and Y chromosomes. Since the ovary and testis make the same hormones, and since all estrogen is made via androgen, two obvious points of control for sex chromosome–mediated sexual identity are (1) the amount of androgen made per day, and (2) the amount of it converted to estrogen. In the male, relatively more androgen is made, and a very tiny (but significant) amount taken to estrogen; in the female, much less androgen is produced, but the fractional conversion to estrogen in the gonad approaches 50%. Minor distortions of the resulting ratio could account for such clinical features as gynecomastia. Evidence of this effect was provided by LaFranchi et al.,[50] and by Lee,[51] both studies finding elevations in the E_2:testosterone ratio in association with the transient gynecomastia of adolescence.

Testosterone is metabolized to the 17-ketosteroids androsterone and etiocholanolone; to the 5 α-reduced compounds (dihydrotestosterones); and, to a minuscule degree, to estrogens. Since other androgens contribute to the same end products, measurement of the urinary 17-ketosteroids is not a satisfactory way to assess testicular function. It has been replaced for this purpose by measurements of serum testosterone and, in certain laboratories, the urinary testosterone glucuronide.

The action of testosterone, like that of other steroid hormones, requires its entry into the cell, combination with a cytosol receptor, translocation to the nucleus, and formation there of a receptor–hormone–chromatin complex. Following this formation, activation of specific gene loci leads to formation of unique messenger RNAs, and ultimately to protein synthesis. These processes were extensively reviewed in the last several years by Liao,[52] Mainwaring and Mangan,[53] and Minguell and Sierralta.[54]

Androgen target tissues must thus be able to bind androgens; this binding capacity appears to involve two kinds of sites. The androgen-binding protein (ABP) is found in the testis and epididymis, among other tissues. Its synthesis is increased by FSH,[55] thus providing at least one mechanism for the role of FSH in spermatogenesis. A second type of androgen-binding is to specific high-affinity androgen receptors in both cytosol and nucleus. This type of binding usually shows higher affinity for testosterone than does the ABP. Most significantly, cyproterone acetate competes with androgen for binding to this receptor, and exerts its antiandrogen effect by preventing the attachment of the native steroid.[56] In one suggestive study of benign prostatic hypertrophy,[57] both types of androgen-binding were demonstrated, and in the 8S (receptor) fraction, there was a particularly high concentration of DHT. The potential significance of this observation can be best appreciated by a brief review of a new disorder known either as the guevodoces syndrome[6] or as familial male incomplete pseudohermaphroditism, type 2.[5]

It had been known that testosterone is unique among steroid hormones in that it is metabolized intracellularly to a more active species of the molecule, DHT. Certain androgen target tissues do not contain the reductase needed for this transformation, raising questions about the importance of this step. A clinical syndrome of hereditary deficiency of the reductase provided the first opportunity to dissect the relative roles of T and DHT in male puberty. This condition, cited above,[5,6] results in male newborns who, despite having testes and male internal genitalia, have an ambiguous external appearance. At puberty, these children undergo secondary male development, including a growth spurt, deepening of the voice, male muscularity, male libido, erectile potency, and spermatogenesis, but they do not develop either male beard growth or significant prostate enlargement. By inference, then, T is adequate for all the changes of male puberty except stimulation of the beard and prostate. DHT is required for the latter, and there is preliminary evidence that elevated levels of DHT may be implicated in the pathogenesis of benign prostatic hypertrophy.[58,59]

5.4.2.2. Spermatogenesis

Although methods for the study of spermatogenesis are improving, the process remains poorly understood. Most approaches involve artificial circumstances from which extrapolation to the natural state of the testis is difficult. Some of the points of agreement include the following:

1. FSH is necessary but not sufficient for full spermatogenesis. It appears to attach selectively to Sertoli cells, and to work via activation of adenylate cyclase.[60] It induces the formation of an ABP, which is then secreted into the epididymal lumen.[61] Depending on the circumstances, FSH contributes to the opening of the tubular cells in early puberty, and to the completion of the process of spermiogenesis.[60,62]
2. FSH alone does not stimulate germinal cells, but does stimulate ABP production by Sertoli cells; the tubule is thus "prepared" for the arrival of testosterone and the initiation of its influence.
3. LH attaches to specific receptors in the Leydig cells, and also acts via cAMP. Testosterone is delivered locally to the testicular tubules, where it initiates the process of spermatogenesis by forming a hormone–protein–chromatin complex.
4. Distinct from ABP are the cytoplasmic and nuclear acceptor proteins that ultimately form the steroid–acceptor–chromatin complex. These proteins have a higher affinity for androgens,

and it is this bond that is inhibited by the antiandrogens such as cyproterone.[57]

5. Both FSH and LH, given over a prolonged period, are necessary for optimal development of spermatogenesis.[63] This point agrees with the observations in normal puberty, in which development of complete spermatogenesis takes about 2 years from the early evidence of gonadotropic activation.

5.4.2.3. Effect of Age on Human Testicular Function

In sharp contrast to the ovary, the testis appears to function throughout adult life. Several recent studies, however, have suggested that beyond age 60, significant decreases in testicular function occur. Stearns et al.[64] found a fall in mean free testosterone after age 50, and in mean total testosterone after age 70. LH and FSH rose gradually after age 40, and more steeply after age 70. Isurugi et al.[65] also found significant differences between the FSH and LH levels of younger men and those of men over 40, with progressive rises in each decade thereafter. The values were not so high, however, as those seen in the menopausal female. Comparing subjects of ages 22–61 and others of ages 67–93, Pirke and Doerr[66] found a 20% fall in total T, a 43% fall in free T, and a curious rise in E_2. Finally, Snyder et al.[67] also observed a decrease in dialyzable ("free") testosterone, and slight increases in FSH and LH, in older males. Although more such studies are needed, these provide the first clear evidence for a decline in testicular function with age. This change is suggestive of that seen in the menopause, but it is less marked, more gradual, more variable in onset, and rarely complete.

5.5. Adult Pathophysiology

5.5.1. Gonadotropin Deficiencies

Hypogonadotropic hypogonadism is perhaps more appropriately considered in Chapter 1, but the significant advances in its understanding bear repetition here. Several syndromes of pubertal failure in the male are known. The most familiar is Kallman's syndrome, in which hypogonadotropinism is associated with reduced or absent sense of smell and a variable congeries of midline somatic defects. Absence of gonadotropin also occurs as a sporadic finding, then making it more difficult to distinguish this syndrome from intrinsic pituitary disease. In both circumstances, failure of puberty is associated with both low testosterone and low gonadotropin. The availability of LH–RH for testing has shown that in a few of these patients, LH–RH releases small amounts of LH and, rather more often, almost normal amounts of FSH. What is more significant, however, is that pretreatment with LH–RH for days to weeks often converts a marginal response to a normal one, thus clearly establishing the diagnosis.[34,68–70] Patients with delayed puberty due to *pituitary* failure usually have growth hormone (GH) impairment as well, but isolated pituitary gonadotropin deficiency occurs, though rarely. Unfortunately, there is still some overlap of response to LH–RH in patients with pituitary tumors, so that unless the sella is enlarged, it may be difficult to definitively separate hypothalamic and pituitary hypogonadotropinism.[71]

Sporadic investigations of the "fertile eunuch" syndrome have been reported. Williams *et al.*[77] found that LH–RH raised both FSH and LH, the latter somewhat more. As in patients with hypothalamic hypogonadotropinism, prior treatment with LH–RH raised the response to the test dose. In the short time of trial, T and DHT did not rise after LH–RH, but did after HCG, administration. The authors interpret their findings to indicate that there must be two gonadotropin-releasing hormones, since FSH is apparently normal, but LH deficient. Incidentally, this patient was azoospermic with a normal FSH; this finding confirms the importance of LH and testosterone in spermatogenesis, and certainly mocks the appellation "fertile eunuch."

A similar case was described by del Pozo *et al.*[73] The patient had low androgen levels, and the testis, although showing complete spermatogenesis in isolated tubules, did not reveal a normal pattern quantitatively. FSH and LH were low normal, and neither responded to clomiphene, but both responded to LH–RH.

Finally, there is a fascinating report of therapy with LH–RH in patients with hypothalamic or pituitary hypogonadism.[74] Prolonged self-administration of LH–RH induced pubertal changes, rises in testosterone, and, after 4 months, spermatogenesis. This important advance could be made more widely available in coming years.

5.5.2. The Testis

5.5.2.1. Steroidogenesis

5.5.2.1a. Defects in Synthesis. The major forms of testicular enzyme deficiency were summarized in Section 5.2.1.2a. Four are manifest in the infant male because of either simultaneous cortisol deficiency (20α-cholesterol hydroxylase, 3β-hydroxysteroid dehydrogenase) or ambiguous genitalia (17-hydroxylase deficiency and 17,20-desmolase deficiency). One presents in adults who have been raised as females, but develop clitoromegaly, primary amenorrhea, and virilization at puberty. In the original reports,[14] gynecomastia was routinely present, but Givens *et al.*[15] described 2 sisters who apparently had the same defect, and yet did not have gynecomastia. Although this disorder is thought to be rare, as Givens and his co-workers point out, it may turn out to be more common than anticipated at present, since it is not a cause of adrenal insufficiency. Goebelsmann and his colleagues have made two valuable contributions to the understanding of this syndrome. In 1973, they pointed out that the plasma testosterone, although lower than male, is higher than female, and over 90% is derived from peripheral (not gonadal) conversion from androstenedione.[75] In 1975, in another study of 2 such patients, he found that the dominant product in testicular homogenates was androstenedione, with very little 17-OH progesterone and even less testosterone.[76] These workers also found that the 17,20-lyase activity was increased in these patients, accounting for the fact that they secrete normal amounts of 17-OH progesterone and progesterone, rather than the increased amounts typical of congenital adrenal hyperplasia (see Fig. 1). Further, they found that conversion of E_1 to E_2 was less impaired than that of androstenedione to testosterone, and that testosterone was back-converted to androstenedione almost normally. They therefore suggest that there may be more than one 17-hydroxysteroid dehydrogenase involved in these reactions.

The deficiency of testosterone in this syndrome is also significant within the testis. Longo *et al.*[77] described the histological and ultrastructural defects that accompany the failure of spermatogenesis.

5.5.2.1b. Defects in Transport, Binding, or Metabolism. A series of elegant studies by Wilson and resonating reports from others in the past three years have clarified a previously confused area in the field of sex differentiation. At issue here are the steps in male differentiation beyond Mullerian suppression; in other words, in the syndromes to be described, genetic males all have adequate MRF, but differ in the nature of the defects in their androgen effect. In the preceding section, we discussed defects in testosterone biosynthesis; here, we detail defects in the transport, action, or intracellular metabolism of testosterone.

The story begins with *testicular feminization,* in which genetic males with normal or high levels of testosterone have no signs of virilization beyond Mullerian suppression. Their testosterone production rates are elevated, as is their production of both E_2 and E_1. Serum gonadotropins are elevated, but are imperfectly responsive to testosterone suppression.[78] The patients therefore have the unusual combination of high T and high LH. The pathogenetic defect is in the testosterone receptor of target tissues.[79] Since testosterone cannot attach normally to this site, it does not reach the chromatin and cannot activate genomic transcription. Feminization occurs because potent estrogens are opposed by ineffective androgen.

A significant advance in understanding the genetics of the testicular feminization defect was reported by Meyer, and his colleagues,[80] who exploited the knowledge that DHT-binding to a specific fibroblast androgen receptor is deficient in testicular feminization.[81] Cultures of skin fibroblasts were made from normal controls and from patients with testicular feminization and their mothers, who are obligate heterozygotes. Binding of DHT in the mothers was intermediate between that in normals and in the patients, with individual values suggestive of two cell populations, as would be predicted by the Lyon hypothesis for an X-linked trait.[82] The bimodility was not sharp, however, and the overlaps were significant. Nevertheless, combined with the comparative evidence of Ohno[83] that traits X-linked in one species are X-linked in all, the data pretty well establish that the locus for androgen sensitivity is on the X-chromosome.

The term *"incomplete" testicular feminization* has been applied to a whole congeries of poorly defined patients who have in common Mullerian suppression and slight or pronounced external virilization. Madden *et al.*[16] recently described one patient who had Wolffian duct development, partial external virilization, and, at the time of puberty, both masculinization and feminization. Plasma testosterone levels and production rates were normal, plasma estrogen levels and production rates were elevated, and gonadotropins were high as well. Since testosterone levels were adequate, but its effect incomplete, the patient was considered an example of incomplete testicular feminization; however, the distinction from familial incomplete male pseudohermaphroditism, type 1, described below, is unclear.

Familial incomplete male pseudohermaphroditism was a term coined by Wilson *et al.*[18] for a family whose pheotypes varied from mildly masculinized "females" to Reifenstein syndrome–like males with only hypospadias as a clue to their abnormality. Plasma levels and production rates of testosterone were greatly elevated; peripheral conversion of testosterone to E_2, and hence to E_1, was also high. LH was high, FSH normal. Since LH was high despite the high testosterone level, and since administered Depo-Provera did not suppress it, Wilson and co-workers inferred that this syndrome was one of androgen insensitivity, rather than androgen lack. The high estrogen levels are presumed to be due to (1) the high LH driving the testis to increased estrogen production, and (2) increased peripheral conversion of androgen to estrogen. Thus, the endocrine evidence and mechanisms of this syndrome and those of incomplete testicular feminization overlap. Wilson's group has tentatively separated them on the basis of distinctive anatomical findings. The patients with incomplete testicular feminization have an introitus with partial labial fusion plus clitoromegaly, mixed feminization and virilization at puberty, and normal rather than elevated testosterone values. An example of the difficulties involved in the separation is the patient with familial male incomplete pseudohermaphroditism described by Perez-Palacios *et al.*[17] It is not yet clear whether the distinction between the two closely similar disorders will prove valid.

The final group in this sequence is the syndrome or syndromes of $5\propto$ -reductase deficiency. Patients have been described from two sources, Santa Domingo and Texas. Those reported by Imperato-McGinley *et al.*[6] had normal Mullerian suppression and Wolffian ducts, but poorly masculinized external genitalia. At puberty, they underwent normal male development, except for beard and prostate. Plasma testosterone was normal, but plasma DHT low. When labeled testosterone was administered, the ratio of $5\beta/5\alpha$-metabolites was increased (and the values in obligate-heterozygote parents were intermediate). Unlike the other syndromes, this one is inherited as an autosomal recessive. Walsh *et al.*[5] described 2 siblings with similar findings. Endocrine studies showed normal male plasma testosterone levels and production rates, normal estrogen levels and production rates, and normal androgen–estrogen fractional conversions. Gonadotropin levels were normal, suggesting that testosterone was effective in its regulation. *In vitro* studies of perineal skin, epididymis, and phallus showed impaired conversion of T to DHT,[84] and this impairment was assumed to be the defect in this syndrome, previously reported as pseudovaginal perineoscrotal hypospadias.[85] The term *familial incomplete male pseudohermaphroditism, type 2,* was proposed for this disorder.

A major conceptual advance has been made in this area of male pseudohermaphroditism. Future work of this nature should help to define the disorders and differentiate among them.

5.5.2.2. Tubular Defects

5.5.2.2a. Klinefelter's Syndrome. The tubular defect in Klinefelter's syndrome remains unexplained, but some interesting new sidelights on the disorder have been revealed. DeBehar *et al.*[86] studied the gonadotropin levels and response to LH–RH in a number of primary gonadal disorders. Before puberty, LH levels were raised in 4 of 10 patients with Turner's syndrome and in 4 of 7 with anorchia, but in none of 18 Klinefelter patients. Similarly, FSH was raised in 8 of 10 Turner patients and in 7 of 7 anorchia patients, but in none of 18 with Klinefelter's syndrome. Thus, in marked contrast to other forms of nonfunctioning gonads, the Klinefelter testis is able to suppress gonadotropin before puberty. This finding accords well with the normal histology of the testis before puberty. Even after puberty, Klinefelter patients raise their FSH in response to LH–RH much less than do patients with primary gonadal failure.[86]

The Leydig cell defect in this disease is also still puzzling. Despite normal or increased numbers and a hyperfunctional appearance, the Leydig cells produce less testosterone than normal. Urinary testosterone is decreased[87]; mean plasma levels and production rates are lower, although both overlap the low normal range; and the response to HCG is less than normal.[88] Some authors had suggested that the adrenal contribution to plasma testosterone in Klinefelter's syndrome is significant, but Smals et al.[89] showed that (1) the diurnal variation in plasma testosterone in this disease is normal in range, and (2) there is no significant change in response to either ACTH or dexamethasone. Pazzagli et al.[90] found that DHT levels were depressed about as much as was testosterone, which matches other reports that the two are parallel in a wide range of conditions.

Wang et al.[91] made a valuable contribution by studying androgen and estrogen dynamics in Klinefelter's syndrome. In summary, these investigators found low values for total and free testosterone, and for the plasma production rate and metabolic clearance rate of testosterone. The metabolic clearance rate of E_2 was also low, but the plasma level was elevated, apparently because of the low clearance *and* increased peripheral conversion of testosterone to E_2. Thus, the ratio of E_2 to testosterone was increased, presumably accounting for some of the feminizing features of the disease. These data are also pertinent to the pituitary function in this disease. Several studies have suggested that the hypothalamic–pituitary regulation of Klinefelter's syndrome may be abnormal. Certain patients are found with elevated plasma LH despite normal plasma testosterone.[88,92] Similarly, attempts at suppression of gonadotropin by estrogens show that higher doses are needed.[93]

Several phenotypic aspects of the diseases have been either confirmed or developed. Thus, Schibler et al.[94] found Klinefelter patients both before and after puberty to be taller than their brothers or fathers, a difference attributed to greater growth of the legs, and not related to the androgen deficiency. Lauder and Milne[92] found the cortical thickness of bone in Klinefelter patients to be more like that of 46,XX women than normal 46,XY men. With time, the full range of the disorder is being recognized, and it is now clear that the mild end of the spectrum includes patients with normal virilization and only small testes as a clue. For this reason, and in view of the possibility of mosaicism, a chromatin negative pattern does not exclude the diagnosis—a karyotype is needed.

To the geneticist, the most challenging variant of Klinefelter's syndrome is the male with a 46,XX karyotype. Over 50 such patients have been reported.[96] They are less tall, show less evidence of retardation, and are normally male in differentiation, but have small testes and may show evidence of inadequate androgen. Various hypotheses have been advanced to explain the differentiation of a testis in the absence of a Y chromosome. The most interesting sidelight on this question is the report from Kasdan *et al.*[97] of a pedigree of 46,XX patients whose pattern was consistent with an autosomal locus. Taken with a number of animal defects, such as the polled mutation in the goat, plus prior reports of familial true hermaphroditism and 46,XX true hermaphroditism, the evidence now strongly suggests that there is an autosomal locus in man controlling sex differentiation. The normal role of this gene is unknown. In the mutant form, the locus codes for differentiation of a testis in XX males. The testis is abnormal, showing the Klinefelter defect after puberty.

5.5.2.2b. Other Tubular Defects. The Sertoli-cell-only syndrome is a disease of unknown origin in which the germinal epithelium of the tubules is severely depleted or absent. Such patients have been thought to have normal Leydig cell function. An interesting study by Christiansen[98] analyzed urinary gonadotropins in 12 patients, and found that FSH was higher than in normals but lower than in castrates. This important observation suggests that something that has a negative feed-back control of FSH is produced in these testes; although Christiansen attributes this control to inhibin produced by Sertoli cells, other hormonal influences from the Leydig cells need to be considered as well. Unfortunately, the test was done only with urinary measurements and bioassay; it would be important to confirm this observation with plasma and immunoassay data.

An important acquired defect of tubular function should also be mentioned at this point—the inhibition of spermatogenesis produced by prolonged use of cyclophosphamide. A valuable short paper by Buchanan *et al.*[99] documented the reversibility of the defect when the period of exposure was less than 18 months, and the slow and partial recovery when it was longer.

5.5.2.2c. Infertility. It was to be hoped that advances in cytogenetics, particularly the subtlety of the banding techniques, would illuminate defects in meiosis that impair reproductive performance. Two interest-ing papers were published in 1974 bearing on these points. Benirschke[100] reviewed the known disorders of sex chromosomes, and concluded that chromosome errors are significant in reproductive fail-ure, but that, except for gross defects such as those of Klinefelter's syndrome, mechanistic explanations are not yet available. Infertile men have shown a 5% incidence of chromosomal defect, half of them in sex chromosomes, but how these may contribute to defects in meiotic pairing is not known. Beatty[101] provided a theoretical and empirical approach to the frequency of diploid spermatozoa and to the origin of triploid zygotes ($n = 69$), which comprise a significant fraction of human fetal wastage. He concluded that some diploid spermatozoa are fertile; that 60% of triploids have two sets of maternal chromosomes and the remaining 40%, two sets of paternal; and that meiotic error in the testis is the cause of the latter. Dispermic fertilization he believes to be close to zero.

Reame and Hafez[102] reviewed the hereditary aspects of subfertility, predominantly in animals, but in man as well. It is ironic that there is so much more understanding and awareness of this problem in other animals than in man. For practical purposes, the subject of male infertility remains an enigma. Aside from the established severe defects of the germinal cells, such as those in Klinefelter's syndrome, the Sertoli-cell-only syndrome, and postpubertal mumps orchitis, there is very limited understanding of almost any of the disorders. Thus, the terms *idiopathic oligospermia* and *subfertility* recur in the clinician's mind as a frustrating and difficult group. Endocrine aspects have been hard to elucidate, partly because satisfactory subclassification has been elusive. Many studies of the correlation of gonadotropin levels with sperm count or testicular biopsy have been done. All studies show strikingly high FSH levels in castrate males, and lesser elevation in Klinefelter's syndrome. Among patients with idiopathic azoospermia, Rastogi *et al.*[103] found FSH levels significantly increased, but not so high as in the aforementioned groups. In oligospermic males, several papers[103-106] confirmed, as Franchimont *et al.*[107] did *not*, the finding of Rosen and Weintraub[108] of an inverse correlation between sperm count and FSH. The depression of sperm count is usually severe before significant deviations are found in individual cases. (LH values are usually normal until severe oligospermia is evident.) Data correlating FSH elevation with testicular biopsy are in general agreement with those of Johnsen[109] indicating that FSH elevation occurs when the late stages of spermatogenesis, particularly the transition to spermatids, are impaired. Confirming this, Franchimont *et al.*[110] found increased basal FSH *and* increased FSH responses to LH–RH in men whose biopsies showed poor spermatid formation. Basal LH levels and responses showed no similar correlation. This laboratory also found a protein in seminal plasma that selectively lowers FSH and the FSH response to LH–RH in the castrate rat. This protein could be a source of the almost legendary inhibin so long postulated but never found.

Improved techniques in other areas may also prove to be helpful, but their use is not yet established. Ultrastructural studies of the testis in infertile males should be able to point to new approaches to meiotic failure of other than endocrine origin.[111]

The lack of understanding on the part of most patients with oligospermia is complemented by unsuccessful approaches to therapy and unimpressive reports of various attempts thereat. Two authors[104,112] have reported increases in sperm motility from androgen therapy, especially where impaired motility was the only defect. Clomiphene has been said to increase sperm production in patients with oligospermia.[113] Lamensdorf et al.[114] recently summarized the treatment of 131 oligospermic patients with large doses of testosterone for 6–12 months; they found a 29% pregnancy rate during the posttreatment rebound period. Mauss et al.[115] detailed the endocrine and seminal responses to long treatment with testosterone enanthate in 7 normal males. Plasma FSH and LH fell and testosterone rose; sperm count fell to 3×10^6. After therapy was discontinued, endocrine recovery was prompt, but in some patients, sperm counts remained depressed. The literature on infertility remains frustrating because of a combination of poor statistics, lack of adequate pretreatment sperm counts, unknown natural history of the disease being studied, and other shortcomings. For these reasons, care must be exercised in evaluating reports.

One area of keen interest has been the role of varicocele and its correction in management of the oligospermic male. Comhaire and Vermeulen[116] found an interesting decrease in testosterone values with age in patients with varicocele and impotence, but not in varicocele patients without impotence or in patients with psychogenic impotence. These authors suggested that varicocele may contribute to decreased potency and seminal quality through impaired Leydig cell function. It is worth noting that although a low testosterone is usually accorded a causal role when accompanied by impotence, the relationship could be the other way, with psychogenic factors producing a lowered LH, and thus diminished testosterone. At any rate, in contrast to the findings of the Comhaire and Vermeulen paper, Swerdloff and Walsh[117] studied 13 subfertile males with varicocele, and were unable to find any abnormality of FSH, LH, testosterone, or E_2. The two studies are different in that Comhaire and Vermeulen selected patients for impotence as well as varicocele.

Regardless of mechanism, Dubin and Amelar[118] reviewed their extensive experience with varicocelectomy. Although this paper did not present the desired details, the high success rate in selected patients seems to make this procedure worth considering in oligospermic patients with varicocele. (Incidentally, the paper points to the need to examine the patient upright to demonstrate the lesion.)

5.5.2.2d. Control of Fertility. The control of male fertility has been investigated from numerous aspects—immunological, endocrinologic, surgical. No reversible, acceptable, and practicable method has yet been demonstrated. Of nonreversible approaches, vasectomy is in increasing use, and two studies have confirmed the lack of endocrine damage.[119,120]

5.6. Influence of Other Disease on Testicular Function

The influence of other, especially chronic, illness on pituitary and testicular function has not received adequate attention. Two areas in which valuable contributions have been made recently are chronic renal failure and hepatic disease, including alcoholism.

5.6.1. Uremia

Sherman[121] found that impotence was more frequent in patients on chronic dialysis than in the general population, although admittedly it is difficult to get good data in either group. He pointed out that neuropathy and psychological factors may both be important, but that endocrine aspects should not be forgotten. Several groups[122-126] have studied various aspects of endocrine function in patients with chronic uremia. A single picture does not yet emerge, but several types of abnormalities have been found. Plasma testosterone levels and production rates tend to be lower than normal, but in at least one study, the metabolic clearance rate was unaltered. Serum LH and FSH varied from normal to high. Sperm counts were low in about half the patients studied. The interpretation at present suggests combined deficiencies at both gonadal and central levels, since not all patients with low sperm counts or plasma testosterone had the expected elevations of gonadotropins. Conforming this view, Stewart-Bentley et al.[125] and Rager et al.[124] found impaired response of the serum testosterone to exogenous gonadotropin. Whatever the underlying mechanism, dialysis appears to be ineffective in correcting it, but transplantation often succeeds dramatically. A very interesting feature found by Lim and Fang[123] was that en route to posttransplantation correction, an already high FSH rose strikingly before spermatogenesis recovered.

5.6.2. Cirrhosis

Clinical features of estrogen excess are common in cirrhosis—gynecomastia, testicular atrophy, spider angiomata, impotence. Clarification of pathogenesis has lagged, however, and recent studies are not in easy agreement. The level of SHBG is usually elevated, and the level of testosterone usually low; the free testosterone, although seldom measured, is probably even lower than one would anticipate from the total value. Estrogen measurements have been extremely variable, but E_2 tends to be elevated, and several studies[127–129] have found elevated E_1 as well. Consistent with the latter finding, there appear to be shifts toward female androgen: estrogen ratios, with increases in androstenedione, in the conversion of androstenedione to E_1 and other metabolites. This difference is enhanced by HCG administration.[129] The increase in E_2 relative to testosterone may thus have complex determinants. Van Thiel and his colleagues[130,131] suggest an intriguing additional mechanism. Retinal is essential for spermatogenesis, and is produced from retinol in the testis by alcohol dehydrogenase. The activity of this enzyme, and thus the production of retinal, is inhibited by alcohol. Similar effects are postulated for androgen and estrogen synthesis and metabolism. The feminizing consequences of alcohol and liver disease may thus be complex results of abnormalities related both to alcohol and to liver disease.

5.7. Conclusions

Most of the recent progress in our understanding of testicular function has been due to better techniques for studying hypothalamic–pituitary interrelationships and steroid hormone biosynthesis. Therapy for patients with gonadotropin deficiency has entered a new era. The treatment of patients with primary testicular disease, however, remains pathetically limited, and awaits a better understanding of the pathophysiology involved.

ACKNOWLEDGMENT

I have had invaluable help from Mrs. Janet Morgan in the preparation of this review.

References

1. Goldstein, J. L., and Wilson, J. D., 1975, Genetic and hormonal control of male sexual differentiation, *J. Cell. Physiol.* **85**(Suppl. 1 Pt. 2):365–377.
2. Blanchard, M.-G., and Josso, N., 1974, Source of the anti-Müllerian hormone synthesized by the fetal testis: Müllerian-inhibiting activity of fetal bovine Sertoli cells in tissue culture, *Pediatr. Res.* **8**:968–971.
3. Josso, N., 1974, Müllerian-inhibiting activity of human fetal testicular tissue deprived of germ cells by *in vitro* irradiation, *Pediatr. Res.* **8**:755–758.

4. Wilson, J. D., and Lasnitzki, I., 1971, Dihydrotestosterone formation in fetal tissues of the rabbit and rat, *Endocrinology* **89:**659–668.
5. Walsh, P. C., Madden, J. D., Harrod, M. J., Goldstein, J. L., MacDonald, P. C., and Wilson, J. D., 1974, Familial incomplete male pseudohermaphroditism, type 2. Decreased dihydrotestosterone formation in pseudovaginal perineoscrotal hypospadias, *N. Engl. J. Med.* **291:**944–949.
6. Imperato-McGinley, J., Guerrero, L., Gautier, T., and Peterson, R. E., 1974, Steroid 5α-reductase deficiency in man: An inherited form of male pseudohermaphroditism, *Science* **186:**1213–1215.
7. Givens, J. R., Wiser, W. L., Summitt, R. L., Kerber, I. J., Andersen, R. N., Pittaway, D. E., and Fish, S. A., 1974, Familial male pseudohermaphroditism without gynecomastia due to deficient testicular 17-ketosteroid reductase activity, *N. Engl. J. Med.* **291:**938–944.
8. Catt, K. J., Dufau, M. L., Neaves, W. B., Walsh, P. C., and Wilson, J. D., 1975, LH-hCG receptors and testosterone content during differentiation of the testis in the rabbit embryo, *Endocrinology* **97:**1157–1165.
9. Payne, A. H., and Jaffe, R. B., 1975, Androgen formation from pregnenolone sulfate by fetal, neonatal, prepubertal and adult human testes, *J. Clin. Endocrinol. Metab.* **40:**102–107.
10. Ahluwalia, B., Williams, J., and Verma, P., 1974, *In vitro* testosterone biosynthesis in the human fetal testis. II. Stimulation by cyclic AMP and human chorionic gonadotropin (hCG), *Endrocrinology* **95:**1411–1415.
11. Brook, C. G. D., Wagner, H., Zachmann, M., Prader, A., Armendares, S., Frenk, S., Aleman, P., Najjar, S. S., Slim, M. S., Genton, N., and Bozic, C., 1973, Familial occurrence of persistent Müllerian structures in otherwise normal males, *Br. Med. J.* **1:**771–773.
12. Morillo-Cucci, G., and German, J., 1971, Males with a uterus and fallopian tubes, a rare disorder of sexual development, *Birth Defects: Orig. Artic. Serv.* **VII**(6):229–231.
13. Zachmann, M., Völlmin, J. A., Hamilton, W., and Prader, A., 1972, Steroid 17,20-desmolase deficiency: A new cause of male pseudohermaphroditism, *Clin. Endocrinol.* **1:**369–385.
14. Saez, J. M., DePeretti, E., Morera, A. M., David, M., and Bertrand, J., 1971, Familial male pseudohermaphroditism with gynecomastia due to a testicular 17-ketosteroid reductase defect. I. Studies *in vivo*, *J. Clin. Endocrinol. Metab.* **32:**604–610.
15. Givens, J. R., Wiser, W. L., Summitt, R. L., Kerber, I. J., Andersen, R. N., Pittaway, D. E., and Fish, S. A., 1974, Familial male pseudohermaphroditism without gynecomastia due to deficient testicular 17-ketosteroid reductase activity, *N. Engl. J. Med.* **291:**938–944.
16. Madden, J. D., Walsh, P. C., MacDonald, P. C., and Wilson, J. D., 1975, Clinical and endocrinologic characterization of a patient with the syndrome of incomplete testicular feminization, *J. Clin. Endocrinol. Metab.* **41:**751–760.
17. Perez-Palacios, G., Ortiz, S., López-Amor, E., Morato, T., Febres, F., Lisker, R., and Scaglia, H., 1975, Familial incomplete virilization due to partial end organ insensitivity to androgens, *J. Clin. Endocrinol. Metab.* **41:**946–952.
18. Wilson, J. D., Harrod, M. J., Goldstein, J. L., Hemsell, D. L., and MacDonald, P. C., 1974, Familial incomplete male pseudohermaphroditism, type 1, *N. Engl. J. Med.* **290:**1097–1103.
19. Forest, M. G., and Cathiard, A. M., 1975, Pattern of plasma testosterone and Δ⁴-androstenedione in normal newborns: Evidence for testicular activity at birth, *J. Clin. Endocrinol. Metab.* **41:**977–980.

20. Forest, M. G., Sizonenko, P. C., Cathiard, A. M., and Bertrand, J., 1974, Hypophyso–gondal function in humans during the first year of life. I. Evidence for testicular activity in early infancy, *J. Clin. Invest.* **53:**819–828.

21. Grumbach, M. M., Grave, G. D., and Mayer, F. E. (eds.), 1974, *Control of the Onset of Puberty,* John Wiley and Sons, New York.

22. Bierich, J. R. (ed.), 1975, Disorders of puberty, *Clin. Endocrinol. Metab.* **4:**1–225.

23. Faiman, C., and Winter, J. S. D., 1974, Gonadotropins and sex hormone patterns in puberty: Clinical data, *in: The Control of the Onset of Puberty* (M. M. Grumbach, G. D. Grave, and F. E. Mayer, eds.), pp. 32–61, John Wiley and Sons, New York.

24. Lee, P. A., Jaffe, R. B., and Midgley, A. R., Jr., 1974, Serum gonadotropin, testosterone and prolactin concentrations throughout puberty in boys: A longitudinal study, *J. Clin. Endocrinol. Metab.* **39:**664–672.

25. Grumbach, M. M., Roth, J. C., Kaplan, S. L., and Kelch, R. P., 1974, Hypothalamic–pituitary regulation of puberty in man: Evidence and concepts derived from clinical research, *in: Control of the Onset of Puberty* (M. M. Grumbach, G. D. Grave, and F. E. Mayer, eds.), pp. 115–181, John Wiley and Sons, New York.

26. Sizonenko, P. C., and Paunier, L., 1975, Hormonal changes in puberty III: Correlation of plasma dehydroepiandrosterone, testosterone, FSH, and LH with stages of puberty and bone age in normal boys and girls and in patients with Addison's disease or hypogonadism or with premature or late adrenarche, *J. Clin. Endocrinol. Metab.* **41:**894–904.

27. Hopper, B. R., and Yen, S. S. C., 1975, Circulating concentrations of dehydroepiandrosterone and dehydroepiandrosterone sulfate during puberty, *J. Clin. Endocrinol. Metab.* **40:**458–461.

28. Lee, P. A., and Migeon, C. J., 1975, Puberty in boys: Correlation of plasma levels of gonadotropins (LH, FSH), androgens (testosterone, androstenedione, dehydroepiandrosterone and its sulfate), estrogens (estrone, and estradiol) and progestins (progesterone and 17-hydroxyprogesterone), *J. Clin. Endocrinol. Metab.* **41:**556–562.

29. Reiter, E. O., Grumbach, M. M., Kaplan, S. L., and Conte, F. A., 1975, The response of pituitary gonadotropes to synthetic LRF in children with glucocorticoid-treated congenital adrenal hyperplasia: Lack of effect of intrauterine and neonatal androgen excess, *J. Clin. Endocrinol. Metabol.* **40:**318–325.

30. Grumbach, M. M., Roth, J. C., Kaplan, S. L., and Kelch, R. P., 1974, Hypothalamic-pituitary regulation of puberty in man: Evidence and concepts derived from clinical research, *in: Control of the Onset of Puberty* (M. M. Grumbach, J. D. Grave, and F. E. Mayer, eds.), Chapt. 6, pp. 136 and 137, John Wiley and Sons, New York.

31. Parker, D. C., Judd, H. L., Rossman, L. G., and Yen, S. S. C., 1975, Pubertal sleep–wake patterns of episodic LH, FSH and testosterone release in twin boys, *J. Clin. Endocrinol. Metab.* **40:**1099–1109.

32. Boyar, R. M., Rosenfeld, R. S., Kapen, S., Finkelstein, J. W., Roffwarg, H. P., Weitzman, E. D., and Hellman, L., 1974, Human puberty. Simultaneous augmented secretion of luteinizing hormone and testosterone during sleep, *J. Clin. Invest.* **54:**609–618.

33. Rowe, P. H., Racey, P. A., Lincoln, G. A., Ellwood, M., Lehane, J., and Shenton, J. C., 1975, The temporal relationship between the secretion of luteinizing hormone and testosterone in man, *J. Endocrinol.* **64:**17–26.

34. Reitano, J. F., Caminos-Torres, R., and Snyder, P. J., 1975, Serum LH and FSH responses to repetitive administration of gonadotropin-releasing hormone in patients with idiopathic hypogonadotropic hypogonadism, *J. Clin. Endocrinol. Metab.* **41:**1035–1042.

35. Jeffcoate, S. L., 1975, The control of testicular function in the adult, *Clin. Endocrinol. Metab.* **4:**521–544.

36. Edmonds, M., Molitch, M., Pierce, J. G., and Odell, W. D., 1975, Secretion of alpha subunits of luteinizing hormone (LH) by the anterior pituitary, *J. Clin. Endocrinol. Metab.* **41:**551–555.

37. Hagen, C., and McNeilly, A. S., 1975, Changes in circulating levels of LH, FSH, LHβ- and α-subunit after gonadotropin-releasing hormone, and of TSH, LHβ- and α-subunit after thyrotropin-releasing hormone, *J. Clin. Endocrinol. Metab.* **41:**466–470.

38. Stewart-Bentley, M., Odell, W., and Horton, R., 1974, The feedback control of luteinizing hormone in normal adult men, *J. Clin. Endocrinol. Metab.* **38:**545–553.

39. Santen, R. J., 1975, Is aromatization of testosterone to estradiol required for inhibition of luteinizing hormone secretion in men? *J. Clin. Invest.* **56:**1555–1563.

40. Bramble, F. J., Houghton, A. L., Eccles, S. S., Murray, M. A. F., and Jacobs, H. S., 1975, Specific control of follicle stimulating hormone in the male: Postulated site of action of inhibin, *Clin. Endocrinol.* **4:**443–449.

41. Zárate, A., Garrido, J., Canales, E. S., Soria, J., and Schally, A. V., 1974, Disparity in the negative gonadal feedback control for LH and FSH secretion in cases of germinal aplasia or Sertoli-cell-only syndrome, *J. Clin. Endocrinol. Metab.* **38:**1125–1127.

42. Jeffcoate, S. L., 1975, The control of testicular function in the adult, *Clin. Endocrinol. Metab.* **4:**537.

43. Rubin, R. T., Gouin, P. R., Lubin, A., Poland, R. E., and Pirke, K. M., 1975, Nocturnal increase of plasma testosterone in men: Relation to gonadotropins and prolactin, *J. Clin. Endocrinol. Metab.* **40:**1027–1033.

44. Rowe, P. H., Lincoln, G. A., Racey, P. A., Lehane, J., Stephenson, M. J., Shenton, J. C., and Glover, T. D., 1974, Temporal variations of testosterone levels in the peripheral blood plasma of men, *J. Endocrinol.* **61:**63–73.

45. Doering, C. H., Kraemer, H. C., Brodie, H. K. H., and Hamburg, D. A., 1975, A cycle of plasma testosterone in the human male, *J. Clin. Endocrinol. Metab.* **40:**492–500.

46. Brooks, R. V., 1975, Androgens, *Clin. Endocrinol. Metabol.* **4:**503–520.

47. Scholler, R., Roger, M., Leymarie, P., Castanier, M., Toublanc, J. E., Canlorbe, P., and Job, J. C., 1975, Evaluation of Leydig-cell function in normal prepubertal and pubertal boys, *J. Steroid Biochem.* **6:**95–99.

48. Fan, D.-F., Oshima, H., Troen, B. R., and Troen, P., 1974, Studies of the human testis. IV. Testicular 20 α-hydroxysteroid dehydrogenase and steroid 17 α-hydroxylase, *Biochim. Biophys. Acta* **360:**88–99.

49. Fan, D.-F., and Troen, P., 1975, Studies of the human testis. VII. Conversion of pregnenolone to progesterone, *J. Clin. Endocrinol. Metab.* **41:**563–574.

50. LaFranchi, S. H., Parlow, A. F., Lippe, B. M., Coyotupa, J., and Kaplan, S. A., 1975, Pubertal gynecomastia and transient elevation of serum estradiol level, *Amer. J. Dis. Child.* **129:**927–931.

51. Lee, P. A., 1975, The relationship of concentrations of serum hormones to pubertal gynecomastia, *J. Pediatr.* **86:**212–215.

52. Liao, S., 1974, Biochemical studies on the receptor mechanisms involved in androgen action, in: *Biochemistry of Hormones* (H. V. Rickenberg, ed.), pp. 153–185, Butterworths, London.
53. Mainwaring, W. I. P., and Mangan, F. R., 1973, A study of the androgen receptors in a variety of androgen-sensitive tissues, *J. Endocrinol.* **59**:121–139.
54. Minguell, J. J., and Sierralta, W. D., 1975, Molecular mechanism of action of the male sex hormones, *J. Endocrinol.* **65**:287–315.
55. Sanborn, B. M., Elkington, J. S. H., Chowdhury, M., Tcholakian, R. K., and Steinberger, E., 1975, Hormonal influences on the level of testicular androgen binding activity: Effect of FSH following hypophysectomy, *Endocrinology* **96**:304–312.
56. Hansson, V., Djøseland, O., Attramadal, A., Trygstad, O., French, F. S., Stumpf, W. E., Sar, M., McLean, W. S., Smith, A. A., Weddington, S. C., Steiner, A. L., Petrusz, P., Nayfeh, S. N., Ritzén, E. M., and Hagenäs, L., 1974, Hormone binding and activation in the testis and epididymis, *Acta Pathol. Microbiol. Scand. Sect. A: Suppl.* **248**:75–88.
57. Rosen, V., Jung, I., Baulieu, E. E., and Robel, P., 1975, Androgen-binding proteins in human benign prostatic hypertrophy, *J. Clin. Endocrinol. Metab.* **41**:761–770.
58. Horst, H.-J., Dennis, M., Kaufmann, J., and Voigt, K. D., 1975, *In vivo* uptake and metabolism of ^{3}H-5-α-androstane-3α, 17β-diol and of ^{3}H-5α-androstane-3β,17β-diol by human prostatic hypertrophy, *Acta Endocrinol.* **79**:394–402.
59. McMahon, M. J., Butler, A. V. J., and Thomas, G. H., 1974, Testosterone metabolism in cultured hyperplasia of the human prostate, *Acta Endocrinol.* **77**:784–793.
60. Dorrington, J. H., and Fritz, I. B., 1974, Effects of gonadotropins on cyclic AMP production by isolated seminiferous tubule and interstitial cell preparations, *Endocrinology* **94**:395–403.
61. Hansson, V., Ritzén, E. M., and French, F. S., 1974, Androgen transport mechanisms in the testis and epididymis, *Acta Endocrinol.* **77**(Suppl. 191):191–198.
62. Steinberger, E., Steinberger, A., and Sanborn, B., 1974, Endocrine control of spermatogenesis, *Basic Life Sci.* **4**(Part A):163–181.
63. Bergadá, C., and Mancini, R. E., 1973, Effect of gonadotropins in the induction of spermatogenesis in human prepubertal testis, *J. Clin. Endocrinol. Metab.* **37**:935–943.
64. Stearns, E. L., MacDonnell, J. A., Kaufman, B. J., Padua, R., Lucman, T. S., Winter, J. S. D., and Faiman, C., 1974, Declining testicular function with age. Hormonal and clinical correlates, *Amer. J. Med.* **57**:761–766.
65. Isurugi, K., Fukutani, K., Takayasu, H., Wakabayashi, K., and Tamaoki, B.-I., 1974, Age-related changes in serum luteinizing hormone (LH) and follicle-stimulating hormone (FSH) levels in normal men, *J. Clin. Endocrinol. Metab.* **39**:955–957.
66. Pirke, K. M., and Doerr, P., 1975, Age related changes in free plasma testosterone, dihydrotestosterone and oestradiol, *Acta Endocrinol.* **80**:171–178.
67. Snyder, P. J., Reitano, J. F., and Utiger, R. D., 1975, Serum LH and FSH responses to synthetic gonadotropin-releasing hormone in normal men, *J. Clin. Endocrinol. Metab.* **41**:938–945.
68. Mortimer, C. H., Besser, G. M., McNeilly, A. S., Marshall, J. C., Harsoulis, P.,

Tunbridge, W. M. G., Gomez-Pan, A., and Hall, R., 1973, Luteinizing hormone and follicle stimulating hormone-releasing hormone test in patients with hypothalamic–pituitary–gonadal dysfunction, *Br. Med. J.* **4:** 73–77.

69. Mortimer, C. H., Besser, G. M., Hook, J., and McNeilly, A. S., 1974, Intravenous, intramuscular, subcutaneous and intranasal administration of LH/FSH–RH: The duration of effect and occurrence of asynchronous pulsatile release of LH and FSH, *Clin. Endocrinol.* **3:**19–25.

70. Yoshimoto, Y., Moridera, K., and Imura, H., 1975, Restoration of normal pituitary gonadotropin reserve by administration of luteinizing-hormone-releasing-hormone in patients with hypogonadotropic hypogonadism, *N. Engl. J. Med.* **292:**242–245.

71. Hashimoto, T., Miyai, K., Uozumi, T., Mori, S., Watanabe, M., and Kumahara, Y., 1975, Effect of prolonged LH-releasing hormone administration on gonadotropin response in patients with hypothalamic and pituitary tumors, *J. Clin. Endocrinol. Metab.* **41:**712–716.

72. Williams, C., Wieland, R. G., Zorn, E. M., and Hallberg, M. C., 1975, Effect of synthetic gonadotropin-releasing hormone (GnRH) in a patient with the "fertile eunuch" syndrome, *J. Clin. Endocrinol. Metab.* **41:**176–179.

73. del Pozo, E., Bolté, E., and Very, M., 1975, Suprasellar disturbance in the syndrome of fertile eunuchoidism: Case report, *Acta Endocrinol.* **80:**165–170.

74. Mortimer, C. H., McNeilly, A. S., Fisher, R. A., Murray, M. A. F., and Besser, G. M., 1974, Gonadotrophin-releasing hormone therapy in hypogonadal males with hypothalamic or pituitary dysfunction, *Br. Med. J.* **4:**617–621.

75. Goebelsmann, U., Horton, R., Mestman, J. H., Arce, J. J., Nagata, Y., Nakamura, R. M., Thorneycroft, I. H., and Mishell, D. R., Jr., 1973, Male pseudohermaphroditism due to testicular 17β-hydroxysteroid dehydrogenase deficiency, *J. Clin. Endocrinol. Metab.* **36:**867–879.

76. Goebelsmann, U., Hall, T. D., Paul, W. L., and Stanczyk, F. Z., 1975, *In vitro* steroid metabolic studies in testicular 17β-reduction deficiency, *J. Clin. Endocrinol. Metab.* **41:**1136–1143.

77. Longo, F. J., Coleman, S. A., and Givens, J. R., 1975, Ultrastructural analysis of the testis in male pseudohermaphrodism due to deficiency of 17-ketosteroid reductase, *Amer. J. Clin. Pathol.* **64:**145–154.

78. Judd, H. L., Hamilton, C. R., Barlow, J. J., Yen, S. S. C., and Kliman, B., 1972, Androgen and gonadotropin dynamics in testicular feminization syndrome, *J. Clin. Endocrinol. Metab.* **34:**229–234.

79. Bardin, C. W., and Bullock, L. P., 1974, Testicular feminization: Studies of the molecular basis of a genetic defect, *J. Invest. Dermatol.* **63:**75–84.

80. Meyer, W. J., III, Migeon, B. R., and Migeon, C. J., 1975, Locus on human X chromosome for dihydrotestosterone receptor and androgen insensitivity, *Proc. Nat. Acad. Sci. U.S.A.* **72:**1469–1472.

81. Keenan, B. S., Meyer, W. J., III, Hadjian, A. J., Jones, H. W., and Migeon, C. J., 1974, Syndrome of androgen insensitivity in man: Absence of 5α-dihydrotestosterone binding protein in skin fibroblasts, *J. Clin. Endocrinol. Metab.* **38:**1143–1146.

82. Lyon, M. F., 1972, X-chromosome inactivation and developmental patterns in mammals, *Biol. Rev.* **47:**1–35.

83. Ohno, S., 1967, Conversion of the original X and homology of the X-linked genes in placental mammals, *in: Sex Chromosomes and Sex-Linked Genes, Monogr. Endocrinol.* **1:**46–72.

84. Wilson, J. D., 1975, Dihydrotestosterone formation in cultured human fibroblasts. Comparison of cells from normal subjects and patients with familial incomplete male pseudohermaphroditism, type 2, *J. Biol. Chem.* **250:**3498–3504.

85. Opitz, J. M., Simpson, J. L., Sarto, G. E., Summitt, R. L., New, M., and German, J., 1972, Pseudovaginal perineoscrotal hypospadias, *Clin. Genet.* **3:**1–26.

86. deBehar, B. R., Mendilaharzu, H., Rivarola, M. A., and Bergadá, C., 1975, Gonadotropin secretion in prepubertal and pubertal primary hypogonadism: Response to LHRH, *J. Clin. Endocrinol. Metab.* **41:**1070–1075.

87. Niermann, H., Lenau, H. Ayi-Bonte, G., and Schultz, H., 1975, Excretion of urinary testosterone in Klinefelter's syndrome, *Humangenetik* **26:**61–70.

88. Smals, A. G. H., Kloppenborg, P. W. C., and Benraad, T. J., 1974, The effect of short and long term human chorionic gonadotrophin (HCG) administration on plasma testosterone levels in Klinefelter's syndrome, *Acta Endocrinol.* **77:**753–764.

89. Smals, A. G. H., Kloppenborg, P. W. C., and Benraad, T. J., 1975, Plasma testosterone in Klinefelter's syndrome: Diurnal variation and response to ACTH and dexamethasone, *Acta Endocrinol.* **78:**604–612.

90. Pazzagli, M., Forti, G., Cappellini, A., and Serio, M., 1975, Radioimmunoassay of plasma dihydrotestosterone in normal and hypogonadal men, *Clin. Endocrinol.* **4:**513–520.

91. Wang, C., Baker, H. W. G., Burger, H. G., deKretser, D. M., and Hudson, B., 1975, Hormonal studies in Klinefelter's syndrome, *Clin. Endocrinol.* **4:**399–411.

92. Paulsen, C. A., Gordon, D. L., Carpenter, R. W., Gandy, H. M., and Drucker, W. D., 1968, Klinefelter's syndrome and its variants: A hormonal and chromosomal study, *Recent Prog. Horm. Res.* **24:**321–363.

93. Smals, A. G. H., Kloppenborg, P. W. C., Lequin, R. M., and Benraad, Th. J., 1974, The effect of oestrogen administration on plasma testosterone, FSH and LH levels in patients with Klinefelter's syndrome and normal men, *Acta Endocrinol.* **77:**765–783.

94. Schibler, D., Brook, C. G. D., Kind, H. P., Zachmann, M., and Prader, A., 1974, Growth and body proportions in 54 boys and men with Klinefelter's syndrome, *Helv. Paediatr. Acta* **29:**325–333.

95. Lauder, I. J., and Milne, J. S., 1975, Bone mass in men with Klinefelter's syndrome and in normal subjects, estimated by the cortical thickness of bone, *Clin. Genet.* **8:**48–54.

96. de la Chappelle, A., 1972, Analytic review: Nature and origin of males with XX sex chromosomes, *Amer. J. Hum. Genet.* **24:**71–105.

97. Kasdan, R., Nankin, H. R., Troen, P., Wald, N., Pan, S., and Yanaihara, T., 1973, Paternal transmission of maleness in XX human beings, *N. Engl. J. Med.* **288:**539–545.

98. Christiansen, P., 1975, Urinary gonadotropins in the Sertoli-cell-only syndrome, *Acta Endocrinol.* **78:**180–191.

99. Buchanan, J. D., Fairley, K. F., and Barrie, J. U., 1975, Return of spermatogenesis after stopping cyclophosphamide therapy, *Lancet* **2:**156–157.

100. Benirschke, K., 1974, Chromosomal errors and reproductive failure, *in: Physiology and Genetics of Reproduction*, Part A (E. M. Coutinho and F. Fuchs eds.), pp. 73–90, Plenum Press, New York.

101. Beatty, R. A., 1974, Genetic aspects of spermatozoa, *in: Physiology and*

Genetics of Reproduction, Part A (E. M. Coutinho and F. Fuchs, eds.), pp. 183–196, Plenum Press, New York.

102. Reame, N. E., and Hafez, E. S. E., 1975, Hereditary defects affecting fertility, *N. Engl. J. Med.* **292:**675–681.

103. Rastogi, G. K., Datta, B. N., Dash, R. J., and Sinha, M. K., 1974, Serum gonadotropin levels in men with hypogonadism; mesterolone in the treatment of oligozoospermia, *in: Gonadotropins and Gonadal Function* (N. R. Moudgal, ed.), pp. 545–550, Academic Press, New York.

104. Christiansen, P., 1975, Studies on the relationship between spermatogenesis and urinary levels of follicle-stimulating hormone and luteinizing hormone in oligospermic men, *Acta Endocrinol.* **78:**192–208.

105. Hunter, W. M., Edmond, P., Watson, G. S., and McLean, N., 1974, Plasma LH and FSH levels in subfertile men, *J. Clin. Endocrinol. Metab.* **39:**740–749.

106. Purvis, K., Brenner, P. F., Landgren, B.-M., Cekan, Z., and Diczfalusy, E., 1975, Indices of gonadal function in the human male. I. Plasma levels of unconjugated steroids and gonadotrophins under normal and pathological conditions, *Clin. Endocrinol.* **4:**237–246.

107. Franchimont, P., Millet, D., Vendrely, E., Letawe, J., Legros, J. J., and Netter, A., 1972, Relationship between spermatogenesis and serum gonadotropin levels in azoospermia and oligospermia, *J. Clin. Endocrinol. Metab.* **34:**1003–1008.

108. Rosen, S. W., and Weintraub, B. D., 1971, Monotropic increase of serum FSH correlated with low sperm count in young men with idiopathic oligospermia and aspermia, *J. Clin. Endocrinol. Metab.* **32:**410–416.

109. Johnsen, S. G., 1970, The stage of spermatogenesis involved in the testicular–hypophyseal feed-back mechanism in man, *Acta Endocrinol.* **64:**193–210.

110. Franchimont, P., Chari, S., Schellen, A. M. C. M., and Demoulin, A., 1975, Relationship between gonadotropins, spermatogenesis and seminal plasma, *J. Steroid Biochem.* **6:**1037–1041.

111. Gould, K. G., and Martin, D. E., 1975, (SEM/EDX): A tool of potential diagnostic value in cases of infertility, *J. Reprod. Med.* **14:**197–200.

112. Brown, J. S., 1975, The effect of orally administered androgens on sperm motility, *Fertil. Steril.* **26:**305–308.

113. Schellen, T. M. C. M., and Beek, J. J. H. M. J., 1974, The use of clomiphene treatment for male sterility, *Fertil. Steril.* **25:**407–410.

114. Lamensdorf, H., Compere, D., and Begley, G., 1975, Testosterone rebound therapy in the treatment of male infertility, *Fertil. Steril.* **26:**469–472.

115. Mauss, J., Börsch, G., Bormacher, K., Richter, E., Levendecker, G., and Nocke, W., 1975, Effect of long-term testosterone oenanthate administration on male reproductive function: Clinical evaluation, serum FSH, LH, testosterone and seminal fluid analyses in normal men, *Acta Endocrinol.* **78:**373–384.

116. Comhaire, F., and Vermeulen, A., 1975, Plasma testosterone in patients with varicocele and sexual inadequacy, *J. Clin. Endocrinol. Metabl.* **40:**824–829.

117. Swerdloff, R. S., and Walsh, P. C., 1975, Pituitary and gonadal hormones in patients with varicocele, *Fertil. Steril.* **26:**1006–1012.

118. Dubin, L., and Amelar, R. D., 1975, Varicocelectomy as therapy in male infertility: A study of 504 cases, *Fertil. Steril.* **26:**217–220.

119. Johnsonbaugh, R. E., O'Connell, K., Engel, S. B., Edson, M., and Sode, J., 1975, Plasma testosterone, luteinizing hormone, and follicle-stimulating hormone after vasectomy, *Fertil. Steril.* **26:**329–330.

120. Varma, M. M., Varma, R. R., Johanson, A. J., Kowarski, A., and Migeon, C. J., 1975, Long-term effects of vasectomy on pituitary–gonadal function in man, *J. Clin. Endocrinol. Metab.* **40:**868–871.
121. Sherman, F. P., 1975, Impotence in patients with chronic renal failure on dialysis: Its frequency and etiology, *Fertil. Steril.* **26:**221–223.
122. Distiller, L. A., Morley, J. E., Sagel, J., Pokroy, M., and Rabkin, R., 1975, Pituitary–gonadal function in chronic renal failure: The effect of luteinizing hormone–releasing hormone and the influence of dialysis, *Metabolism* **24:**711–720.
123. Lim, V. S., and Fang, V. S., 1975, Gonadal dysfunction in uremic men: A study of the hypothalamo–pituitary–testicular axis before and after renal transplantation, *Amer. J. Med.* **58:**655–662.
124. Rager, K., Bundschu, H., and Gupta, D., 1975, The effect of HCG on testicular androgen production in adult men with chronic renal failure, *J. Reprod. Fertil.* **42:**113–120.
125. Stewart-Bentley, M., Gans, D., and Horton, R., 1974, Regulation of gonadal function in uremia, *Metabolism* **23:**1065–1072.
126. Zadeh, J. A., Koutsaimanis, K. G., Roberts, A. P., Curtis, J. R., and Daly, J. R., 1975, The effect of maintenance haemodialysis and renal transplantation on the plasma testosterone levels of male patients in chronic renal failure, *Acta Endocrinol.* **80:**577–582.
127. Gordon, G. C., Olivo, J., Rafii, F., and Southren, A. L., 1975, Conversion of androgens to estrogens in cirrhosis of the liver, *J. Clin. Endocrinol. Metab.* **40:**1018–1026.
128. Van Thiel, D. H., Gavaler, J. S., Lester, R., Loriaux, D. L., and Braunstein, G. D., 1975, Plasma estrone, prolactin, neurophysin, and sex steroid-binding globulin in chronic alcoholic men, *Metabolism* **24:**1015–1019.
129. Kley, H. K., Nieschlag, E., and Krüskemper, H. L., 1975, Estrone, estradiol and testosterone in patients with cirrhosis of the liver: Effect of HCG, *Horm. Metab. Res.* **7:**99, 100.
130. Van Thiel, D. H., and Lester, R., 1974, Sex and alcohol, *N. Engl. J. Med.* **291:**251–253.
131. Van Thiel, D. H., Gavaler, J., and Lester, R., 1974, Ethanol inhibition of vitamin A metabolism in the testes: Possible mechanism for sterility in alcoholics, *Science* **186:**941, 942.

The Adrenal Cortex

Robert L. Ney

6.1. Introduction

The initial portions of this chapter will focus on some recent advances in our understanding of corticosteroid biosynthesis, in particular on some of the mechanisms of the mitochondrial enzyme systems involved in the rate-limiting reactions of the biosynthetic pathways. These considerations will lead to an examination of current concepts as to how ACTH regulates the steroid biosynthetic mechanisms. In addition, some consideration will be given to the adrenal growth–promoting effects of ACTH.

The final portions of the chapter will focus on diseases of the adrenal cortex. While the basic hypothalamic and pituitary mechanisms involved

ROBERT L. NEY • Departments of Medicine and Physiology, University of North Carolina, Chapel Hill, North Carolina.

in ACTH secretion, as well as abnormalities of ACTH secretion, are considered in other chapters, discussion of disorders of the adrenal necessitates some consideration of these ACTH secretory disorders here, as well as of diseases in which the primary defect lies within the adrenal cortex itself.

6.2. Corticosteroid Biosynthesis

Cholesterol serves as the precursor for the corticosteroid hormones. While the adrenal has the capability to synthesize cholesterol from acetate, in some species at least (the rat, man), the main portion of precursor cholesterol is derived by uptake from plasma.[1,2] The cholesterol synthesized or taken up by the gland may potentially be utilized directly for corticosteroid biosynthesis. Alternatively, the gland possesses the enzymatic mechanisms for esterifying cholesterol,[3,4] with the cholesterol esters being stored in lipid droplets that are evident under the light microscope. These stores of esterified cholesterol may be drawn on during periods of active steroidogenesis. Thus, the adrenal possesses enzymes capable of cleaving cholesterol esters.[5,6] Precisely how free cholesterol reaches the mitochondrial sites that are the locus for the first steps in steroid synthesis remains an enigma. It is uncertain whether the cholesterol is transported from lipid droplets or other loci within the cell to mitochondria in association with proteins that serve as cholesterol carriers.[7,8] It may also be that cholesterol is transferred from lipid droplets to mitochondria through direct contact between these particles. Recently, it has been shown that agents such as colchicine that affect microtubules can stimulate steroidogenesis in cultured adrenal cells.[9,10] It may be that microtubules play an important role in orienting lipid droplets spatially in relation to mitochrondria, thereby regulating the flow of substrate cholesterol to mitochondria. It is furthermore of interest that in the disrupted cells of adrenal homogenates, it is no longer possible to increase steroidogenesis by agents such as ACTH and AMP, again emphasizing the importance of the structural relationships among the components of the steroidogenic system.

Once cholesterol is taken up by mitochondria, it can be converted to pregnenolone by these organelles. The formation of pregnenolone appears to be rate-limiting in the overall steroid biosynthetic pathway; once pregnenolone is formed, it is converted rapidly and almost completely to steroid hormones in normal adrenal cells.[11] Several intermediates have been identified in the conversion of cholesterol to pregnenolone, including 22R-hydroxycholesterol, 20α,22R-dihydrocholesterol, and, in a few studies, small quantities of 20α-hydroxycholesterol.[12,13] Although the precise mechanism of the formation of these intermediates en route to pregnenolone is not fully elucidated, it appears that the formation of pregnenolone involves hydroxylation and cleavage of the cholesterol side chain, yielding pregnenolone and isocaproaldehyde.[14]

This cholesterol side chain–cleavage system, as well as steroid 18- and 11β-hydroxylations, represent mitchondrial mixed function oxidations. The reactions depend on the transfer of electrons from NADPH to oxygen through the successive action of a flavoprotein and a nonheme iron protein (adrenodoxin), with mitochondrial cytochrome P-450 serving as the terminal oxidase to which the substrate is bound.[15,16] The binding of cholesterol to P-450 is associated with a change in the energy state of the electrons of the heme iron of P-450, which can be measured by changes in the so-called "spin-state" of the P-450 by optical and electron paramagnetic resonance (EPR) methods. Thus, when cholesterol binds to P-450, it changes from a low-spin to a high-spin state.[17,18] The conversion of cholesterol to pregnenolone (involving the formation of hydroxylated intermediates as discussed above) results in reversion of the P-450 to a low-spin state.[19] These techniques have proved to be useful in examining the flow of cholesterol to the site where it serves as a steroidogenic substrate under various physiological conditions.[20,21]

Although not proved, it seems possible that the same basic mechanisms apply in the formation of pregnenolone in differing species, and in all the cells of the adrenal cortex of a given species, regardless of the final steroid that is principally produced (e.g., cortisol, aldosterone). Subsequent to the formation of pregnenolone, the steroid biosynthetic pathways begin to diverge according to species, and according to differentiation into cells with differing enzymatic mechanisms in various adrenal zones (e.g., glomerulosa, fasciculata, reticularis) of a given species. Thus, the human adrenal possesses 17α-hydroxylase activity, which is needed for the biosynthesis of cortisol, while the rat adrenal is essentially devoid of this activity, and produces corticosterone as its principal glucocorticoid. Furthermore, aldosterone-producing cells of the human adrenal, located predominantly in the zona glomerulosa, lack 17α-hydroxylase activity, but possess the 18-hydroxylase activity needed for aldosterone formation, while cortisol-producing cells, located predominantly in the zona fasciculate, possess the needed 17α-hydroxylase, but lack 18-hydroxylase. A detailed consideration of the steroid biosynthetic pathways in differing species and in different adrenal cell types is beyond the scope of this discussion, but can be found in several excellent reviews published elsewhere.[22-24]

6.3. Mechanism of Action of ACTH

The work of Haynes first established that ACTH increases adrenal cAMP levels, and that cAMP in turn could stimulate adrenal steroidogenesis.[25,26] Subsequent investigations by Grahame-Smith *et al.*[27] with rat adrenals *in vivo* and *in vitro* established temporal and quantitative relationships between cAMP levels and rates of steroidogenesis during ACTH stimulation. These investigations were interpreted as indicating that cAMP serves as the intracellular mediator of ACTH action in the adrenal. Recent investigations employing incubations of isolated rat adrenal cells have revealed that low concentrations of ACTH are capable of stimulating steroidogenesis without a concomitant increase in the cellular content of cAMP.[28] These studies could mean that cAMP is not an obligatory intermediate in the action of ACTH on steroidogenesis, or that at very low doses, ACTH produces small increases in cAMP at critical intracellular sites that are not measurable against the background of the total cellular cAMP. Thus, although a considerable body of evidence supports the concept of cAMP as a mediator of ACTH action, some questions remain concerning this hypothesis.

It is clear that ACTH increases adrenal cAMP levels largely by stimulating the enzyme adenylate cyclase.[27] The bulk of this enzyme activity in adrenals is associated with plasma membranes.[29] The work of Lefkowitz *et al.*[30] first suggested that ACTH binds to the outer surface of adrenal cells. The enzyme adenylate cyclase is most likely situated on the inner portion of the cell membrane, where it can be accessible to substrate ATP. The hormone-responsive adenylate cyclase system can thus be conceived of as possessing an ACTH-binding receptor accessible to the exterior of the plasma membrane and thereby to circulating ACTH, and a catalytic component oriented toward the inner surface of the plasma membrane, where it can bind substrate ATP and release formed cAMP into the intracellular environment. It appears that a number of factors such as membrane phospholipids[31] and optimal concentrations of cations[32,33] are needed for the translation of the signal of hormone–receptor interaction into stimulation of adenylate cyclase activity. It has also recently been shown that certain nucleotides, particularly those containing guanine, bind to adrenocortical plasma membrane preparations and modulate ACTH-sensitive adenylate cyclase activity of such preparations.[34] It has been possible to solubilize adenylate cyclase from adrenal membranes using nonionic detergents,[35] but such solubilized enzyme preparations lose their hormone responsiveness, perhaps due to separation of the enzyme from hormone receptors, but probably more importantly due to removal of factors present in the membrane needed for hormone activation of the enzyme. Recently, Glossman has solubilized both adrenal membrane adenylate cyclase and guanyl nucleotide binding sites, and has separated these activities by chromatographic procedures.[35]

In addition to investigations focusing on the mechanisms of activation of adenylate cyclase by ACTH, much attention has been devoted to examining how cAMP, once formed through the action of this enzyme, effects the stimulation of steroidogenesis. Like other tissues, the adrenal possesses protein kinase activity that is stimulated by cAMP. The protein kinase catalyzes the transfer of the terminal phosphate of ATP to protein substrates, offering a potential mechanism for altering the properties or activities of enzymes or structural proteins that might serve as physiological substrates. Detailed studies by Gill and associates have clarified the properties of adrenal cAMP–dependent protein kinase.[36] The enzyme is composed of two units, one a receptor protein that binds cAMP, the other a catalytic unit. In the absence of cAMP, the receptor binds to the catalytic unit. When the receptor binds cAMP, it dissociates from the catalytic unit. Although there has been considerable clarification of the properties of the adrenal cAMP–dependent protein kinase, the adrenal proteins that are phosphorylated by this enzyme activity remain to be identified, and although it seems a likely possibility, it is still not established whether the protein kinase is involved in the stimulation of steroidogenesis by cAMP, or whether some entirely different mechanism is involved.

As noted in Section 6.2, the formation of pregnenolone appears to be rate-limiting in the overall steroid biosynthetic pathway. When ACTH rapidly stimulates steroidogenesis, an effect that is measurable in a matter of minutes, it appears to do so by increasing the formation of pregnenolone.[37] While it seemed possible that ACTH and its mediator cAMP might act by stimulating the mitochondrial enzymes involved in the conversion of cholesterol to pregnenolone, some studies have failed to confirm such an effect.[38] On the other hand, ACTH treatment appears to increase the amount of cholesterol bound to mitochondrial cytochrome P-450,[17,18] suggesting either that ACTH has altered the P-450 itself and enhanced its capacity to bind cholesterol or that ACTH has increased the flux of substrate cholesterol from other sites, such as the lipid droplets, into adrenal mitochondria. Recent studies have suggested that the latter mechanism may be operative.[20,21] Other experiments have made use of the inhibitor aminoglutethimide, which blocks the mitochondrial conversion of cholesterol to pregnenolone, some studies have failed to confirm such ACTH treatment brings about mitochondrial accumulation of cholesterol.[39] As one possible source of this cholesterol, it has been noted that ACTH treatment results in cleavage of cholesterol esters within adrenal lipid droplets,[40] and it has been shown that cholesterol esterase activity is increased under these circumstances.[41] It has furthermore been suggested that cholesterol esterase is a substrate for cAMP-dependent protein kinase,[42] providing a potential mechanistic link between cAMP and an enzyme that may play a role in regulating the availability of substrate cholesterol for steroidogenesis. In addition, as noted in Section 6.2, colchicine and other drugs that affect microtubules have been shown to stimulate steroidogenesis in isolated adrenal cells,[9,10] and it seems possible that alterations in such structural elements might be a means for regulating the availability of cholesterol substrate for steroidogenesis. Thus, while it was initially believed that ACTH and cAMP regulate the mitochondrial enzymes that convert cholesterol to pregnenolone, more recent work has focused on the regulation of the flux of cholesterol to mitochondria, and more particularly on the binding of cholesterol to cytochrome P-450. In addition to adrenal lipid droplets serving as an immediate potential source of substrate cholesterol, in some species, ACTH treatment over several hours brings about an increased uptake of cholesterol from plasma,[43] some of this cholesterol perhaps being esterified and stored in lipid droplets, but some perhaps being directly used for steroidogenesis.

Inhibitors of protein synthesis have been shown to block the steroidogenic effect of ACTH.[44,45] These drugs, including puromycin and cycloheximide, appear to block the formation of pregnenolone. It has been suggested that ACTH stimulates steroidogenesis by stimulating formation of proteins that regulate steroidogenesis, and that puromycin and cycloheximide prevent this hormone effect. However, such regulatory proteins remain to be identified, and it also seems possible that the drugs inhibit steroidogenesis through some effect other than their inhibition of protein synthesis.

In addition to the effect of ACTH in rapidly stimulating steroidogenesis within a matter of minutes, the hormone also exerts effects that are manifest only over longer periods of time—hours to days. Most striking is the decrease in adrenal weight that occurs after hypophysectomy and that can be prevented by the administration of ACTH. While ACTH is considered to play a major role in maintaining the mass of the adrenal gland, the possibility remains that growth hormone (GH) and other as yet unidentified pituitary factors may also play a role in this phenomenon. When ACTH maintains or increases adrenal weight, this effect is first accompanied by an increase in total adrenal RNA and protein, and after a lag phase, adrenal DNA increases also.[46] Thus, adrenal cells appear at first to accumulate components such as RNA and protein, but ultimately there is an increase in adrenal cell number—in other words, adrenal hyperplasia. The mechanisms of this effect of ACTH have been the subject of great interest, not only because they may increase understanding of the regulation of the adrenal, but also because of broader ramifications for the understanding of cell replication and its hormonal regulation.

It is known that ACTH increases adrenal blood flow, and it is possible that an increased supply of needed substrates is at least a needed corollary in the adrenal growth–promoting effect of ACTH, if not a causative mechanism. It is true that it has been very difficult to show stimulatory effects of ACTH on adrenal protein synthesis or other growth-related phenomena *in vitro*.[47]

One question that might be raised is whether cAMP can be implicated as a mediator of the adrenal growth–promoting effects of ACTH, as it has been in the steroidogenic actions of the hormone. It has been shown, for example, that ACTH can produce dramatic increases in adrenal cAMP levels, levels of this nucleotide far beyond those needed for the stimulation of steroidogenesis.[27] During ACTH-induced adrenal hyperplasia, the adrenal maintains very high levels of cAMP. It is of interest that adrenal cGMP levels fluctuate in a manner opposite to cAMP levels, both acutely and chronically.[48] Thus, after hypophysectomy, adrenal cAMP levels fall, while those of cGMP rise. ACTH treatment produces converse results. Furthermore, administration of dibutyryl cAMP to hypophysectomized rats produces a decrease in the elevated adrenal cGMP levels of such animals, suggesting that cAMP may play some role in the regulation of cGMP levels in this tissue.[48] Immunocytochemical technics have revealed that cGMP is largely localized in nuclear sites in the rat adrenal,[48] while cAMP is predominantly extranuclear in location. Finally, dibutyryl cAMP is capable of at least partially maintaining adrenal weight and content of DNA, RNA, and protein in hypophysectomized rats.[49] Thus, a certain amount of evidence points to a role for cAMP in the growth-promoting effects of ACTH, and cGMP may also be involved. Much more work is needed to clarify this question, however, and it remains possible that entirely different mechanisms are operative.

The activities of a number of growth-related enzymes, including DNA and RNA polymerases and ornithine decarboxylase,[50,51] are increased in the adrenal during ACTH treatment, and some of these effects are reproduced when dibutyryl cAMP is given to hypophysectomized animals. However, there is uncertainty not only as to the causative role of cyclic nucleotides in these phenomena, but also as to which is the primary or initiating event in bringing about the growth-promoting effect of ACTH. In addition, it should be noted that in most cell culture systems employing transformed or neoplastic cells, cAMP exerts an inhibitory effect on cell replication.[52] In cell cultures of a mouse adrenal tumor, both ACTH and cAMP exert such an effect,[53] in contrast to the trophic effects of ACTH on normal adrenals *in vivo*.

In addition to effecting long-term changes in adrenal growth and mass, ACTH also effects more chronic changes in the steroid-producing capacity of the adrenal, changes that are distinguishable from the acute effects of the hormone in activating steroidogenesis. Thus, when rats are studied at varying time periods after hypophysectomy, the adrenal steroid-ogenic response to pulse doses of ACTH progressively decreases,[11] and this defect can be prevented by the continuing administration of ACTH to the hypophysectomized animals. After hypophysectomy, the activity of the adrenal mitochondrial cholesterol side chain–cleavage system decreases,[54] as does the activity of later steps in the steroid biosynthetic pathway.[11] It seems possible that the decrease in adrenal protein content that occurs after hypophysectomy also includes enzymes involved in steroid biosynthesis, limiting the capacity of the gland to respond to acute pulses of ACTH.

6.4. Diseases of the Adrenal Cortex

6.4.1. Enzymatic Defects in Steroidogenesis

Congenital defects in virtually every step in the cortisol biosynthetic pathway have been described,[55] and these disorders are often grouped together under the heading *congenital adrenal hyperplasia*. Impairment in cortisol biosynthesis due to a defect in one or another of the needed enzymes leads to reflex increases in pituitary ACTH secretion and hyper-plasia of the adrenal glands. In some cases, in which the enzyme defect is not complete, these compensatory mechanisms may maintain reasonably adequate cortisol levels, but at the expense of hyperplastic adrenals driven by large quantities of ACTH. Specific enzyme defects in 21-hydroxylase, 11β-hydroxylase, 17α-hydroxylase, and Δ^5-isomerase-3β-hydroxysteroid dehydrogenase activities have been described. In addition, a form of the disease referred to as *lipoid adrenal hyperplasia* has been described in which the adrenal cells are filled with lipid droplets; the precise enzymatic defect or defects in this disease are unknown. The clinical and biochemical manifestations of these disorders are quite diverse, and have been reviewed in considerable detail elsewhere.[55] Their recognition depends on the clinical manifestations, and on the measurement in blood and urine of steroid precursors and their metabolites, which accumulate in excess prior to the enzymatic block in steroidogenesis and are released from the adrenal glands. Estimation of the nature of the enzymatic defect has generally been indirect and based on which precursors are detectable in excess in blood and urine, since adrenal tissue has not been available for direct enzymatic studies.

6.4.2. Adrenal Hypofunction

Reference is made here to Addison's disease and to adrenocortical hypofunction associated with hypopituitarism, while selective disorders of aldosterone secretion are considered in Chapter 7. Diagnostic tests for adrenal insufficiency have not changed substantially in recent years, and continue to be based largely on the plasma cortisol and urinary 17-hydroxycorticosteroid responses to administered ACTH. These ACTH-stimulated tests are used to document primary adrenal disease and to distinguish it from hypopituitarism in patients with frank adrenal insufficiency. Patients with pituitary disease may have normal baseline hypothalamic–pituitary–adrenal function, but may have impaired pituitary ACTH "reserve," which can be detected with the metyrapone test or other stimuli that provoke ACTH secretion, such as insulin-induced hypoglycemia. All these tests of the hypothalamic–pituitary–adrenal axis that are used in the diagnosis of adrenal insufficiency can be referred to in a recent detailed review.[56] Although assays are not available in all institutions, measurement of plasma ACTH levels can distinguish primary from secondary insufficiency.[57]

6.4.3. Cushing's Syndrome

Tests for the diagnosis of Cushing's syndrome have not changed drastically in recent years, and are discussed in detail in a recent review.[56] Measurement of urinary free cortisol is useful in detecting the presence of hypercortisolism, while dexamethasone suppression tests continue to be the best discriminator in distinguishing the pathophysiological basis for the hypercortisolism. Plasma ACTH assays may be necessary in some cases to distinguish between the ectopic ACTH syndrome and adrenocortical neoplasms.

There has been considerable interest in whether pituitary ACTH hypersecretion in Cushing's disease is due to an intrinsic defect in the anterior pituitary itself, or to an abnormality in hypothalamic regulatory centers. It is believed that neural impulses converging on the hypothalamus are conveyed by neurotransmitters to hypothalamic neurosecretory cells. These cells secrete corticotropin-releasing factor (CRF) into the pituitary portal circulation, which delivers the CRF to anterior pituitary cells, bringing about ACTH release. In experimental animals, stimulation of ACTH secretion is brought about by serotoninergic, cholinergic, and adrenergic pathways, while dopaminergic pathways inhibit ACTH release.[58] The well-established circadian rhythmicity of pituitary–adrenal function may well depend on neural pathways linked to visual stimuli. This rhythmicity is usually lost in patients with pituitary Cushing's disease.[56]

It is of interest that studies of adrenal function in patients with serotonin-secreting carcinoid tumors revealed certain abnormalities in pituitary–adrenal function.[59] These patients had greater responses to metyrapone than normal subjects, but these responses were reduced when the patients were given the serotonin antagonist cyproheptadine. Furthermore, the administration of cyproheptadine to a small number of patients with pituitary Cushing's disease has been associated with amelioration of clinical and biochemical evidences of hypercortisolism.[60] These studies have been interpreted as favoring the concept that Cushing's disease is due primarily to a defect in the hypothalamic–neural mechanisms regulating ACTH secretion.

On the other hand, some patients with pituitary Cushing's disease are known to harbor pituitary adenomas. While these adenomas may originally be incited by hypothalamic overstimulation of pituitary cells, these observations are generally taken to indicate a primary defect within the pituitary itself. Furthermore, removal of such an adenoma completely restores pituitary–adrenal function to normal,[61] a result that would not be expected if a persistent hypothalamic defect was present.

The ectopic ACTH syndrome is another form of Cushing's syndrome that has been the subject of continuing investigation. This disorder is found in conjunction with a varied group of neoplasms, but it is most common with pulmonary neoplasms, more specifically with oat cell carcinoma of the lung. Although hypercortisolism is present in only a minority of patients with lung cancer, the true incidence of ectopic ACTH has been the subject of interest, since it seemed possible that some tumors might produce small amounts of ACTH that were insufficient to induce adrenal hyperfunction, while others might produce biologically inactive fragments or precursors of ACTH. Gewirtz and Yalow[62] studied tumor tissue from 15 patients with primary carcinoma of the lung (the exact cell type was not specified), and found immunoreactive ACTH in 14 cases. The preponderant form of ACTH was "big" ACTH, a larger precursor of the ACTH molecule. Furthermore, in 83 patients with lung cancer, more than half had elevated afternoon blood levels of immunoreactive ACTH, again predominantly of the "big" ACTH variety. Orth et al.[63] found that tumors from patients with the ectopic ACTH syndrome contain, in addition to ACTH that is biologically and immunologically undistinguishable from pituitary ACTH, N-terminal and C-terminal fragments of the ACTH molecule, presumably resulting from proteolytic digestion of ACTH within the tumor tissue.

From physiological studies performed in patients with the various disorders, it appears that the regulation of ACTH secretion by tumors producing ectopic ACTH, the regulation by pituitaries of patients with Cushing's disease, and the regulation by the normal pituitary are all quite different. With few exceptions, glucocorticoids fail to suppress ectopic ACTH secretion even in large doses, while large doses suppress pituitary

ACTH secretion in Cushing's disease, and only small physiological doses are needed for suppression of the normal pituitary. However, recent *in vitro* studies of tumors producing ectopic ACTH suggests that their regulatory mechanisms may not be entirely different from those of the pituitary.[64] In several such tumors, median eminence extracts from the rat stimulated release of ACTH as well as of β-MSH, a concomitant tumor product in most cases of the ectopic ACTH syndrome. CAMP also brought about release of both these hormones. Some of the difference in the regulation of ACTH secretion by tumors producing the hormone in an ectopic manner in comparison to the pituitary may therefore be due to the remote location of the tumor in terms of exposure to hypothalamic regulatory factors.

6.4.4. Adrenocortical Neoplasms

Adrenal neoplams may be adenomas or carcinomas, and may secrete cortisol, producing Cushing's syndrome, or 17-ketosteroids, producing virilization in the female, or aldosterone (a subject considered in Chapter 7). Cortisol or 17-ketosteroid production by adrenal neoplasms is nonsuppressible by even large quantities of glucocorticoids,[56] and in the case of cortisol-producing neoplasms is associated with decreased plasma levels of ACTH. In the case of cortisol-producing adenomas, the diagnosis may be complicated in some cases by the fluctuating activity of the tumor.[65,66]

Recently, interest has focused on the regulation of the function of adrenocortical tumors, and how this regulation resembles or differs from that of the normal adrenal. Leichter and Daughaday[67] have described a patient with an adrenal adenoma producing massive quantities of 17-ketosteroids. This patient had hypocholesterolemia, which reverted to normal soon after removal of the tumor, suggesting that the tumor, like the normal human adrenal, derives much of its precursor cholesterol for steroidogenesis by uptake from plasma. Some adrenal adenomas exhibit steroidogenic responses to ACTH, while most carcinomas show little or no response. Schorr *et al.*[68] studied a rat adrenocortical carcinoma that did not increase steroid production in response to ACTH. This tumor did possess an ACTH-sensitive adenylate cyclase, however, and this cyclase also showed unexpected responses to catecholamines and TSH. Saez *et al.*[69] failed to show such aberrant adenylate cyclase hormone responses in human adrenocortical tumors. However, in these studies, several other abnormalities were found in the tumor adenylate cyclase system, including in some cases alterations in the ACTH receptor binding sites, and in another a defect in adenylate cyclase catalytic activity.

The treatment of adrenocortical neoplasms continues to be centered around surgical removal. Nonresectable adrenocortical carcinomas may be responsive to therapy with o,p'-DDD, which inhibits both cortisol and 17-ketosteroid production (although it has little effect on aldosterone), and may induce regression of tumor masses. Several long-term survivals have recently been described in patients receiving this drug.[70]

ACKNOWLEDGMENTS

The author wishes to acknowledge the assistance of Mrs. Darien Mahaffee and Mrs. Glenda Foushee in the preparation of this chapter.

References

1. Dexter, R. N., Fishman, L. M., and Ney, R. L., 1970, Stimulation of adrenal cholesterol uptake from plasma by adrenocorticotropin, *Endocrinology* **87:**836–846.
2. Shima, S., and Pincus, G., 1969, Effects of adrenocorticotropic hormone on rat adrenal corticosteroidogenesis *in vivo, Endocrinology* **84:**1048–1054.
3. Longcope, C., and Williams, R. H., 1963, Esterification of cholesterol by homogenates of rat adrenal tissue, *Endocrinology* **72:**735–741.
4. Shyamala, G., Lossow, W. J., and Chaikoff, I. L., 1966, Esterification of cholesterol by rat adrenal gland homogenates and subcellular components, *Biochim. Biophys. Acta* **116:**543–554.
5. Trzeciak, W. H., and Boyd, G. S., 1974, Activation of cholesteryl esterase in bovine adrenal cortex, *Eur. J. Biochem.* **46:**201–207.
6. Boyd, G. S., and Trzeciak, W. H., 1973, Cholesterol metabolism in the adrenal cortex: Studies on the mode of action of ACTH, *Ann. N.Y. Acad. Sci.* **212:**361–376.
7. Kan, K. W., Ritter, M. C., Zengar, F., and Dempsey, M. E., 1972, The role of a carrier protein in cholesterol and steroid hormone synthesis by adrenal enzymes, *Biochem. Biophys. Res. Commun.* **48:**423–429.
8. Kan, K. W., and Ungar, F., 1973, Characterization of an adrenal activator for cholesterol side chain cleavage, *J. Biol. Chem.* **248:**2868–2875.
9. Temple, R., and Wolff, J., 1973, Stimulation of steroid secretion by antimicrotubular agents, *J. Biol. Chem.* **248:**2691–2698.
10. Temple, R., Williams, J. A., Wilberg, J. F., and Wolff, J., 1972, Colchicine and hormone secretion, *Biochem. Biophys. Res. Commun.* **46:**1454–1461.
11. Ney, R. L., Dexter, R. N., Davis, W. W., and Garren, L. D., 1967, A study of the mechanisms by which adrenocorticotropic hormone maintains adrenal steroidogenic responsiveness, *J. Clin. Invest.* **46:**1916–1924.
12. Solomon, S., Levitan, P., and Lieberman, S., 1956, Possible intermediates between cholesterol and pregnenolone in corticosteroidogenesis, *Rev. Can. Biol.* **15:**282.
13. Burstein, S., Middleditch, B. S., and Gut, M., 1975, Mass spectrometric study of the enzymatic conversion of cholesterol to (22R)-22-hydroxycholesterol, (20R,22R)-20,22-dihydroxycholesterol and pregnenolone, and of (22R)-22-hydroxycholesterol to the glycol and pregnenolone in bovine adrenocortical preparations, *J. Biol. Chem.* **250:**9028–9037.

14. Staple, E., Lynn, W. S., and Gurin, S., 1956, An enzymatic cleavage of the cholesterol side chain, *J. Biol. Chem.* **219:**845–851.

15. Simpson, E. R., and Boyd, G. S., 1967, The cholesterol side-chain cleavage system of bovine adrenal cortex, *Eur. J. Biochem.* **2:**275–285.

16. Jefcoate, C. R., Simpson, E. R., and Boyd, G. S., 1973, The detection of different states of the P-450 cytochromes in adrenal mitochondria, changes induced by ACTH, *Ann. N.Y. Acad. Sci.* **212:**243–261.

17. Brownie, A. C., and Paul, D. P., 1974, Further studies on the effect of ACTH on cholesterol side chain cleavage cytochrome P-450 in rat adrenal mitochondria, *Endocrine Res. Commun.* **3:**321–330.

18. Brownie, A. C., Simpson, E. R., Jefcoate, C. R., and Boyd, G. S., 1972, Effect of ACTH on cholesterol side-chain cleavage in rat adrenal mitochondria, *Biochem. Biophys. Res. Commun.* **46:**483–490.

19. Simpson, E. R., Jefcoate, C. R., and Boyd, G. S., 1971, Spin state changes in cytochrome P-450 associated with cholesterol side chain cleavage in bovine adrenal cortex mitochondria, *FEBS Lett.* **15:**53–58.

20. Bell, J. J., Cheng, S. C., and Harding, B. W., 1973, Control of substrate flux and adrenal cytochrome P-450, *Ann. N.Y. Acad. Sci.* **212:**290–305.

21. Bell, J. J., and Harding, B. W., 1974, The acute action of adrenocorticotropic hormone on adrenal steroidogenesis, *Biochim. Biophys. Acta* **348:**285–298.

22. Griffiths, K., and Cameron, E. H. D., 1970, Steroid biosynthetic pathways in the human adrenal, *Adv. Steroid Biochem. Pharmacol.* **2:**223–265.

23. Vinson, G. P., and Whitehouse, B. J., 1970, Comparative aspects of adrenocortical function, *Adv. Steroid Biochem. Pharmacol.* **1:**163–342.

24. Grant, J. K., 1968, The biosynthesis of adrenocortical steroids, *J. Endocrinol.* **41:**111–135.

25. Haynes, R. C., Jr., 1958, The activation of adrenal phosphorylase by the adrenocorticotropic hormone, *J. Biol. Chem.* **233:**1220–1222.

26. Haynes, R. C., Jr., Koritz, S. B., and Peron, F. G., 1959, Influence of adenosine 3′,5′-monophosphate on corticoid production by rat adrenal glands, *J. Biol. Chem.* **234:**1421–1423.

27. Grahame-Smith, D. G., Butcher, R. W., Ney, R. L., and Sutherland, E. W., 1967, Adenosine 3′,5′-monophosphate as the intracellular mediator of the action of adrenocorticotropic hormone on the adrenal cortex, *J. Biol. Chem.* **242:**5535–5541.

28. Beall, R. S., and Sayers, G., 1972, Isolated adrenal cells: Steroidogenesis and cyclic AMP accumulation in response to ACTH, *Arch. Biochem. Biophys.* **148:**70–76.

29. Finn, F. M., Widnell, C. C., and Hofman, K., 1972, Localization of an adrenocorticotropic hormone receptor in bovine adrenal cortical membranes, *J. Biol. Chem.* **247:**5695–5702.

30. Lefkowitz, R. S., Roth, J., Pricer, W., and Pastan, I., 1970, ACTH receptors in the adrenals: Specific binding of ACTH-^{125}I and its relation to adenyl cyclase, *Proc. Nat. Acad. Sci. U.S.A.* **65:**745–752.

31. Levey, G. S., 1971, Restoration of glucagon responsiveness of solubilized myocardial adenyl cyclase by phosphatidylserine, *Biochem. Biophys. Res. Commun.* **43:**108–113.

32. Lefkowitz, R. S., Roth, J., and Pastan, I., 1970, Effects of calcium on ACTH stimulation of the adrenal: Separation of hormone binding from adenyl cyclase activation, *Nature London* **228:**864–866.

33. Lefkowitz, R. S., Roth, J., and Pastan, I., 1971, ACTH–Receptor interaction

in the adrenal: A model for the initial step in the action of hormones that stimulate adenyl cyclase, *Ann. N.Y. Acad. Sci.* **185**:195–209.

34. Londos, C., Salomon, Y., Lin, M. C., Harwood, J. P., Schramm, M., Wolff, J., and Rodbell, M., 1974, 5'-Guanylylimidodiphosphate, a potent activator of adenylate cyclase systems in eukaryotic cells, *Proc. Nat. Acad. Sci. U.S.A.* **71**:3087–3090.

35. Glossman, H., 1975, Adrenal cortex adenylate cyclase. Solubilization of adenylate cyclase and guanyl nucleotide binding sites, *Naunyn-Schmiedeberg's Arch. Pharmacol.* **291**:89–100.

36. Gill, G. N., 1972, Mechanism of ACTH action, *Metabolism* **21**:571–588.

37. Karaboyas, G. C., and Koritz, S. B., 1965, Identity of the site of action of 3',5'-adenosine monophosphate and adrenocorticotropic hormone in corticosteroidogenesis in rat adrenal and beef adrenal cortex slices, *Biochemistry* **4**:462–468.

38. Cohen, M. P., and Moriwaki, K., 1969, 3',5'-cyclic AMP and the adrenal desmolase system, *Proc. Soc. Exp. Biol. Med.* **131**:1267–1271.

39. Mahaffee, D., Reitz, R. C., and Ney, R. L., 1974, The mechanism of action of adrenocorticotropic hormone, *J. Biol. Chem.* **249**:227–233.

40. Garren, L. D., Gill, G. N., Masui, H., and Walton, G. M., 1971, On the mechanism of action of ACTH, *Recent Prog. Horm. Res.* **27**:433–478.

41. Trzeciak, W. W., and Boyd, G. S., 1973, The effect of stress induced by ether anesthesia on cholesterol content and cholesteryl–esterase activity in rat adrenal cortex, *Eur. J. Biochem.* **37**:327–333.

42. Trzeciak, W. W., and Boyd, G. S., 1974, Activation of cholesteryl esterase in bovine adrenal cortex, *Eur. J. Biochem.* **46**:201–207.

43. Dexter, R. N., Fishman, L. M., Ney, R. L., and Liddle, G. W., 1967, An effect of adrenocorticotrophic hormone on adrenal cholesterol accumulation, *Endocrinology* **81**:1185–1187.

44. Davis, W. W., and Garren, L. D., 1968, On the mechanism of action of adrenocorticotropic hormone: The inhibitory site of cycloheximide in the pathway of steroid biosynthesis, *J. Biol. Chem.* **243**:5153–5157.

45. Ferguson, J. J., Jr., 1963, Protein synthesis and adrenocorticotropin responsiveness, *J. Biol. Chem.* **238**:2754–2759.

46. Farese, R. V., and Reddy, W. J., 1963, Observations on the interrelations between adrenal protein, RNA and DNA during prolonged ACTH administration, *Biochim. Biophys. Acta* **76**:145–148.

47. Farese, R. V., 1969, Effects of ACTH and cyclic AMP *in vitro* on incorporation of ³H-leucine and ¹⁴C-orotic acid into protein and RNA in the presence of an inhibitor of cholesterol side chain cleavage, *Endocrinology* **85**:1209–1212.

48. Whitley, T. H., Stowe, N. W., Ong, S. H., Ney, R. L., and Steiner, A. L., 1975, Control and localization of rat adrenal cyclic guanosine 3',5'-monophosphate: Comparison with adrenal cyclic adenosine 3',5'-monophosphate, *J. Clin. Invest.* **56**:146–154.

49. Ney, R. L., 1969, Effects of dibutyryl cyclic AMP on adrenal growth and steroidogenic capacity, *Endocrinology* **84**:168–170.

50. Masui, H., and Garren, L. D., 1970, On the mechanism of action of adrenocorticotropic hormone: Stimulation of deoxyribonucleic acid polymerase and thymidine kinase in adrenal glands, *J. Biol. Chem.* **245**:2627–2632.

51. Richman, R., Dobbins, C., Voina, S., Underwood, L., Mahaffee, D., Gitel-

man, H. J., Van Wyk, J., and Ney, R. L., 1973, Regulation of adrenal ornithine decarboxylase by adrenocorticotropic hormone and cyclic AMP, *J. Clin. Invest.* **52:**2007–2015.

52. Anderson, W. B., Russell, T. R., Corchman, R. A., and Pastan, I., 1973, Interrelationship between adenylate cyclase activity, adenosine 3',5'-cyclic monophosphate phosphodiesterase activity, adenosine 3',5'-cyclic monophosphate levels, and growth of cells in culture, *Proc. Nat. Acad. Sci. U.S.A.* **70:**3802–3805.

53. Masui, H., and Garren, L. D., 1971, Inhibition of replication in functional mouse adrenal tumor cells by adrenocorticotropic hormone mediated by adenosine 3',5'-cyclic monophosphate, *Proc. Nat. Acad. Sci. U.S.A.* **68:**3206–3210.

54. Mostafapour, M. K., and Tchen, T. T., 1973, Capacity for steroidogenesis of adrenals in hypophysectomized and adrenocorticotropic hormone–treated hypophysectomized rats, *J. Biol. Chem.* **248:**6674–6678.

55. Bongiovanni, A. M., Eberlein, W. R., Goldman, A. S., and New, M., 1967, Disorders of adrenal steroid biogenesis, *Recent Prog. Hormone Res.* **23:**375–449.

56. Gwinup, B., and Johnson, B., 1975, Clinical testing of the hypothalamic–pituitary–adrenocortical system in states of hypo- and hypercortisolism, *Metabolism* **24:**777–791.

57. Liotta, A., and Krieger, D. T., 1975, A sensitive bioassay for the determination of human plasma ACTH levels, *J. Clin. Endocrinol. Metab.* **40:**268–277.

58. Frohman, L. A., and Stachura, M. E., 1975, Neuropharmacological control of neuroendocrine function in man, *Metabolism* **24:**211–234.

59. Plonk, J., and Feldman, J. M., 1975, Adrenal function in the carcinoid syndrome: Effects of the serotonin antagonist and cyproheptadine, *Metabolism* **24:**1035–1046.

60. Krieger, D. T., Amorosa, L., and Linick, F., 1975, Cyproheptadine-induced remission of Cushing's disease, *N. Engl. J. Med.* **293:**893–896.

61. Lagerquist, L. G., Meikle, A. W., West, C. D., and Tyler, F. H., 1974, Cushing's disease with cure by resection of a pituitary adenoma, *Amer. J. Med.* **57:**826–830.

62. Gewirtz, G., and Yalow, R. S., 1974, Ectopic ACTH production in carcinoma of the lung, *J. Clin. Invest.* **53:**1022–1032.

63. Orth, D. N., Nicholson, W. E., Mitchell, W. M., Island, D. P., and Liddle, G. W., 1973, Biological and immunological characterization and physical separation of ACTH and ACTH fragments in the ectopic ACTH syndrome, *J. Clin. Invest.* **52:**1756–1769.

64. Hirata, Y., Yamamoto, H., Matsukura, S., and Imura, H., 1975, *In vitro* release and biosynthesis of tumor ACTH in ectopic ACTH producing tumors, *J. Clin. Endocrinol. Metab.* **41:**106–114.

65. Blau, N., Miller, W. E., Miller, E. R., Jr., and Cervi-Skinner, S. J., 1975, Spontaneous remission of Cushing's syndrome in a patient with an adrenal adenoma, *J. Clin. Endocrinol. Metab.* **40:**659–663.

66. Green, J. R. B., and Van't Hoff, W., 1975, Cushing's syndrome with fluctuation due to adrenal adenoma, *J. Clin. Endocrinol. Metab.* **41:**235–240.

67. Leichter, S. B., and Daughaday, W. H., 1974, Massive steroid excretion and hypocholesterolemia with an adrenal adenoma, *Ann. Intern. Med.* **81:**638–640.

68. Schorr, I., Rathnam, P., Saxena, B. B., and Ney, R. L., 1971, Multiple specific hormone receptors in the adenylate cyclase of an adrenocortical carcinoma, *J. Biol. Chem.* **246:**5806–5811.
69. Saez, J. M., Dazord, A., and Gallet, D., 1975, ACTH and prostaglandin receptors in human adrenocortical tumors: Apparent modification of a specific component of the ACTH-binding site, *J. Clin. Invest.* **56:**536–547.
70. Becker, D., and Schumacher, O. P., 1975, *o,p'*-DDD Therapy in invasive adrenocortical carcinoma, *Ann. Intern. Med.* **82:**677–679.

Aldosterone and the Renin–Angiotensin System

Edward G. Biglieri

7.1. Introduction

The renin–angiotensin system is recognized as the major regulator of aldosterone production in determining both the level of basal aldosterone secretion and the changes in secretion observed following intravascular volume changes effected by alterations in sodium intake and posture.[1-6] The roles of adrenocorticotropin,[7-9] potassium concentration,[10,11] and possibly sodium concentration, are of varying importance in the presence of an active renin–angiotensin system, but assume greater significance as modulators of aldosterone production in the absence of the renin–angiotensin system.

The relationships between the state of activation of the renin–angi-

EDWARD G. BIGLIERI • Endocrinology Division of the Medical Service and the Clinical Study Center, San Francisco General Hospital; and the Department of Medicine, University of California, San Francisco, California.

otensin system and the secretion of aldosterone and other mineralocorticoid hormones are examined herein mainly according to the plasma aldosterone concentration (PAC). The quantitative measurement of PAC by both double-isotope dilution derivative[12] and radioimmunoassay techniques[13,14] is providing new insight into circadian patterns of both aldosterone and renin activity and into the interrelationships of other regulators. The more subtle and sophisticated interrelationships between aldosterone and the renin–angiotensin system have been better probed and characterized with the advent of both this measurement and other new techniques. Consequently, we are now more aware of the complexities of the renin–angiotensin–aldosterone system in its critical role in maintaining electrolyte and volume homeostasis.

7.2. Increased Aldosterone Production

7.2.1. Renin Suppressed

7.2.1.1. Syndrome of Primary Hyperaldosteronism

The syndrome of primary hyperaldosteronism (Conn's syndrome) is an established disorder resulting from excessive secretion of aldosterone. Thus, in the presence of normal cortisol levels, increased aldosterone production leads to the signs and symptoms of mineralocorticoid hormone excess: hypertension, potassium wasting (hypokalemia), and almost totally suppressed plasma renin activity (PRA).[15] The adrenal pathological lesions that result in these findings are now clearly related to four types of hyperaldosteronism.[15] The identification of the exact pathological lesion has an important bearing on the precise form of treatment recommended.

To establish a biochemical basis for distinction between an adenoma and hyperplasia, various maneuvers have been employed. Lack of suppression of aldosterone production or PAC by challenging the expanded extracellular fluid volume with large doses of deoxycorticosterone acetate[16] or intravenous saline[17] is considered useful in identifying a nonsuppressible presumably unilateral adenoma. Although these maneuvers are informative, examination of the circadian rhythm of PAC now provides a more discriminating means of identifying the adrenal lesion.

7.2.1.1a. Adrenocortical Aldosterone-Producing Adenoma. A unilateral adrenal adenoma accounts for approximately 75% of patients with the syndrome of primary hyperaldosteronism. The unique characteristic of an adenoma is that in patients with this lesion, there occurs an anomalous fall of PAC with upright posture.[14,18] Studying the circadian rhythm of PAC in continuously recumbent normal subjects as well as in patients with an aldosterone-producing adenoma eliminates the effect of upright posture in activating the renin–angiotensin system, thus providing a baseline for subsequent comparison. Over a 24-hr period of recumbency, PAC correlates well with the characteristic circadian pattern of cortisol,[19,20] with peak levels occurring during the early morning hours in both groups and correlates with PRA in normal subjects.[8] Thus, PAC is of no discriminating value in these patients when studied in the recumbent position.

In normal subjects, however, assumption of upright posture for 4 hr after overnight recumbency causes an endogenous stimulus that increases PRA and angiotensin II and effects a 2- to 4-fold increase in PAC. In patients with an aldosterone-producing adenoma, who have virtually no PRA, upright posture fails to activate the renin–angiotensin system sufficiently, and PAC shows a paradoxical fall or blunted increase in most patients.[14,18]

Intrinsic factors in the adenoma define the level of increased aldosterone production, but the modulator of the plasma aldosterone level is adrenocorticotropin. This conclusion is based on the significant correlation of PAC with the plasma cortisol level, regardless of postural changes. In patients with such an adenoma, PAC is greater than 20 ng/dl at 08:00 hours after overnight recumbency (6–8 hr) while on a 7–8 g/24 hr sodium chloride diet. After 4 hr in the upright posture (at 12:00 hours), PAC usually decreases; in the normal subject studied under the same conditions, it increases. Further evidence that adrenocorticotropin is the modulator of the circadian pattern in patients with an aldosterone-producing adenoma is the transient suppression of this pattern by suppressive doses of dexamethasone given for 6–24 hr.[18–20] The continued treatment with dexamethasone reveals that mineralocorticoid escape occurs, and that elevated levels resume in a chaotic pattern similar to the patterns observed in patients with an adrenal carcinoma associated with hyperaldosteronism. Thus, the inherently chaotic pattern of secretion of the adenoma is unmasked by removing adrenocorticotropin.

The combination of precise biochemical identification and techniques for lateralizing the lesion, plus normalization of blood pressure after surgical removal, make unilateral adrenalectomy the treatment of choice. Amelioration or complete normalization of high blood pressure and hypokalemia can be achieved with spironolactone therapy (200–600 mg/day for 4–6 weeks); this is an effective preoperative preparation. Prolonged treatment with spironolactone is used only for inoperable patients, or possibly when the dosage required is small (50–100 mg/24 hr).[21] Infrequently, spironolactone may inhibit aldosterone synthesis directly by retarding 11-β-hydroxylation or later steps in aldosterone synthesis.[22] Instead of the increases in aldosterone production and PRA that usually accompany spironolactone treatment, a patient with an aldosterone-producing adenoma was reported[22] in whom this drug reduced the increased aldosterone production to normal levels, with subsequent normalization of serum potassium concentration and PRA. In this patient, a more general effect on adrenal steroid production was suggested by the limited increase in cortisol production after exogenous administration of adrenocorticotropin.

Spironolactone can be used as preoperative treatment to prevent postoperative hypoaldosteronism. In most patients from whom an adenoma is removed, transient hypoaldosteronism occurs, but it is brief, and temporary treatment with 9α-fludrocortisone is rarely required. Complete recovery of the renin–angiotensin–aldosterone system invariably occurs, however. Although pretreatment with spironolactone can prevent the period of postoperative hypoaldosteronism, and can normalize blood pressure and potassium concentration, the effect of spironolactone on the suppressed renin–angiotensin system and on the uninvolved zona glomerulosa is not clear. Over long periods (6–72 months), spironolactone increases PRA and further elevates an already increased aldosterone production (adenomatous in origin). However, the increases in PRA are only into the normal range, and may not be high enough to stimulate uninvolved zona glomerulosa that has been suppressed for long periods. Thus, the low normal levels of aldosterone observed after adenoma removal in patients pretreated with spironolactone may still be related more to inadequate renin response than to the inhibition of the late synthesis of aldosterone by spironolactone,[23] as suggested in the case just described.[22]

7.2.1.1b. Adrenocortical Hyperplasia

Idiopathic Hyperaldosteronism (Pseudo-Primary Aldosteronism). This type of adrenocortical hyperplasia is the cause of the syndrome of primary hyperaldosteronism in approximately 15% of patients. The diagnosis is usually suspected when hypertension is more severe, potassium depletion is less severe, PRA is suppressed but not obliterated, and elevated urinary excretion of aldosterone is not so great as in patients with an adenoma. However, there is considerable overlap of these values in hyperplasia and adenoma. Various statistical techniques have been applied to an analysis of the deviation of these factors from normal in order to predict the pathological lesion.[24-26] Although such methods are effective, direct biochemical measurements of PAC are diagnostically more accurate and can be reinforced by suppressive maneuvers that corroborate the diagnosis. PAC after overnight recumbency is usually elevated (9–19 ng/dl; normal is 4–14) during sodium intake of 7–8 g/24 hr.[14] The conditions for measuring PAC are critical, because multiple factors in a dynamic system influence this single measurement. After overnight recumbency, PAC is increased 2- to 4-fold in patients with idiopathic hyperaldosteronism[14,26] who assume the upright posture. Administration of deoxycorticosterone acetate, 20 mg i.m./day for 3 days, does not suppress aldosterone levels (confirming autonomous production) in patients with either an aldosterone-producing adenoma or idiopathic hyperaldosteronism.

Whether or not hyperplasia represents a primary adrenal disorder is uncertain. An insight into the factors that may cause this type of hyperplasia was provided by the demonstration that peripheral plasma from such a patient, when injected into the arterial blood supply of an adrenal gland autotransplanted into the neck of a sheep, evoked an increase in adrenal venous aldosterone production, whereas plasma from a patient with adenoma showed no increase.[27] This finding provides gross but suggestive evidence that adrenal stimulators are present. Subtotal or total adrenalectomy results in inconsistent, unpredictable, and infrequent improvement of the hypertension in patients with idiopathic hyperaldosteronism.[28] Hence, this form of therapy is not recommended for these patients.[15,27] Spironolactone corrects potassium depletion, but additional antihypertensive agents are required to reduce blood pressure.

Indeterminate Hyperaldosteronism. In contrast to the two foregoing types, this variant of hyperaldosteronism is characterized by suppressibility of increased aldosterone production by deoxycorticosterone acetate.[15] The clinical features are milder than those in patients with idiopathic hyperaldosteronism or an aldosterone-producing adenoma, and the biochemical findings are borderline. Aldosterone production is increased, but less than in the idiopathic and adenoma types. PRA is suppressed but measurable, and increases after 4 h in upright posture. Overlap of all laboratory values between indeterminate and idiopathic adrenocortical hyperplasia and adenoma is great. The distinguishing features of this type of hyperplasia and adenoma is great. The distinguishing features of this type of hyperplasia are: (1) normal to borderline elevated PAC that increases with upright posture, (2) slightly elevated aldosterone production that is suppressed by deoxycorticosterone acetate, and (3) hypertension and hypokalemia that can be normalized by spironolactone. This third response is also characteristic of patients with an adenoma; thus, patients with indeterminate hyperaldosteronism may be a pivotal group in a possible continuum of primary hyperaldosteronism between the normal or low-renin state and the patients with established adenoma. These patients may eventually develop either idiopathic hyperaldosteronism or an adrenocortical adenoma. Because of the questionable benefit from surgery, mildness of hypertension, and excellent control of blood pressure with spironolactone, adrenalectomy is a dubious treatment at best. Patients in this group are similar in many ways to low-renin hypertensive patients, except for the increased aldosterone production and its metabolic consequences.

Glucocorticoid-Remediable Hyperaldosteronism. Although glucocorticoid-remediable hyperaldosteronism is a very rare form of hyperaldosteronism, it is an established and recognizable entity. Subsequent reported cases differ little from the original patient[29]: they have the clinical and biochemical findings of the other hyperplastic disorders associated with the syndrome of primary hyperaldosteronism, but the hyperaldosteronism, hypertension, and hypokalemia can be normalized by administration or replacement doses of glucocorticoid hormones. The ability of the glucocorticoid hormones to correct the hyperaldosteronism and its metabolic consequences suggests the existence of a glucocorticoid-sensitive aldosterone-stimulatory factor.

7.2.1.2. Location of Adrenocortical Adenoma with [131I]19-Iodocholesterol

Biochemical identification of the pathological lesion causing hyperaldosteronism can be corroborated by the use of [131I]19-iodocholesterol adrenal imaging. This noninvasive technique holds great promise for identifying precisely the type of adrenal pathological lesion and determining its localization in the case of adenoma. [131I]19-Iodocholesterol is taken up and esterified by the adrenal gland. Adequate blockade of thyroid uptake of iodine is a necessary condition for this procedure: saturated solution of potassium iodide should be administered before and for 3 weeks after administration of the isotope.[30] Care must be exercised not to misinterpret uptake by the gallbladder and colon as uptake by the adrenal gland, and repeated imaging may be necessary to allow disappearance of such activity. The usefulness and effectiveness of this technique are already apparent in patients who were proved to have this lesion. In two large series of patients, the presence of an adenoma was demonstrated in 83%[30] and 77%.[31] Determination of the type of pathological lesion may be possible by preliminary and continued administration of dexamethasone (0.5–1 mg every 6 hr): asymmetrical adrenal uptake within 5 days suggests a unilateral adrenal adenoma; earlier bilateral adrenal uptake, nodular hyperplasia; and no uptake, microscope hyperplasia[31] or adrenal carcinoma.[30] Adenomas from 0.9 to 2.0 cm in diameter can be identified.

7.2.2. Renin Increased

7.2.2.1. Malignant or Accelerated Hypertension

In patients with accelerated hypertension, often regardless of cause, peripheral levels of PRA and angiotensin II are elevated and are associated with increased aldosterone production. The trigger for the activation of the renin–angiotension–aldosterone system is not always clear. Intense intrarenal arteriolar spasm or degeneration, as well as sodium depletion, could in part or in concert effect the activation of the renin system.[6]

It is of great interest that when effective antihypertensive therapy is carried out, the increased activity of the renin–angiotensin system is normalized. However, aldosterone levels frequently remain elevated; nevertheless, the presence of an aldosterone-producing adenoma is very unusual.[32] The possibility that the continued endogenous elevation of angiotensin II may exert a tropic action on the zona glomerulosa to alter its responses to other stimuli is intriguing.[33] The continued examination of the importance of angiotensin II in these disorders will be enhanced by the use of the nonapeptide-converting enzyme inhibitor (SQ20881) (angiotensin I to angiotensin II). Several reports indicate a dramatic and prompt reduction of these severe hypertensive states with the intravenous administration of 1–4 mg/kg.[34–36]

7.2.2.2. Unilateral Renovascular Disease

Increases in both renin and aldosterone should occur early in the genesis of the hypertension that results from unilateral renal arterial narrowing. However, detection is infrequent. During the more chronic state of hypertension, the renin and aldosterone production are within the normal range, possibly due to volume expansion. The only clinically useful abnormality is the difference in renal venous plasma renin concentration (PRC) of the two kidneys. A PRC ratio in the affected/noninvolved kidney greater than 1.5 and a ratio approaching 1 between the noninvolved kidney and the inferior vena cava provide excellent prognostic information for surgical improvement or cure of the renal lesion.[37] No provocative maneuvers, such as sodium depletion or administration of diuretics or hydralazine, are necessary.

The cause of sustained hypertension in an originally renin-mediated hypertensive state is still conjectural to a great degree. In rats with a single kidney, and in which the remaining renal artery has been constricted to produce hypertension ("one-kidney" model), angiotensin II increases early, but then diminishes as hypertension persists, suggesting that changes occur that increase vascular sensitivity to circulating angiotensin II. Support for increased sodium and volume expansion as a partial explanation of this phenomenon was obtained in two models[38,39] in rats, using either angiotensin II antagonists[40] or inhibitors of converting enzyme,[34,41] which is responsible for the conversion of angiotensin I to angiotensin II in the lungs and vascular beds. When blood pressure was sustained mainly by the sodium-volume component (in the one-kidney hypertensive rat model), the angiotensin II antagonists (Saralasin® 1-sar-8-ala angiotensin II) had little effect. When sodium-volume increases were prevented or corrected, blood pressure decreased in response to the angiotensin II antagonists. In the presence of sodium retention and volume increases, a lesser level of angiotensin II was required to sustain the increased blood pressure. In contrast, in the experimental "two-kidney" rat model (one renal artery constricted, contralateral renal artery not constricted) with hypertension and high plasma renin and angiotensin II, the angiotensin II antagonist was effective in reducing the elevated blood pressure. Although they are still in a developmental stage, such powerful tools may provide crucial information on the dependence of certain hypertensive states on the renin–angiotensin system.

7.2.2.3. Renin-Secreting Tumors

The rare concurrence of a high PAC and high PRA in the absence of a renovascular lesion is *per se* almost pathognomonic of a renin-secreting tumor. Such tumors dramatically identify angiotensin II as a potent vasopressive peptide that can produce hypertension even in the absence of excessive production of aldosterone; in the case reported,[42] aldosterone production was low and fixed as a result of subtotal adrenalectomy. A case of a Wilms' tumor producing excess renin has also been observed. In the circulating plasma, an "inactive" larger molecule of renin–prorenin was extracted and was activated to renin by acidification.[43] The role of pro-renin and other renin zymogens[44] is still speculative, but they may be potential markers of clinical disorders.

7.2.2.4. "Bartter's Syndrome"

The syndrome originally reported by Bartter included hypokalemia, metabolic alkalosis, and urinary potassium wasting with hypertrophy of the juxtaglomerular complex.[45] However, there are many variants of this syndrome. Nonhypertensive hyperaldosteronism with hyperreninemia and pressor insensitivity to angiotensin II and reduced potassium levels can be ascribed to a multitude of causes, from the iatrogenic disorders of laxative and diuretic abuse to the disturbed behavioral patterns of patients with anorexia nervosa and surreptitious vomiting. In the patient who wastes potassium, both normal sodium[46] and diminished sodium conservation have been documented.[47,48] Although a renal defect in potassium transport is strongly suspected in these patients, it has not been documented. Impaired sodium reabsorption in the proximal nephron might result in secondary hyperaldosteronism and augmented sodium–potassium exchange in the distal nephron without limiting the level of renal sodium conservation.[47] A defect in chloride transport has been suggested as the primary abnormality,[49] the suggestion being based on the recent observations that active chloride transport occurs in the ascending limb of the loop of Henle, with sodium and potassium passively following. Thus, the chloride defect could result in potassium wasting augmented by, but not dependent on, secondary hyperaldosteronism. A primary renal tubular defect in potassium transport is supported by the complexity and difficulty of the treatment required to retard renal potassium loss: spironolactone, aminoglutethemide, sodium restriction, propranolol,[46,50] and potassium supplementation are often required to effect acceptable serum potassium concentrations. Even adrenalectomy has failed to correct the potassium wasting.[51]

Another unique feature of this syndrome is the lack of a pressor response to angiotensin II infusion. The controversy continues as to whether or not rapid volume expansion of the extracellular fluid volume with either saline or albumin[48] corrects this insensitivity. Other alternatives proposed consist of either changes in intracellular ion concentration, or the conversion of angiotensin II to angiotensin III (heptapeptide), which can produce a specific aldosterone-stimulating effect without vascular pressor effects, or both.

An intriguing preliminary report documents sustained correction of Bartter's syndrome by treatment with 150 mg p.o./24 hr indomethacin (an inhibitor of prostaglandin synthesis).[52]

7.3. Normal Aldosterone Production—Low-Renin Hypertension

The 20–30% of hypertensive patients with low PRA but normal aldosterone production constitute a heterogeneous group with regard to mechanism of renin suppression; this heterogeneity stems, in part, from inconsistency in the definition and in the conditions under which PRA is measured. The consistency of a low-renin state and its periodicity must be questioned. In such patients, circadian rhythms of plasma aldosterone and PRA in the recumbent position can show a normal midnight to early morning rise.[53] Hence, the failure of the stimuli of posture and sodium depletion to increase plasma renin in low-renin hypertensive patients does not necessarily imply that the nocturnal increase is abolished.[54] Retesting of many patients classified as having low-renin hypertension shows that 22–33% of the patients have a normal renin profile.[55] One must question the use of stimulating maneuvers, such as posture, sodium depletion, and diuretics, as effective ways to standardize a very dynamic system. Much of the response to a pharmacological agent is dependent on the state of sodium balance. Even the suppressed PRA in patients with primary aldosteronism caused by an adenoma may show an increase if the stimulus is great enough. It is surprising to observe, however, that 20–30% of hypertensive patients with normal aldosterone levels, when tested with a variety of testing techniques, repeatedly have subnormal PRA.[56]

This identifiable group of hypertensive patients poses a number of provocative questions: (1) Does this hormonal profile indicate that the patient has a reduced risk of having the complications of hypertension? (2) Why is aldosterone production maintained at a normal level in the presence of suppressed renin activity? (3) Could this circumstance be a stage of the syndrome of primary hyperaldosteronism? Clear answers to these questions are not currently available.

With all other cardiovascular–renal risk factors being constant (which is difficult to imagine because they can change independently and continuously), the original idea of reduced risk[57] of stroke or heart attack in patients with low-renin hypertension has been challenged repeatedly on many grounds, and remains at best controversial.[58,59] Prolonged prospective studies are required to resolve the proposal convincingly.

Whether or not all hypertensive patients require an assessment of PRA is moot. The measurement peripheral PRA is of *proved value* in establishing the diagnosis of hyporeninemic hypoaldosteronism and renin-secreting tumors and in corroborating the diagnosis of an aldosterone-producing tumor. Bilateral renal vein renin levels locate renin-secreting tumors and identify and confirm unilateral renal disease. Peripheral renin measurements *may be helpful* in various forms of hypertension, such as the intractable hypertension of chronic renal failure, accelerated hypertension, secondary hyperaldosteronism, and in identification of other mineralocorticoid hormones in hypokalemic hypertensives with reduced aldosterone production.

The enigma of normal aldosterone production in the presence of suppressed PRA in the patient with low-renin hypertension continues. Attention was first focused on the suppressed renin activity because of earlier observations of an increase in extracellular fluid volume[56] and exchangeable sodium[60] in such patients, together with a decrease in blood pressure after treatment with spironolactone[61] or aminoglutethemide.[60] These observations suggested that a mineralocorticoid hormone could be the effector of the suppressed renin formation. However, the increases in extracellular fluid volume[62] and exchangeable sodium,[63] and the specificity of the blood pressure–lowering response to spironolactone,[64] have not been observed in other patients and remain controversial. In addition, mineralocorticoid activity in human plasma can be assessed *in vitro* by using an aldosterone receptor from rat kidney slices[65]; no apparent increase in steroids that interact with this receptor was observed in plasma from low-renin hypertensive patients.[65]

In the search for unusual mineralocorticoid hormones, 18-hydroxy-deoxycorticosterone has been found in both hypertensive rat and man[66] and has been shown to possess weak mineralocorticoid properties. 16β-hydroxydihydroepiandrosterone has also been identified in the urine of some patients with low-renin hypertension.[67] The mineralocorticoid potency of both these steroids is limited, and their singular role in patients with low-renin hypertension is uncertain. Secretion and excretion of deoxycorticosterone are within normal limits in these patients. The slight elevations of plasma deoxycorticosterone concentration observed in 6 of 21 low-renin patients in the presence of normal values for other steroids[68] bear no similarity to the high levels (greater than 200 ng/dl) found in patients with the syndromes of deoxycorticosterone excess (11- and 17-hydroxylation deficiency syndromes) with increased blood pressure, reduced serum potassium levels, and suppressed renin activity. In patients with the endogenous deoxycorticosterone excess, and in normal subjects during administration of deoxycorticosterone acetate, PRA and aldosterone secretion are both suppressed. Sufficient secretion of a cryptic mineralocorticoid hormone to suppress renin should also reduce aldosterone levels, not merely maintain aldosterone at normal levels.[69]

It is just as likely either that another adrenal stimulator exists or that the adrenal gland is responding in a unique manner to established regulatory factors, such as adrenocorticotropin and potassium. The normal aldosterone levels with suppressed renin activity could also be the result of other, less well defined mineralocorticoid hormones, or the consequence of a more fundamental renal defect in patients with primary hypertension.

Whether or not the low-renin hypertensive patients represent part of the continuum of primary aldosteronism is not established. Adrenal abnormalities consisting primarily of adrenocortical hyperplasia have been reported. Whether these pathological findings are a cause or an effect is not known.

7.4. Reduced Aldosterone Production

7.4.1. Renin Suppressed

7.4.1.1. Hyporeninemic Hypoaldosteronism

The most common form of diminished aldosterone production is that associated with reduced renin activity. The recognition of hypoaldosteronism is based on the demonstration of hyperkalemia.[70] One must, of course, rule out other primary adrenal causes of reduced or absent aldosterone production, e.g., primary adrenal disease, such as Addison's disease, and disorders of the late synthesis of aldosterone (18-hydroxyla-tion or 18-dehydrogenation), in which renal sodium wasting results in volume depletion and thus increased PRA. Other causes of hyperkalemia must be considered, such as severe acidosis and the action of drugs such as spironolactone, triamterene, amiloride, and heparin.

Although some evidence of renal disease is frequently present, it is not sufficient to explain the hyperkalemia[71,72]; in fact, some degree of renal disease may be a necessary component of the occurrence of the clinical manifestations of the aldosterone deficiency. Patients with hypo-reninemic hypoaldosteronism frequently have such disorders as pyelone-phritis, gout, nephrolithiasis, previous hyperparathyroidism, postopera-tive hypoaldosteronism after removal of an aldosterone-producing adenoma, or diabetes. Diabetes may, in time, be the disorder most fre-quently associated with this syndrome. The segmental hyalinization of juxtaglomerular cells commonly observed in patients with diabetes may be responsible for the decreased renin secretion.

Hyporeninemic hypoaldosteronism, often called *selective hypoaldoster-onism*,[70] is most likely due to a defect in the stimulation or the release of renin, or to both.[71] The bulk of evidence suggests that renin deficiency is most likely due to destructive lesions in the juxtaglomerular cells. In patients with these lesions, production of the remaining glucocorticoid and mineralocorticoid hormones (zona fasciculata steroids) is normal. The responses of cortisol, deoxycorticosterone, and corticosterone to intrave-nous administration of adrenocorticotropin are normal.[71] This explains, in part, the lack of sodium wasting and the frequent improvement of hypokalemia during aggressive stimulation with adrenocorticotropin. Excretion of the metabolite of 18-hydroxycorticosterone is normal, thus excluding the possibility of an enzymatic defect in late aldosterone synthesis.

The maneuvers that elicit activation of the renin system, such as sodium restriction, upright posture, and intravenous administration of furosemide, fail to produce normal stimulation of the low renin level.[71] Direct stimulation with angiotensin II has not uniformly stimulated adre-nal production of aldosterone,[73] in part because of the limited amounts that can be administered and because of the chronic lack of the tonic stimulation of the renin–angiotensin system. The hypoaldosterone state, even in the presence of hyperkalemia, indicates that in the presence of a deficient or suppressed renin–angiotensin system, hyperkalemia *per se* is not a sufficient stimulus to maintain normal secretion of aldosterone.

The management of patients with this disorder is variable and must be tailored to the individual patient. The etiology and degree of renal insufficiency often dictate the treatment modalities. Often, mineralocorti-coid replacement at physiological levels alone does not correct the hyperkalemia, particularly in patients with chronic renal insufficiency. In such cases, tubular insensitivity to mineralocorticoid hormones must also be considered as a possible cause. Potassium restriction, correction of alkalosis, mineralocorticoid hormone replacement, and furosemide all are part of the potential therapeutic armamentarium. With such multiple etiologies, the clinical manifestations of this disorder can be quite variable. The moderate to severe protein restriction practiced by patients with renal failure can prevent the hyperkalemia expected in the syndrome because of the concomitant limitation of potassium intake. An interesting report of a patient with deficiencies of both aldosterone and insulin further demonstrates the complexity of this disorder[74]; intravenous administration of glucose produced hyperkalemia because the insufficient aldosterone and insulin levels did not reverse the transfer of potassium to the extracellular fluid. Though treatment with deoxycorticosterone acetate improved and blunted the effect of the glucose, the expected hypokalemic effect of the intravenous glucose occurred only after insulin was administered.

ACKNOWLEDGMENTS

This work was supported in part by U.S. Public Health Service Research Grants HE-11046 from the National Heart Institute and AM-06415 from the National Institute of Arthritis and Metabolic Diseases. The studies were carried out in the General Clinical Research Center (RR-00083) at San Francisco General Hospital, with support by the Division of Research Resources, National Institutes of Health.

References

1. Oparil, S., and Haber, E., 1974, The renin–angiotensin system, *N. Engl. J. Med.* **291**:389–401, 446–457.
2. Davis, J. O., 1973, The control of renin release, *Amer. J. Med.* **55**:333–350.
3. Liddle, G. W., Duncan, L. E., Jr., and Bartter, F. C., 1956, Dual mechanism regulating adrenocortical function in man, *Amer. J. Med.* **21**:414–430.
4. Ganong, W. F., Biglieri, E. G., and Mulrow, P. J., 1966, Mechanisms regulating adrenocortical secretion of aldosterone and glucocorticoids, *Recent Prog. Horm. Res.* **22**:381–414.
5. Hollenberg, N. K., Chenitz, W. R., Adams, D. F., and Williams, G. H., 1974, Reciprocal influence of salt intake on adrenal glomerulosa and renal vascular responses to angiotensin II in normal man, *J. Clin. Invest.* **54**:34–42.
6. Beevers, D. G., Brown, J. J., Fraser, R., Lever, A. F., Morton, J. J., Robertson, J. I. S., Semple, P. F., and Tree, M., 1975, The clinical value of renin and angiotensin estimations, *Kidney Int.* **8**:S181–S201.

7. Michelakis, A. M., and Horton, R., 1970, The relationship between plasma renin and aldosterone in normal man, *Circ. Res. Suppl.* **26–27:**I185–I194.
8. Katz, F. H., Romfh, P., and Smith, J. A., 1975, Diurnal variation of plasma aldosterone, cortisol and renin activity in supine man, *J. Clin. Endocrinol. Metab.* **40:**125–134.
9. Williams, G. H., Rose, L. I., Dluhy, R. G., Dingman, J. F., and Lauler, D. P., 1971, Aldosterone response to sodium restriction and ACTH stimulation in panhypopituitarism, *J. Clin. Endocrinol. Metab.* **32:**27–35.
10. Himathongkam, T., Dluhy, R. G., and Williams, G. H., 1975, Potassium–aldosterone–renin interrelationships, *J. Clin. Endocrinol. Metab.* **41:**153–159.
11. Dluhy, R. G., Axelrod, L., Underwood, R. H., and Williams, G. H., 1972, Studies of the control of plasma aldosterone concentration in normal man. II. Effect of dietary potassium and acute potassium infusion, *J. Clin. Invest.* **51:**1950–1957.
12. Brodie, A. H., Shimizu, N., Tait, S. A. S., and Tait, J. F., 1967, A method for the measurement of aldosterone in peripheral plasma using ^{3}H-acetic anhydride, *J. Clin. Endocrinol. Metab.* **27:**997–1011.
13. Bayard, F., Beitins, I. Z., Kowarski, A., and Migeon, C. J., 1970, Measurement of plasma aldosterone by radioimmunoassay, *J. Clin. Endocrinol. Metab.* **31:**1–6.
14. Biglieri, E. G., Schambelan, M., Brust, N., Chang, B., and Hogan, M., 1974, Plasma aldosterone concentration. Further characterization of aldosterone-producing adenomas, *Circ. Res. Suppl. I* **34–35:**I183–I191.
15. Biglieri, E. G., Stockigt, J. R., and Schambelan, M., 1972, Adrenal mineralocorticoids causing hypertension, *Amer. J. Med.* **52:**623–632.
16. Slaton, P. E., Jr., Schambelan, M., and Biglieri, E. G., 1969, Stimulation and suppression of aldosterone secretion in patients with an aldosterone-producing adenoma, *J. Clin. Endocrinol. Metab.* **29:**239–250.
17. Cain, J. P., Tuck, M. L., Williams, G. H., Dluhy, R. G., and Rosenoff, S. H., 1972, The regulation of aldosterone secretion in primary aldosteronism, *Amer. J. Med.* **53:**627–637.
18. Ganguly, A., Melada, G. A., Luetscher, J. A., and Dowdy, A. J., 1973, Control of plasma aldosterone in primary aldosteronism: Distinction between adenoma and hyperplasia, *J. Clin. Endocrinol. Metab.* **37:**765–775.
19. Kem, D. C., Weinberger, M. H., Gomez-Sanchez, C., Kramer, N. J., Lerman, R., Furuyama, S., and Nugent, C. A., 1973, Circadian rhythm of plasma aldosterone concentration in patients with primary aldosteronism, *J. Clin. Invest.* **52:**2272–2277.
20. Vetter, H., Berger, M., Armbruster, H., Siegenthaler, W., Werning, C., and Vetter, W., 1974, Episodic secretion of aldosterone in primary aldosteronism: Relationship to cortisol, *Clin. Endocrinol. Oxford* **3:**41–48.
21. Biglieri, E. G., and Schambelan, M., 1973, Management of primary hyperaldosteronism, *in: Hypertension: Mechanisms and Management* (G. Onesti, K. E. Kim, and J. H. Moyer, eds.) pp. 493–498. Grune and Stratton, New York.
22. Sundsfjord, J. A., Marton, P., Jørgensen, H., and Aakvaag, A., 1974, Reduced aldosterone secretion during spironolactone treatment in primary aldosteronism: Report of a case, *J. Clin. Endocrinol. Metab.* **39:**734–739.
23. Bravo, E. L., Dustan, H. P., and Tarazi, R. C., 1975, Selective hypoaldosteronism despite prolonged pre- and postoperative hyperreninemia in primary aldosteronism, *J. Clin. Endocrinol. Metab.* **41:**611–617.
24. Stockigt, J. R., Collins, R. D., and Biglieri, E. G., 1971, Determination of

plasma renin concentration by angiotensin I immunoassay. Diagnostic import of precise measurement of subnormal renin in hyperaldosteronism, *Circ. Res. Suppl. II* **28**:II175–II191.

25. Aitchison, J., Brown, J. J., Ferriss, J. B., Fraser, R., Kay, A. W., Lever, A. F., Neville, A. M., Symington, T., and Robertson, J. I. S., 1971, Quadric analysis in the preoperative distinction between patients with and without adrenocortical tumors in hypertension with aldosterone excess and low plasma renin, *Amer. Heart J.* **82**:660–671.

26. Luetscher, J. A., Ganguly, A., Melada, G. A., and Dowdy, A. J., 1974, Preoperative differentiation of adrenal adenoma from idiopathic adrenal hyperplasia in primary aldosteronism, *Cir. Res. Suppl. I* **34–35**:I175–I182.

27. Nicholls, M. G., Espiner, E. A., Hughes, H., Ross, J., and Stewart, D. T., 1975, Primary aldosteronism. A study in contrasts, *Amer. J. Med.* **59**:334–342.

28. Ferriss, J. B., Brown, J. J., Fraser, R., Haywood, E., Davies, D. L., Kay, A. W., Lever, A. F., Robertson, J. I. S., Owen, K., and Peart, W. S., 1975, Results of adrenal surgery in patients with hypertension, aldosterone excess, and low plasma renin concentration, *Br. Med. J.* **1**:135–138.

29. Salti, I. S., Stiefel, M., Ruse, J. L., and Laidlaw, J. C., 1969, Non-tumorous "primary" aldosteronism: I. Type relieved by glucocorticoid (glucocorticoid remediable aldosteronism), *Can. Med. Assoc. J.* **101**:1–10.

30. Hogan, M. J., McRae, J., Schambelan, M., and Biglieri, E. G., 1976, Location of aldosterone-producing adenomas with ^{131}I-19-iodocholesterol, *N. Engl. J. Med.* **294**:410–414.

31. Seabold, J. E., Cohen, E. L., Beierwaltes, W. H., Hinerman, D. L., Nishiyama, R. H., Bookstein, J. J., Ice, R. D., and Balachandran, S., 1976, Adrenal imaging with ^{131}I-19-iodocholesterol in the diagnostic evaluation of patients with aldosteronism, *J. Clin. Endocrinol. Metab.* **42**:41–51.

32. McAllister, R. G., Van Way, C. W., III, Dayani, K., Anderson, W. J., Temple, E., Michelakis, A. M., Coppage, W. S., and Oates, J. A., 1971, Malignant hypertension: Effect of therapy on renin and aldosterone, *Circ. Res. Suppl. II* **28–29**:II160–II173.

33. Oelkers, W., Schöeneshöfer, M., Schultze, G., Brown, J. J., Fraser, R., Morton, J. J., Lever, A. F., and Robertson, J. I. S., 1975, Effect of prolonged low-dose angiotensin II infusion on the sensitivity of adrenal cortex in man, *Circ. Res. Suppl. I* **36–37**:I49–I56.

34. Gavras, H., Brunner, H. R., Laragh, J. H., Sealey, J. E., Gavras, I., and Vukovich, R. A., 1974, An angiotensin converting–enzyme inhibitor to identify and treat vasoconstrictor and volume factors in hypertensive patients, *N. Engl. J. Med.* **291**:817–821.

35. Johnson, J. G., Black, W. D., Vukovich, R. A., Hatch, F. E., Jr., Friedman, B. I., Blackwell, C. F., Shenouda, A. N., Share, L., Shade, R. E., Acchiardo, S. R., and Muirhead, E. E., 1975, Treatment of patients with severe hypertension by inhibition of angiotensin-converting enzyme, *Clin. Sci. Mol. Med. Suppl. 2* **48**:53S–56S.

36. Gavras, H., Brunner, H. R., Laragh, J. H., Gavras, I., and Vukovich, R. A., 1975, The use of angiotensin-converting enzyme-inhibitor in the diagnosis and treatment of hypertension, *Clin. Sci. Mol. Med. Suppl. 2* **48**:57S–60S.

37. Stockigt, J. R., Collins, R. D., Noakes, C. A., Schambelan, M., and Biglieri, E. G., 1972, Renal-vein renin in various forms of renal hypertension, *Lancet* **1**:1194–1198.

38. Pals, D. T., Masucci, F. D., Denning, G. S., Jr., Sipos, F., and Fessler, D. C.,

1971, Role of the pressor action of angiotensin II in experimental hypertension, *Circ. Res.* **29:**673–681.

39. Brunner, H. R., Kirschman, J. D., Sealey, J. E., and Laragh, J. H., 1971, Hypertension of renal origin: Evidence for two different mechanisms, *Science* **174:**1344–1346.

40. Streeten, D. H. P., Anderson, G. H., Freiberg, J. M., and Dalakos, T. G., 1975, Use of an angiotensin II antagonist (Saralasin) in the recognition of "angiotensinogenic" hypertension, *N. Engl. J. Med.* **292:**657–662.

41. Davis, J. O., 1975, The use of blocking agents to define the functions of the renin–angiotensin system, *Clin. Sci. Mol. Med. Suppl. 2* **48:**3S–14S.

42. Schambelan, M., Howes, E. L., Jr., Stockigt, J. R., Noakes, C. A., and Biglieri, E. G., 1973, Role of renin and aldosterone in hypertension due to a renin-secreting tumor, *Amer. J. Med.* **55:**86–92.

43. Day, R. P., and Luetscher, J. A., 1974, Big renin: A possible prohormone in kidney and plasma of a patient with Wilms' tumor, *J. Clin. Endocrinol. Metab.* **38:**923–926.

44. Skinner, S. L., Cran, E. J., Gibson, R., Taylor, R., Walters, W. A. W., and Catt, K. J., 1975, Angiotensins I and II, active and inactive renin, renin substrate, renin activity, and angiotensinase in human liquor amnii and plasma, *Amer. J. Obstet. Gynecol.* **121:**626–630.

45. Bartter, F. C., Pronove, P., Gill, J. R., Jr., and MacCardle, R. C., 1962, Hyperplasia of the juxtaglomerular complex with hyperaldosteronism and hypokalemic alkalosis, *Amer. J. Med.* **33:**811–828.

46. Solomon, R. J., and Brown, R. S., 1975, Bartter's syndrome. New insights into pathogenesis and treatment, *Amer. J. Med.* **59:**575–583.

47. Cannon, P. J., Leeming, J. M., Sommer, S. C., Winters, R. W., and Laragh, J. H., 1968, Juxtaglomerular cell hyperplasia and secondary hyperaldosteronism (Bartter's syndrome): A reevaluation of the pathophysiology, *Medicine* **47:**107–131.

48. Goodman, A. D., Vagnucci, A. H., and Hartroft, P. M., 1969, Pathogenesis of Bartter's syndrome, *N. Engl. J. Med.* **281:**1435–1439.

49. Kurtzman, N. A., and Gutierrez, L. F., 1975, Hypothesis. The pathophysiology of Bartter syndrome, *J. Amer. Med. Assoc.* **234:**758–759.

50. Modlinger, R. S., Nicolis, G. L., Krakoff, L. R., and Gabrilove, J. L., 1973, Some observations on the pathogenesis of Bartter's syndrome, *N. Engl. J. Med.* **289:**1022–1024.

51. Trygstad, C. W., Mangos, J. A., Bloodworth, J. M. B., Jr., and Lobeck, C. C., 1969, A sibship with Bartter's syndrome: Failure of total adrenalectomy to correct the potassium wasting, *Pediatrics* **44:**234–242.

52. Verberckmoes, R., Clement, J., Michielsen, P., and van Damme, B., 1975, Bartter's syndrome with hyperplasia of renomedullary interstitial cells. Successful treatment with indomethacin, *Program, International Society of Nephrology*, Abstract No. 558 (June 1975).

53. Grim, C., Winnacker, J., Peters, T., and Gilbert, G., 1974, Low renin, "normal" aldosterone and hypertension: Circadian rhythm of renin, aldosterone, cortisol and growth hormone, *J. Clin. Endocrinol. Metab.* **39:**247–256.

54. Modlinger, R. S., and Gutkin, M., 1975, Normal plasma renin activity in low renin hypertension, *J. Clin. Endocrinol. Metab.* **40:**380–382.

55. Dunn, M. J., and Tannen, R. L., 1974, Editorial review: Low-renin hypertension, *Kidney Int.* **5:**317–323.

56. Jose, A., Crout, J. R., and Kaplan, N. H., 1970, Suppressed plasma renin activity in essential hypertension. Roles of plasma volume, blood pressure, and sympathetic nervous system, *Ann. Intern. Med.* **72:**9–16.

57. Brunner, H. R., Laragh, J. H., Baer, L., Newton, M. A., Goodwin, F. T., Krakoff, L. R., Bard, R. H., and Bühler, F. R., 1972, Essential hypertension: Renin and aldosterone, heart attack and stroke, *N. Engl. J. Med.* **286:**441–449.

58. Hickler, R. B., Lauler, D. P., Gleason, R. E., and Christlieb, R., 1975, Plasma-renin activity and cardiovascular disease, *Clin. Sci. Mol. Med. Suppl. 2* **48:**131S–133S.

59. Mroczek, W. J., Finnerty, F. A., and Catt, K. J., 1973, Lack of association between plasma-renin and history of heart-attack or stroke in patients with essential hypertension, *Lancet* **2:**464–468.

60. Woods, J. W., Liddle, G. W., Stant, E. G., Michelakis, A. M., and Brill, A. B., 1969, Effect of an adrenal inhibitor in hypertensive patients with suppressed renin, *Arch. Intern. Med.* **123:**366–370.

61. Crane, M. G., and Harris, J. J., 1970, The effect of spironolactone in hypertensive patients, *Amer. J. Med. Sci.* **260:**311–330.

62. Schalekamp, M. A., Lebel, M., Beevers, D. G., Fraser, R., Kolsters, G., and Birkenhäger, W. H., 1974, Body-fluid volume in low-renin hypertension, *Lancet* **2:**310–311.

63. Lebel, M., Schalekamp, M. A., Beevers, D. G., Brown, J. J., Davies, D. L., Fraser, R., Kremer, D., Lever, A. F., Morton, J. J., Robertson, J. I. S., Tree, M., and Wilson, A., 1974, Sodium and the renin–angiotensin system in essential hypertension and mineralocorticoid excess, *Lancet* **2:**308–310.

64. Vaughan, E. D., Laragh, J. H., Gavras, I., Bühler, F. R., Gavras, H., Brunner, H. R., and Baer, L., 1973, Volume factor in low and normal renin essential hypertension. Treatment with either spironolactone or chlorthalidone, *Amer. J. Cardiol.* **32:**523–532.

65. Baxter, J. D., Matulich, D. T., Spindler, B. J., Schambelan, M., Kawasaki, T. K., and Bartter, F. C., 1975, Aldosterone receptors and mineralocorticoid activity in hypertension, *Clin. Res.* **23:**386A.

66. Melby, J. C., Dale, S. L., Grekin, R. J., Gaunt, R., and Wilson, T. E., 1972, 18-Hydroxy-11-deoxycorticosterone (18-OH-DOC) secretion in experimental and human hypertension, *Recent Prog. Horm. Res.* **28:**287–351.

67. Sennett, J. A., Brown, R. D., Island, D. P., Yarbro, L. R., Watson, J. T., Slaton, P. E., Hollifield, J. W., and Liddle, G. W., 1975, Evidence for a new mineralocorticoid in patients with low-renin essential hypertension, *Circ. Res. Suppl. I* **36–37:**12–19.

68. Brown, J. J., Fraser, R., Love, D. R., Ferriss, J. B., Lever, A. F., Robertson, J. I. S., and Wilson, A., 1972, Apparently isolated excess deoxycorticosterone in hypertension, *Lancet* **2:**243–247.

69. Shade, R. E., and Grim, C. E., 1975, Suppression of renin and aldosterone by small amounts of DOCA in normal man, *J. Clin. Endocrinol. Metab.* **40:**652–658.

70. Michelis, M. F., and Murdaugh, H. V., 1975, Selective hypoaldosteronism. An editorial revisited after 15 years, *Amer. J. Med.* **59:**1–5.

71. Schambelan, M., Stockigt, J. R., and Biglieri, E. G., 1972, Isolated hypoaldosteronism in adults: A renin-deficiency syndrome, *N. Engl. J. Med.* **287:**573–578.

72. Weidmann, P., Reinhart, R., Maxwell, M. H., Rowe, P., Coburn, J. W., and Massry, S. G., 1973, Syndrome of hyporeninemic hypoaldosteronism and hyperkalemia in renal disease, *J. Clin. Endocrinol. Metab.* **36:**965–977.
73. Brown, J. J., Chinn, R. H., Fraser, R., Lever, A. F., Morton, J. J., Robertson, J. I. S., Tree, M., Waite, M. A., and Park, D. M., 1973, Recurrent hyperkalaemia due to selective aldosterone deficiency: Correction by angiotensin infusion, *Br. Med. J.* **1:**650–654.
74. Goldfarb, S., Strunk, B., Singer, I., and Goldberg, M., 1975, Paradoxical glucose-induced hyperkalemia. Combined aldosterone-insulin deficiency, *Amer. J. Med.* **59:**744–750.

8

Catecholamines and the Sympathoadrenal System

Lewis Landsberg

8.1. Introduction

In 1895, Oliver and Shafer demonstrated that extracts of adrenals contained a substance that raised the blood pressure. The active ingredient, epinephrine (E), was isolated and characterized at the turn of the century, and was therefore the first hormone with a known chemical structure. Since that time, investigations involving catecholamines have been at the forefront of experimental medicine and endocrinology. The theory of neurohumoral transmission was derived in large part from the obvious similarity in the physiological effects of infused catecholamines and sympathetic nerve stimulation. Current concepts of stimulus secretion coupling, and the mechanisms involved in hormone release by exocytosis, were developed in significant degree from studies involving catecholamine

LEWIS LANDSBERG   •   Harvard Medical School, Boston, Massachusetts.

release from the adrenal medulla. Receptor theory, such an integral part of current thinking about the mechanism of action of hormónes and drugs, blossomed after Ahlquist's description, in 1948, of two categories of catecholamine response, each mediated by a distinct receptor. Thus, research involving catecholamines, in addition to establishing the biological functions of the sympathoadrenal system, has helped elucidate general principles applicable to many areas of endocrinology.

The sympathetic nervous system and the adrenal medulla, together, comprise the sympathoadrenal system. This system differs from the other endocrine glands in one important respect: catecholamine release from the sympathetic nerve endings and the adrenal medulla is under the direct control of the CNS. The system is thus ideally suited to respond rapidly to internal and external environmental changes. Similarly, the physiological responses mediated by catecholamines occur rapidly and are dissipated quickly, unlike the slower, more prolonged effects of other hormones. Since Cannon's original description of "flight or fight," the sympathoadrenal system has been popularly associated with mobilization of the body's resources in the face of extreme conditions; indeed, the organization of the system is geared for extensive discharge as a result of both the amplification of preganglionic impulses in the sympathetic ganglia and the simultaneous release of catecholamines from the adrenal medulla. Accordingly, the manifestations of sympathoadrenal discharge are often widespread and spectacular. It should be emphasized, however, that the sympathoadrenal system is not necessarily activated in all-or-none fashion; sympathetic outflow to different regions is not homogeneous, and the adrenal medulla and sympathetic nervous system are usually regulated independently. For example, upright posture selectively activates the sympathetic innervation of the vasculature, while hypoglycemia stimulates the adrenal medulla. Like the other neural and endocrine systems, the sympathoadrenal system labors continuously in the support of a constant internal environment, and the less spectacular "tonic" regulation of vegetative functions by the sympathoadrenal system is of major physiological importance.

Catecholamine biosynthesis and storage are, for practical purposes, limited to the sympathoadrenal system and the CNS. The biologically important, naturally occurring catecholamines are dopamine, norepinephrine (NE), and E. NE is the adrenergic neurotransmitter; it is synthesized and stored in the peripheral sympathetic nerve endings, and released in response to sympathetic nerve impulses. NE released from the sympathetic nerves exerts its physiological effect in the innervated tissue in the immediate vicinity of release. E is the hormone of the adrenal medulla; it is synthesized and stored in the adrenal medullary chromaffin cells, and released in response to preganglionic impulses in the splanchnic nerves. The physiological effects of E are exerted in tissues far removed from the site of release.

Catecholamine biosynthesis begins with tyrosine, which is *m*-hydroxylated to 3,4-dihydroxyphenylalanine (DOPA), decarboxylated to dopamine, β-hydroxylated to NE, and *N*-methylated to E (Fig. 1). The formation of E is limited to the adrenal medulla. NE is also found in the adrenal medulla, but in man, 85% of the adrenal catecholamine store is E. Dopamine is a precursor of NE and E in the sympathetic nerves and the adrenal medulla, but is not present in appreciable amounts in these tissues; dopamine is, however, a transmitter in the CNS.

Catecholamines influence most bodily processes. The physiological effects of catecholamines are mediated by two relatively distinct adrenergic receptors: The alpha receptor mediates vasoconstriction, intestinal relaxation, and pupillary dilation, in addition to a variety of other responses; it is blocked selectively by phentolamine or phenoxybenza-

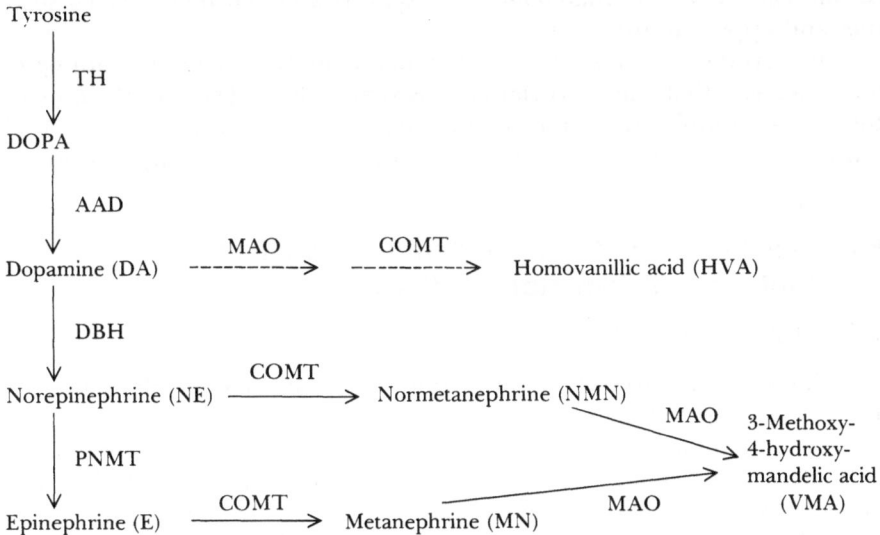

Fig. 1. Biosynthesis and metabolism of the catecholamines. Hydroxylation of tyrosine by tyrosine hydroxylase (TH) is rate-limiting. Aromatic-L-amino acid decarboxylase (AAD) is a widespread pyridoxal phosphate enzyme. Dopamine-β-hydroxylase (DBH) is associated with the subcellular particles that store catecholamines in the sympathetic nerve endings and adrenal medulla; it is released along with the catecholamines, and can be assayed in blood. Phenylethanolamine-*N*-methyl transferase (PNMT) is localized in adrenal medulla. Catechol-*O*-methyl-transferase (COMT) metabolizes circulating catechols predominantly in liver and kidney. Monamine oxidase (MAO) is widespread, but the highest activity is found in liver. TH and DBH are found only in tissues that synthesize catecholamines (sympathetic nerve endings, adrenal medulla, and brain).

mine. The beta receptor mediates cardiac stimulation, lipolysis, intestinal relaxation, vasodilation, and bronchodilation, as well as many other responses; it is blocked selectively by propranolol.

The physiological effects of catecholamines are terminated rapidly. NE released from the sympathetic nerve endings is inactivated predominantly by reuptake into the sympathetic nerves; that portion of released neurotransmitter that escapes reuptake and metabolism in the innervated tissue enters the general circulation and comprises the bulk of the circulating pool of plasma NE. Circulating catecholamines (NE from the sympathetic nerve endings and E from the adrenal medulla) have a rapid half-life in plasma (approximately 30 secs); plasma catecholamines are cleared from the circulation by metabolism, uptake into the sympathetic nerve endings, and renal excretion. The metabolic transformations include m-O-methylation, oxidative deamination, and sulfate and glucuronide conjugation; these metabolic transformations are carried out in the liver, gut, and kidney, with the formation of 3-methoxy-4-hydroxy mandelic acid (VMA) and the metanephrines (see Fig. 1). Free catecholamines and certain catecholamine metabolites are actively secreted by the renal tubules and appear in the urine.

Important recent advances of general interest to endocrinologists and internists that will be reviewed this year include: (1) pheochromocytoma and multiple endocrine adenomatosis; (2) the clinical assessment of sympathoadrenal activity; and (3) catecholamines and hyperthyroidism.

8.2. Familial Pheochromocytoma and Multiple Endocrine Adenomatosis (MEA)

8.2.1. Incidence and Importance

Pheochromocytomas are rare lesions; it is likely that less than 0.1% of hypertensive patients harbor a chromaffin tumor as a cause of the increased blood pressure. The rarity of these tumors, however, should not belie their importance: correctly diagnosed and properly treated, pheochromocytoma is completely curable; misdiagnosed or improperly treated, it is inexorably fatal. The tumors themselves are not aggressive, and clearly less than 10% are malignant. Pheochromocytomas are dangerous because of their capacity to store and release catecholamines in large amounts, with the subsequent production of alarming and occasionally spectacular syndromes. The potential pharmacological effects of the released catecholamines constitute a major surgical and medical therapeutic challenge. That 30–60% of pheochromocytomas are found unexpectedly at autopsy[1] indicates that many potentially curable cases are going undiagnosed.

Although familial pheochromocytomas have been recognized for some time,[2,3] only recently has an association with other endocrine neoplasms become clear. The traditional estimate that only 5% of cases of pheochromocytoma are familial[3] was developed before the recognition of MEA-II and MEA-III (see below), and probably grossly underestimates the familial incidence. More than 30 families with inherited pheochromocytomas with over 100 affected individuals have been reported.[4-7] In many of these families, it is clear that the pheochromocytoma is part of a syndrome associated with the inheritance of other abnormalities as well; since many of these syndromes have been described only recently, it is not clear how often, if at all, pheochromocytoma is inherited as an isolated genetic defect. In the 1968 review of Steiner *et al.*,[4] 11 of 29 families had associated thyroid carcinoma (2 with mucosal neuromas), 2 were associated with phakomatoses, and 16 were not identified with any other defect. Familial pheochromocytoma, alone or in combination with other defects, is inherited as an autosomal dominant trait.

The familial endocrine neoplastic syndromes are summarized in Table I. The first of these syndromes to be described (Wermer's syndrome, MEA-I, MEN Type 1) involves the parathyroids, the pancreatic islets, and the pituitary; intractable peptic ulceration and carcinoid tumors are commonly associated.[8-14] Pheochromocytoma has not been reported in kindreds with MEA-I. Pheochromocytoma is, however, a central part of the other disorders shown in Table I. The incidence of pheochromocytoma in kindreds with inherited phakomatosis, especially von Recklinghausen's neurofibromatosis and von Hippel-Lindau's cerebellar hemangioblastomatosis, is uncertain, but in one large series, less than 1% of patients with von Recklinghausen's disease had pheochromocytoma.[15] On the other hand, in the older literature, about 5% of the reported cases of pheochromocytomas were in association with neurofibromatosis.[2,3,16] In some patients in these families, the pheochromocytoma may dominate the clinical picture, with only subtle signs of neuroectodermal dysplasia.[16] Multiple endocrine adenomatosis II and III are considered in detail below.

8.2.2. Sipple's Syndrome (MEA-II)

8.2.2.1. Background

In 1961, Sipple called attention to an association of pheochromocytoma and thyroid carcinoma.[17] In 1962, a case of familial pheochromocytoma with multiple thyroid carcinomas was described.[18] By 1966, it was clear that the one type of thyroid carcinoma associated with pheochromocytoma was the newly described medullary carcinoma with amyloid pro-

Table I. Inherited Pheochromocytoma: MEA Syndromes

Tissue	MEA-I (Wermer's)	MEA-II (Sipple's)	MEA-III (Mucosal neuroma syndrome)	Phakomatosis (von Recklinghausen's and von Hippel-Lindau's)
Adrenal	—	PHEO	PHEO	PHEO
Thyroid	—	Medullary carcinoma	Medullary carcinoma	—
Parathyroid	Hyperplasia or adenomas	Hyperplasia or adenomas	—	—
Nervous system	—	—	Neuromas, ganglioneuromas	Neurofibromas, retinal–cerebellar hemangioblastomas
Pancreas	Islet cell tumors (β and non-β cell)	—	—	—
Pituitary	Adenomas	—	—	—
Gut	Carcinoids	—	—	—

duction.[19-22] The association of hyperparathyroidism had been present in one of Sipple's original cases, and was subsequently confirmed as an integral part of the syndrome.[18,23,24] Inheritance of the syndrome was defined as an autosomal dominant trait with variable penetrance.

In 1966, Williams[25] proposed that medullary carcinoma of the thyroid originated from the parafollicular or C cells of the thyroid. The association of the parafollicular cells with thyrocalcitonin production led to the important finding of Tashjian and Melvin[26] that tumor and plasma of patients with medullary carcinoma contained large amounts of thyrocalcitonin, as determined by bioassay. Thyrocalcitonin activity was subsequently identified in metastatic deposits of medullary carcinoma in liver.[27] The development of Tashjian and co-workers of a sensitive radioimmunoassay for human thyrocalcitonin[28] led directly to the demonstration of increased basal or stimulated calcitonin levels in the blood of patients with medullary carcinoma, and it soon became clear that calcitonin levels would serve as a useful tumor marker in the early diagnosis[29,30] and follow-up[31] of affected family members.

8.2.2.2. Presentation

Studies of large kindreds have revealed that men and women are affected equally, and that the age of onset varies from early childhood to late middle age; often, the disease becomes manifest in the second or third decade. Presentation is in one of four ways: (1) thyroid nodule; (2) nephrolithiasis, nephrocalcinosis, or hypercalcemia; (3) paroxysmal or malignant hypertension; or (4) identification on family screening (asymptomatic). Among members of known kindreds, presentation with a neck mass has been most common; new kindreds, however, have usually been first identified by the appearance of a propositus with pheochromocytoma or hyperparathyroidism.

In most reported kindreds, medullary carcinoma of the thyroid (MCT) is the most frequently encountered lesion. Some patients may have pheochromocytomas without MCT, but most will have the thyroid tumor at the time the pheochromocytoma is diagnosed. Virtually all patients with hyperparathyroidism have medullary carcinoma, but the MCT may be small, and hyperparathyroidism may dominate the clinical picture. Many affected patients have all three lesions.

8.2.2.3. Pheochromocytoma in MEA-II

Inherited pheochromocytomas differ from the sporadic variety in a number of important ways. Most of the information has been obtained from patients who probably have had Sipple's syndrome; it is not clear whether there are significant differences in pheochromocytoma inherited as part of the different syndromes outlined in Table I. In general, it seems that pheochromocytomas in MEA-II and MEA-III are very similar.

8.2.2.3a. Location. In sporadic pheochromocytoma, 80% of the tumors are single and occur in or about one adrenal gland; 10% are bilateral, 10% extraadrenal.[32] Extraadrenal pheochromocytomas are usually located in or about the sympathetic ganglia, predominantly in the abdomen. Less than 10% of pheochromocytomas are malignant. In familial pheochromocytoma, the incidence of bilateral and multiple adrenal tumors is markedly increased. Of the reported cases, well over 50% are bilateral, and, if patients are followed long enough, it is likely that most, if not all, will eventually involve both adrenals. Some evidence has been advanced that the adrenal lesion begins as bilateral adrenal medullary hyperplasia, with the subsequent formation of distinct tumors.[33] Interestingly enough, extraadrenal pheochromocytoma appears to be distinctly uncommon in familial cases; only 1 reported case of extraadrenal pheochromocytoma in association with medullary carcinoma has been noted,[34] and that was in a patient with the mucosal neuroma syndrome who had bilateral pheochromocytomas and two preaortic extraadrenal tumors. The incidence of malignant pheochromocytoma is not increased in the familial syndromes.

8.2.2.3b. Catecholamine Metabolism. Pheochromocytomas resemble normal human adrenal medulla in many respects. In both normal adrenal chromaffin cells and pheochromocytoma cells, the catecholamines are stored in chromaffin granules. These subcellular storage particles contain, in addition to the catecholamine, ATP, and specific soluble proteins, the chromogranins and dopamine-B-hydroxylase (DBH). The physical properties of the granules from pheochromocytoma cells are normal.[1] In some tumors, the catecholamine:ATP ratio, usually 4:1, is increased, indicating a possible defect in catecholamine storage, since ATP appears to be involved in catecholamine storage by reversibly binding to the catecholamine. This alteration of the 4:1 ratio has not been found uniformly, however.[1] In the normal adrenal medullary chromaffin cells, tyrosine hydroxylase (TH) is subject to feedback inhibition by catechols; in some pheochromocytomas, TH is not inhibited by catechols,[35,36] but in others, the TH activity is normal in all respects.[37] The normal adrenal medullary chromaffin cell is innervated, and releases its catecholamines in response to acetylcholine liberated from the splanchnic nerves by preganglionic nerve impulses; in pheochromocytomas, the mechanism of release is unknown, since pheochromocytomas are not innervated.[1] There is no information available on whether familial pheochromocytomas differ from the sporadic type in any of these characteristics.

Most pheochromocytomas contain predominantly NE (unlike the normal adrenal medulla, which, in man, contains 85% E), and patients with this disorder excrete predominantly increased amounts of NE in the urine.[38] Familial tumors are much more likely to contain large amounts of E, and may excrete predominantly E in the urine; in some patients, a small increase in urinary E is the only biochemical abnormality.[39] Since a significant rise in urinary E may be easily missed, this difference has implications for the diagnosis of pheochromocytoma in MEA-II, as described below.

8.2.2.3c. Symptoms. The paroxysm is the classic manifestation of pheochromocytoma. The typical paroxysm (headache, sweating, palpitation, chest or abdominal pain, apprehension, facial pallor followed by flush) is the obvious expression of the interaction of released catecholamines with adrenergic receptors. About 55% of patients with pheochromocytoma have paroxysms of some sort; 45% have no paroxysmal episodes. Of patients with pheochromocytoma, 90% are hypertensive: in 35%, the hypertension is sustained without crises; in 30%, the hypertension is sustained, but paroxysmal crises occur; in 25%, the hypertension is truly paroxysmal. In 10%, the tumors are asymptomatic (discovered incidentally).[3] The symptoms in familial pheochromocytoma are similar to those in the sporadic variety, except for a far greater incidence of asymptomatic, normotensive patients (40–60% in some series),[39,40] a finding that may reflect earlier diagnosis as a result of family screening. Furthermore, those patients that are hypertensive are much more likely to have paroxysmal hypertension than patients with the sporadic variety[4,39–41]; less than 50% of patients with pheochromocytoma in the MEA-II syndrome appear to have sustained hypertension. It should be noted that the asymptomatic patient with normal blood pressure is at risk of having dangerous and possible fatal paroxysms during operative stress if an unsuspected pheochromocytoma is present.[42]

8.2.2.3d. Diagnosis. The diagnosis of pheochromocytoma in the usual sporadic case depends on the demonstration of increased amounts of catecholamines or catecholamine metabolites in urine. The three tests in common clinical usage involve the measurement of free catecholamines, VMA, or the metanephrines (see Fig. 1). When carefully performed, all these tests are equivalent in their ability to detect pheochromocytoma.[43] The advantage of determining E and NE separately is that formation of E greatly favors an intraadrenal lesion, and thus helps with localization, but well-documented cases of extraadrenal pheochromocytomas secreting E have been described.[44]

It is believed that over 90% of patients with pheochromocytoma will be diagnosed by a single, properly performed assay for catecholamines or metabolites. Those cases that are missed are usually those with paroxysmal symptoms who are not hypertensive at the time the collection is made. The classic pharmacological tests (adrenolytic—phentolamine; provocative—histamine, glucagon, or tyramine) have limited usefulness, and should be employed only by physicians with experience in the use of adrenergic agonists and blockers. The phentolamine test is useful when a patient presents with malignant hypertension and something in the clinical picture suggests the possibility of a pheochromocytoma; a significant blood pressure reduction with phentolamine under these circumstances not only helps with diagnosis, but also indicates the appropriate therapy. Provocative tests are potentially hazardous, and have a significant number (25%) of false negative reactions.[45] Tyramine differs from glucagon and histamine in that it causes a dose-related release of catecholamines from the sympathetic nerve endings; it is therefore probably safer than glucagon or histamine, which release catecholamines from the tumor in an unpredictable manner. The release of catecholamines from pheochromocytomas, either spontaneously or in response to these provocative agents, is poorly understood; spontaneous paroxysms are often the result of physical manipulations, such as lifting or straining, but it is hazardous to try to provoke a paroxysm by these maneuvers. It is of note in this regard that a glucagon receptor has recently been demonstrated in pheochromocytoma tissue.[46] Whether this receptor is related to glucagon-induced release of catecholamines by the tumor is not clear. In general, provocative tests should be used only when paroxysmal symptoms are present, when urine analyses are normal, when a spontaneous paroxysm cannot be observed, and when it is crucial to make the diagnosis quickly. Angiography (see Section 8.2.2.6b) may be even more useful than the standard provocative tests under these circumstances, particularly in the familial cases.

The diagnosis of familial pheochromocytoma is more difficult than the diagnosis of the sporadic tumor. As was noted in Section 8.2.2.3b, these tumors often secrete mainly E[39]; this being so, they may not elevate the total catecholamines, and the VMA has often been normal in patients who have gotten into difficulty during surgical intervention.[42] Furthermore, a high percentage of these tumors secrete paroxysmally.[4,40] Hence, even specific assays for E may be within the normal range on occasion. Finally, provocative tests have shown unreliable results with familial pheochromocytomas; tyramine and glucagon in particular have regularly been associated with false negative responses.[4,5,38,40,41,47]

In summary, familial pheochromocytoma should be diagnosed by analysis of the urine for catecholamines or their metabolites. Experience has indicated that analysis of E specifically is most helpful in confirming or ruling out the diagnosis. If urine assays for catecholamines are persistently and unequivocally negative, and the patient is normotensive and has no paroxysms, the likelihood of pheochromocytoma causing trouble during an operative procedure is small. Where urinary analyses are negative, but the patient is hypertensive or has paroxysms, or when urinary catecholamine analyses are borderline or equivocal, arteriography (after adrenergic blockade; see Section 8.2.2.6b) should probably be undertaken to establish or exclude the diagnosis.

8.2.2.4. Medullary Carcinoma of the Thyroid

Medullary carcinoma of the thyroid (MCT) accounts for 7–9% of all thyroid carcinomas.[5,40,48] It was first described as a distinct entity in 1959 by Hazard *et al.*[49]; these workers noted the regular occurrence of amyloid, distinguished anaplastic thyroid carcinoma, and suggested the name the lesion now bears. Familial medullary carcinoma of the thyroid has been reported to comprise from 4.5 to 38% of the total MCT cases[5,40,48]; in the large series from the Mayo Clinic,[40] about 20% of the MCT cases were familial. Familial and sporadic cases are similar in age of presentation (first to seventh decade) and sex incidence (approximately equal).

8.2.2.4a. Presentation. Medullary thyroid carcinomas are bilateral in virtually 100% of familial cases,[40,48] and in over 50% of the sporadic cases.[48] In the familial cases, the development of distinct tumors is preceded by bilateral C-cell hyperplasia.[50] The parafollicular cells are located predominantly in the upper two-thirds of the lateral lobes,[50,51] the area in which hyperplasia and tumor formation develop. Interestingly, the ^{131}I scan is often normal even when a palpable tumor is present.

Symptoms of MCT may be due to either (1) local tumor growth, (2) metastases, or (3) hormonal products. The tumor tends to mestastasize largely to local cervical nodes and liver, and eventually to lung and bone.[5,39,40,48] Long-term survival is good despite early metastases,[40] with an average 10-year survivorship of 67% in the Mayo Clinic series. In addition to calcitonin, the tumor makes a variety of other substances. Histaminase[52] activity is increased in the blood of patients with metastatic disease, but assay of this enzyme has little to offer clinically. Kallikreins, prostaglandins, and serotonin have been found in excessive quantities in the blood of patients with MCT,[53,54] and the classic carcinoid syndrome has been described[54] in a patient with MCT. The ectopic ACTH syndrome is a well-recognized complication of MCT as well,[55,56] and most of the cases of Cushing's syndrome in association with MEA-II are the result of ACTH secretion by the medullary thyroid tumor.

Diarrhea is a prominent complaint in about 30% of patients with MCT.[5,40,48] The cause is uncertain, but prostaglandins have been implicated by some workers. Diarrhea is most common in patients with advanced disease and large tumor mass; resection often results in amelioration. Many patients with advanced disease also complain of severe flushing attacks and crises not explicable in terms of serotonin or catecholamines. The cause of these symptoms is not known, but prostaglandins, kinins, or other as yet unrecognized products of the tumor may be at fault. An increased incidence of peptic ulcer disease in patients with MCT has been suggested, but it is not certain that this is real.[5,48]

8.2.2.4b. Thyrocalcitonin. Most, but not all, patients with medullary carcinoma have demonstrably increased plasma thyrocalcitonin levels. Often, the basal levels are elevated; in some cases, basal levels are normal, but hyperresponsiveness to stimulation by calcium or pentagastrin is present. A normal resting level, therefore, is not sufficient to rule out MCT. The abnormal calcitonin response to calcium[6,28–31] or pentagastrin infusion[57,58] is the important diagnostic test in establishing the diagnosis and following the course of medullary carcinoma.[30,31] Pentagastrin appears to be more sensitive,[57] as some patients with tumors who have normal responses to calcium are clearly abnormal in their response to pentagastrin. It is important to note that an abnormal calcitonin response to calcium or pentagastrin in a member of an affected family is an indication for total thyroidectomy. Glucagon[6,59] and ethanol[60] also stimulate calcitonin, but the response is less marked than with pentagastrin, and these agents are not useful clinically. Interestingly, magnesium infusion lowers calcitonin levels in patients with MCT, apparently by an effect independent of the calcium level.[61] The importance or significance of this finding is not yet clear. It should be noted that despite very high calcitonin levels in some patients with metastatic MCT, hypocalcemia is rare.

8.2.2.5. Hyperparathyroidism

The incidence of hyperparathyroidism in Sipple's syndrome is not known with certainty. In most kindreds, it is present less often than MCT or pheochromocytoma. The plasma calcium is normal in at least 50% of the MEA-II patients with parathyroid hyperplasia,[39,40] so the reported incidence of hyperparathyroidism often reflects the intensity of the search at the time of thyroid exploration. An incidence of 20%[4] to 90%[40] has been described. It would seem that in most MEA-II kindreds, 50% of affected patients have parathyroid disease, and in 50% of these, there is hypercalcemia or other evidence of hyperparathyroidism, such as nephrolithiasis or nephrocalcinosis. Some patients in an affected kindred without evidence of either MCT or pheochromocytoma have isolated, elevated parathyroid hormone (PTH) levels[6,7]; the significance of this finding is uncertain, and it is not clear whether, in the absence of elevated calcitonin levels, it is evidence that these patients are affected. Hypercalciuria is common in MEA-II patients, but it usually correlates best with MCT rather than hyperparathyroidism (Landsberg and Young, unpublished observations). The cause is unknown, but may be the direct effect of calcitonin. (See Chapter 9 for a thorough discussion of the physiological effects of calcitonin)

Patients with MCT have recently been shown to have a paradoxical increase in plasma PTH levels during calcium infusion.[62] This finding suggests that the rise in endogenous calcitonin stimulates PTH in these patients, and raises the question of the role of calcitonin in inducing parathyroid disease. Porcine calcitonin has been shown to cause secondary hyperparathyroidism in animals.[63]

Involvement of more than one parathyroid gland is common in Sipple's syndrome, and it is presumed that hyperplasia affecting all the glands is usually present.[5,40] Although many patients with "adenomas" have been described, these descriptions have been attributed to failure to recognize hyperplasia in the cases reported in the older literature. The situation is really unclear, however, and occasionally a single adenoma is found even today. Multiple gland involvement is the usual parathyroid lesion.

No well-documented cases of hyperparathyroidism have been noted in MEA-II patients without coexisting MCT, although in many patients, the evidence of parathyroid disease goes back 20-odd years, the clinical development of MCT occurring years after the onset of clinical hyperparathyroidism.[64] Other cases with documented hyperparathyroidism have been noted to have only microscopic foci of MCT.[64]

8.2.2.6. Management of Patients and Families with MEA-II (Sipple's Syndrome)

8.2.2.6a. Family Screening. It is essential that careful study at regular intervals be performed on all members of a kindred affected with MEA-II. It is reasonable to carry out the screening on a yearly basis beginning in children age 7 or under. The screening battery should include:

1. A 24-hr urine collection for catecholamines or catecholamine metabolites (fractionated free catecholamines with specific mea-

surement of E is probably best); calcium excretion can be determined on the same collection.

2. Blood for calcium, phosphorous, BUN, creatinine, electrolytes, and PTH level.
3. Thyrocalcitonin levels in response to calcium infusion (15 mg/kg elemental Ca as calcium gluconate over 4 hr with blood samples for calcitonin and PTH at 1, 2, 3, and 4 hr), or pentagastrin infusion (0.5 μg/kg over 1 min, with blood for calcitonin at 1, 2, 5, 10, and 20 min).

Although precise data are lacking, the most effective screening may involve both tests, with administration of pentagastrin at the end of the calcium infusion. Once an individual member in a kindred is identified as having the trait, therapy should be advised at once. This will involve, in all cases, total thyroidectomy. If pheochromocytoma is present at the time the diagnosis is made, it should be removed first, but thyroidectomy should be performed shortly thereafter. If hyperparathyroidism is present, total thyroidectomy should be performed at the time of the parathyroid exploration.

8.2.2.6b. Management of Pheochromocytomas. Once the diagnosis of pheochromocytoma is established by urinary catecholamine determination, the patient should be placed on α-adrenergic blocking agents. Oral phenoxybenzamine, 10 mg b.i.d., is the usual initial dose. Increments of 10 mg may be made every few days until control of the blood pressure is achieved and the paroxysms disappear. Intravenous phentolamine (2.5–5.0 mg i.v. after the response to a test dose of 0.5 mg is established) should be used to control individual paroxysms before the phenoxybenzamine blockade is effective. α-adrenergic blockade is essential before surgery or angiography; indeed, the best preoperative preparation is a 10-day to 2-week course of phenoxybenzamine, which restores the blood volume and reverses the vascular changes consequent to the hypertension.[65,66] MEA-II patients with pheochromocytoma are much more likely to be normotensive than patients with the sporadic form of the disease, and the management of adrenergic blockade in these patients is more difficult, since a clear endpoint is not available. If paroxysms have been present, α-blockade should completely eliminate them. Even the normotensive, asymptomatic patients should be given phenoxybenzamine prior to surgery or angiography. The usual dose in this situation is about 0.5–1.0 mg/kg, but this dosage must be attained gradually. Examination for orthostatic hypotension should be performed several times per day, and if it is present, the dose should be reduced.

Propranolol is a useful adjunct, and will be required in most patients to control the tachycardia that develops during the α-blockade; it should be given only after α-blockade has begun to take effect, since by blocking β-mediated vasodilation, it can cause an increase in blood pressure in patients with pheochromocytoma in whom α-blockade has not been established. Propranolol is also useful in controlling arrhythmias, particularly those induced by anesthesia. Small doses are usually satisfactory, and 10 mg q.i.d. is the usual starting dose, with titration upward as needed to control tachycardia.

Once the patient is adequately blocked, adrenal arteriography is helpful in locating the pheochromocytomas. Phentolamine and propranolol should be on hand during the procedure, but untoward events are rare in an adequately blocked patient. The demonstration of bilateral adrenal tumors is helpful in planning the surgical approach; similarly, if one adrenal can be cleared completely by a good selective arteriographic study of the superior, middle, and inferior adrenal arteries, a unilateral approach may be undertaken.

The preferred anesthetic regimen is scopolamine and pentobarbital premedication, thiopental induction, and nitrous oxide and narcotics as the prime agents. Both adrenals should be examined, unless angiography has unequivocally demonstrated one normal side. Total adrenalectomy on the involved side is always required.

Intraoperative hypotension should be treated aggressively with volume expansion. Failure of the blood pressure to fall after the removal of one affected adrenal is usually evidence of involvement of the other side. A transient episode of increased blood pressure in the immediate postoperative period is not unusual, and probably reflects fluid shifts and autonomic instability.

Urinary catecholamines return to normal about 1 week after operation. If only one adrenal has been removed, MEA-II patients require continued surveillance for the development of pheochromocytoma in the remaining adrenal. This can be done by yearly check of blood pressure and analysis of urine for catecholamines.

8.2.2.6c. Treatment of Medullary Carcinoma of the Thyroid and Hyperparathyroidism. If management of the pheochromocytoma is the immediate short-term problem in patients with MEA-II, management of the MCT is the major long-term concern. Once a member of an MEA-II kindred is known to have any of the manifestations of the syndrome, total thyroidectomy is indicated. Thus, an elevated calcitonin level in response to calcium or pentagastrin infusion is an indication for total thyroidectomy, even with a normal physical exam and normal ^{131}I scan.

Furthermore, the presence of pheochromocytoma or hyperparathyroidism is an indication for total thyroidectomy even if the calcitonin response is normal, although the neck exploration should follow removal of the pheochromocytoma. Borderline calcitonin responses should be viewed with great suspicion, and should be repeated frequently; if an upward trend is present, thyroidectomy should be performed, and often, bilateral C-cell hyperplasia will be found.[50] Early hepatic metastases have been noted frequently in the absence of extrathyroidal disease in the neck,[7,39,67] so early removal of the thyroid in affected members is critical. Calcitonin responses to calcium and pentagastrin should be studied post-operatively; elevation is diagnostic of residual disease in the neck or elsewhere. Hepatic metastases have been found on blind liver biopsy in such cases when liver function tests and liver scan have been completely normal. The long-term survival in these cases with early hepatic metastases appears to be reasonably good, and no specific treatment is available at the present time.

Management of the hyperparathyroidism is more complex. At the time of thyroidectomy, all the glands should be visualized. If hypercalcemia has been present and hyperplasia is found at exploration, 3½ glands should be removed. If an adenoma is present, a normal-appearing gland should be biopsied to rule out hyperplasia. If the patient has not been hypercalcemic and no adenomas are seen, it is probably best to leave the parathyroids alone, even if they look a little hyperplastic. Periodic surveillance for the development of hyperparathyroidism should be carried out postoperatively, although it is not clear how great the risk is for the development of hyperparathyroidism once the MCT has been removed.

8.2.3. Mucosal Neuroma Syndrome (MEA-III)

Although there is a suggestion in the literature that mucosal neuromas, ganglioneuromas, and marfanoid habitus are part of the fully developed MEA-II syndrome,[6,42] it now appears clear that the mucosal neuroma syndrome (MEA-III) is genetically and phenotypically distinct.[40,41,68–70] Both sporadic and familial cases of this syndrome have been reported.[41] Although parathyroid hyperplasia has been described in patients with this syndrome,[71] some of the reported cases are not convincing, and the incidence of parathyroid disease is certainly less than in Sipple's syndrome (MEA-II).[40,41] The implications for screening families, and the guidelines for diagnosis and treatment of pheochromocytoma and medullary carcinoma of the thyroid, are the same in the mucosal neuroma syndrome as in Sipple's syndrome.

8.2.4. Multiple Endocrine Adenomatosis—Theories of Pathogenesis

8.2.4.1 The APUD Cell Concept

8.2.4.1a. APUD Cells—Properties and Functions. Pearse has called attention to the fact that many endocrine cells in different tissues have similar histochemical and electron-microscopic characteristics.[72,73] The major histochemical characteristics of the group relate to the storage of biogenic amines in specific secretion granules. The mnemonic term *APUD* that has been applied to these cells derives from their histochemical properties: *A*mine content, amine *P*recursor *U*ptake, and amino acid *D*ecarboxylase activity. The stored amine is usually dopamine or serotonin; the amine precursor is the amino acid L-DOPA or 5-hydroxytryptophan (5-HTP); the decarboxylase activity reflects the presence of the enzyme aromatic amino acid decarboxylase. Electron microscopy reveals characteristic membrane-bound secretion vesicles (Fig. 2). An additional property of these cells is the production of specific polypeptides, which in the case of many cells are recognized hormones. The amines and the polypeptide hormones are believed to be stored together in the secretion vesicles. The protein products can be identified in the cell by specific immunofluorescence. Table II lists the APUD cells and their polypeptide products.

Table II. APUD Cells[a]

Site	Polypeptide
Pituitary	
corticotroph	ACTH
melanotroph	MSH
?somatotroph	HGH
Pancreatic islets	
beta cells	insulin
alpha cells	glucagon
delta cells	gastrin
Thyroid	
C cells	calcitonin
Gut	
stomach	gastrin
small bowel	secretin, enteroglucagon, CCK-PZ, vasoactive intestinal peptide, gastric inhibitory peptide
Adrenal	
medulla	chromogranin

[a]Modified from Pearse.[72,73]

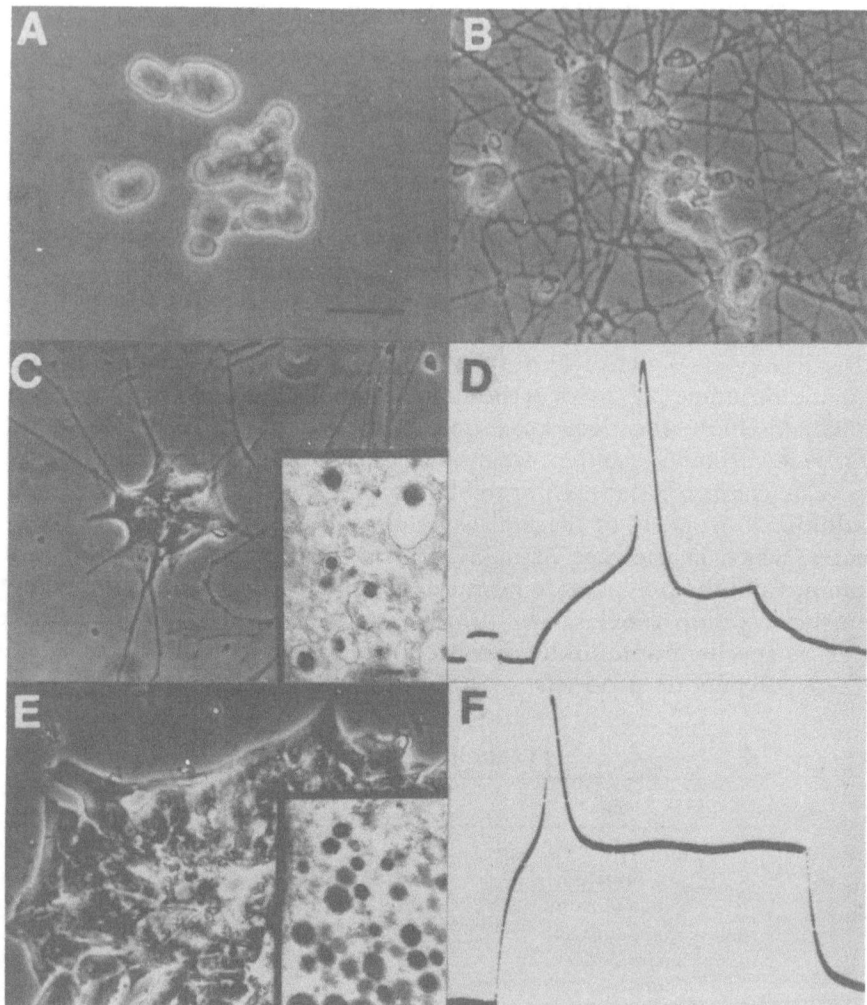

Fig. 2. Neuroendocrine tumors in dissociated cell culture. (A) Cells from a clonal rat pheochromocytoma line (PC12) grown without nerve growth factor (NGF). (B) Same cells as in A grown in the presence of NGF (50 ng/ml). Note the extensive development of processes. (C) Human pheochromocytoma cells grown in NGF (50 ng/ml), showing similar process formation in culture. Inset illustrates typical chromaffin granules as seen in the electron microscope. (D) Intracellular microelectrode recording from human pheochro-mocytoma cell demonstrating large action potential triggered by depolarizing current pulse. (E) Cluster of cells from human medullary carcinoma of thyroid. Inset (EM) illustrates secretory granules in these cells. (F) Intracellular recording from MCT cell demonstrating action potential triggered by depolarizing current pulse. Calibration: Bar in A is 25 μm for A and B, 20 μm for C and E; inset bars at 0.2 μm; square pulse in D is 10 mV and 5 msec for D and F. (Courtesy of Drs. A. Tischler and M. Dichter.)

Pearse and co-workers have provided evidence that the APUD cells are of neural crest origin. Using histochemical fluorescence techniques based on the amine-storing capabilities of these cells, they have demonstrated ventral migration of amine-containing cells from the neural crest, with invasion of the primitive foregut and its derivatives,[74,75] including the ultimobranchial body (thyroid C cells in mammals) and the pancreas. Specific immunofluorescence has demonstrated the polypeptide hormones in some of these cells.[75]

The role of the amines in these cells is not entirely clear. Dopamine or serotonin can be demonstrated in most of them.[76] Pearse speculates that the entire diffuse endocrine system (see Table II) encompassed by the APUD cells is phylogenetically very old. Originally, according to this concept, the amines functioned as neurotransmitters, the polypeptides as storage proteins. In some cells, (most notably the adrenal medulla, and perhaps some of the serotonin-producing cells of the gut), the amines have remained the major secretion product. In most APUD cells, the storage proteins have been modified to the hormones we now recognize, with the function of the amines in doubt (see Owman *et al.*[76]). Direct proof of the theory is lacking, but recent studies strongly support the neural origin of these endocrine cells.

8.2.4.1b. Neural Properties of Certain Endocrine Cells. It has recently been demonstrated that animal and human pheochromocytomas maintained in tissue culture develop typical neural processes when exposed to nerve growth factor (see Section 8.2.4.2), as shown in Fig. 2.[77,78] Furthermore, action potentials have been observed in normal rodent adrenal,[79] as well as pheochromocytoma, medullary carcinoma of the thyroid, and bronchial carcinoids, all of which are derived from APUD cells.[80,81] These findings support the neural origin of these cells, and raise the question as to the role of action potentials in the mechanism of catecholamine release from the adrenal medulla, and possibly in the release of other hormones from other endocrine cells of neural origin.

8.2.4.1c. APUD Cell Tumors and MEA Syndromes. A relationship between the APUD cells and the MEA syndromes is suggested by a comparison of Tables I and II. Many of the endocrine tumors shown in Table I are derived from APUD cells or non-APUD neural ectoderm. This circumstance has led to the suggestion that a single genetic defect in neural ectoderm is responsible for the endocrine hyperplasia and tumor formation characteristic of the MEA syndromes. Since the syndromes shown in Table I are genetically discrete, a different genetic defect or a defect affecting different tissues must be present. There is no information available on what the molecular basis of such a defect might be. Furthermore, the parathyroid glands do not fit conveniently into the APUD theory. It seems reasonably clear[73] that the parathyroids are of endodermal origin. The APUD concept requires that parathyroid involvement be reactive, rather than primary or genetic. The usual explanation for a reactive parathyroid response is calcitonin stimulation of parathormone, either in defense of the serum calcium or, as recently described, by a direct effect.[62] This facile explanation, however, is inconsistent with a large body of clinical experience: (1) hyperparathyroidism is not common in sporadic medullary carcinoma or medullary carcinoma in MEA-III, despite similarly elevated calcitonin levels; (2) clinical hyperparathyroidism may antedate clinical medullary carcinoma of the thyroid more than 20 years; (3) only microscopic medullary carcinoma may be present with overt aggressive hyperparathyroidism; and (4) hyperplasia often does not involve the parathyroids equally, and occasionally single or multiple adenomas are found. Thus, the simple "reactive" theory is inconsistent with a large body of evidence; if parathyroid disease is a primary genetic part of the syndrome, the single defect in neural ectoderm is not tenable. It is conceivable, however, since C cells are known to be present in the parathyroid glands of some species,[73] that increased calcitonin production by hyperplasia of the intraparathyroid C cells causes local hyperplasia of the involved parathyroid. This would explain the patchy involvement of the parathyroids sometimes seen in Sipple's syndrome. The difference between MEA-II and MEA-III might be explicable by the extent of involvement of the parathyroids with C-cell hyperplasia, with greater parathyroid involvement in MEA-II. This, however, is only speculation; there is no evidence for C-cell hyperplasia in affected parathyroid glands, but the appropriate studies have apparently not yet been done.

8.2.4.2. Nerve Growth Factor

Nerve growth factor (NGF) is a protein discovered in rodent tumors; it stimulates the growth of sympathetic nerves and sensory ganglia in a variety of species. Subsequently found in much larger amounts in snake venom and the submaxillary glands of male mice, the protein has been isolated and characterized, and its effects well studied.[82,83] It is a 13,000 mol. wt. polypeptide with a remarkable structural resemblance to proinsulin.[83] When purified factor from mouse salivary gland is administered to animals, it stimulates the growth of the sympathetic ganglia, sympathetic nerve endings and, to a much lessor degree, the sensory ganglia. The individual nerve cells enlarge and demonstrate intense basophilia and increased fibrils, and impressive hyperinnervation of most sympathetically innervated tissues develops. Increased tissue NE levels corresponding to the increase in nerve-cell volume are noted as well.[82] The proinsulinlike molecule binds to specific receptors in sympathetically innervated tissues[83] and ganglia.[84] It stimulates a variety of biological processes in nerves, and some of its effects, such as stimulation of protein and lipid synthesis, and enhancement of glucose utilization resemble those of insulin. It also causes microtubule polymerization,[83] and, as noted above, causes pheochromocytoma cells to develop processes like neurons[81] (see Fig. 2). Specific antisera to NGF cause abrupt degeneration of the sympathetic nervous system when injected into newborn mice or other mammals.

The function of NGF is unknown; it appears to be present in the plasma of many species, including man. In male mice, removal of the submaxillary gland, the major source of NGF, causes no demonstrable impairment in adrenergic function.[82] At the very least, NGF seems to exert a stimulatory effect on immature nerve cells that is needed for the normal development of adrenergic structures.

The neural crest origin of some of the tumors found in MEA-II and MEA-III, coupled with the known stimulating effects of NGF on pheochromocytoma in tissue culture, raises the question of a possible role for NGF in the pathogenesis of the MEA syndromes. Indeed, a recent report indicates very high levels of NGF in an MEA patient with MCT and pheochromocytoma.[85] Further work needs to be done in this area, especially in view of the therapeutic implications of anti-NGF sera.

8.2.4.3. Nesidioblastosis

The presence of hyperplasia preceding tumor formation in both the thyroid and the adrenal in MEA-II, and the frequency of hyperplasia of the parathyroid glands, is compatible with chronic stimulation by a driving force. Unfortunately, no driving force has been identified to account for the hyperplasia in any of the MEA syndromes. It has been suggested that hyperplasia of the islet cells (nesidioblastosis) may be responsible for the glandular tumors in some of the kindreds with the MEA-I syndrome.[86] Glucagon has been implicated in parathyroid hyperplasia by some workers,[87] with or without the intervention of calcitonin, but glucagon levels are not elevated in MEA-II, and are not known to be elevated in MEA-I. Although the pancreatic islets are centrally involved in the MEA-I syndrome, there is no evidence that the islets control the development of the other associated tumors in MEA-I patients. No driving force has been discovered that adequately explains MEA-II.

8.3. Clinical Assessment of the Functional State of the Adrenal Medulla and the Sympathetic Nervous System

8.3.1. The Nature of the Problem

The accurate assessment of adrenal medullary function depends on a reasonable estimate of E secretion. Plasma or urinary levels of E measured under appropriate conditions are usually sufficient to achieve this estimate. As discussed in detail in Section 8.3.2, however, the rapid clearance of E from plasma, the episodic nature of E secretion, the extreme technical difficulty in measuring the small amounts of E in plasma, and the possibility of alterations in E clearance with subtle changes in renal function are all factors that must be considered.

The accurate assessment of the functional state of the sympathetic nervous system is far more difficult, given the limits of current technology. Such an assessment requires a reasonable estimate of the rate of NE release at the sympathetic nerve endings all over the body. Precise measurement of NE levels in plasma or urine may not suffice, since as much as 75–80% of released NE may be recaptured by the sympathetic nerve endings.[88] Furthermore, there is evidence that the percentage of released transmitter that is recaptured is not constant, but is dependent on the level of impulse traffic,[89] blood flow,[90] and perhaps other factors. The level of NE in plasma thus represents that fraction of released NE that escapes both reuptake at the sympathetic nerve endings and local metabolism in the tissue of release. These limitations notwithstanding, there is evidence that NE in plasma does in fact reflect sympathetic nervous activity. A recent study,[91] for example, shows that when the cardiac nerves of dogs are stimulated, the level of NE in coronary sinus blood is a linear function of stimulation frequency at low levels of stimulation. Other recent studies[92–94] indicate that plasma NE levels accurately reflect drug-induced changes in NE release from the sympathetic nerve endings. Nonetheless, the relationship between plasma levels of NE and sympathetic stimulation must be considered tangential rather than direct because of the presence of significant local factors that affect transmitter overflow into the circulation. Incidentally, the contribution to the plasma pool of NE from the adrenal medulla is believed to be small and insignificant.

It should also be emphasized that plasma NE levels reflect NE release from all the adrenergic nerve endings; differential rates of release in different tissues cannot be assessed in man by noninvasive methods. In experimental animals, dynamic measurements of NE turnover in different tissues can be made with the use of tracer NE.[95–97] The steady-state level of NE is reasonably constant despite greatly varying degrees of sympathetic activity; hence, tissue levels of NE cannot be used to assess adrenergic activity in animals or man.

8.3.2. Assay of Catecholamines in Plasma and Urine

Despite the limitations imposed by the theoretical considerations described above, catecholamine levels in urine and plasma have been widely used in assessing sympathoadrenal activity, and, under appropriate circumstances, have provided meaningful data. It is worth emphasizing that analysis of catecholamine metabolites in urine, although it is useful in the diagnosis of pheochromocytoma, has a limited role in the study of sympathoadrenal function in the pathophysiology of disease in man. The metanephrines (see Fig. 1) cannot be measured with sufficient accuracy in the physiological ranges to provide meaningful data. VMA, although it is present in large amounts and easily measurable in urine, is far too heterogenous in origin to give a useful measure of sympathoadrenal acitivity; a large portion of the urinary VMA originates from intraneuronal metabolism of catecholamines in the peripheral and central nervous systems, and a substantial portion of the catecholamine that appears in the urine as VMA has never been released from the nerve endings in a physiologically active form.[32]

8.3.2.1. Plasma Catecholamines

The concentration of NE in plasma is less than 1 ng/ml, with an average in most laboratories of about 0.3 ng/ml. The concentration of E in plasma is only $\frac{1}{10}$ as great, with average concentrations usually below 0.05 ng/ml plasma.[98,99] Catecholamines in plasma are partially bound to serum proteins, particularly albumin. Although studies of catecholamine-binding to plasma proteins are in their infancy, it seems likely that a low-capacity, high-affinity system is involved,[100] with about 50–60% of plasma catecholamine bound to albumin at physiological catecholamine levels.[100–103] The physiological role of protein binding is unknown; catecholamines, unlike the steroid and thyroid hormones, are freely soluble in. water, and hence do not depend on protein-binding for transport in the aqueous phase of blood. It is possible that protein-binding contributes to the inactivation of circulating catecholamines.[103]

A considerable methodological problem with regard to measuring the low levels of catecholamines normally found in plasma still exists. Fluorescent assay, long the mainstay in the quantitative analysis of catecholamines, although it is quite adequate for urine, is generally pushed beyond the limits of usable sensitivity in the measurement of catecholamines in plasma. With meticulous attention to detail and a sizable sample of blood, quantitative results can occasionally be obtained.[104,105] In general, however, measurements of plasma catecholamines by fluorescent assay (particularly with fractionation into E and NE) should be regarded with considerable skepticism. To date, no radioimmunoassay or radioreceptor assay has been developed to the point of general usefulness.

An important advance in methodology was the application of isotope derivative techniques employing radiometric enzymatic assays.[98,106] Engelman *et al.*[98] first described an isotope derivative technique with sufficient sensitivity to measure NE and E in plasma accurately. This method involves the use of purified catechol-*O*-methyltransferase to catalyze the transfer of a ^{14}C-labeled methyl group from *S*-adenosylmethionine to the *m*-hydroxyl position of the catechol group (see Fig. 1), with the formation of ^{14}C-normetanephrine from plasma NE and ^{14}C-metanephrine from plasma E. The labeled metanephrines can be separated chromatographically and then oxidized to ^{14}C-vanillin, which is extracted and counted. This method has proved satisfactory in several laboratories for the precise estimation of plasma catecholamines, but it is technically exacting and, at present, remains a research tool available in only a few centers. The values given above for normal catecholamine levels in plasma were derived from this assay procedure. Another isotope derivative technique involves the use of phenylethanolamine-*N*-methyl transferase (see Fig. 1) and labeled *S*-adenosylmethionine. In this assay, labeled E is formed from plasma NE, and the labeled product is isolated chromatographically and extracted for counting.[93,107] This method is highly sensitive, but cannot be used for the measurement of E; as yet it has not been extensively used in studies involving patients.

The half-life of catecholamines in plasma is very brief. Although precise data in man are lacking, studies with tritiated catecholamines in experimental animals indicate that a bolus of catecholamines is cleared from plasma with a half-life of less than 1 min.[107] Clearance from plasma is via hepatic metabolism, renal excretion, uptake into sympathetic nerve endings throughout the body, and metabolism in the gut.[108]

The major drawbacks to the use of plasma catecholamines in the assessment of sympathoadrenal activity may thus be summarized as follows: (1) theoretical considerations relating to the adequacy of plasma NE as a measure of NE turnover at the sympathetic nerve endings; (2) the short half-life of catecholamines in plasma, which necessitates frequent sampling; (3) the episodic nature of catecholamine secretion; and (4) the technical difficulty of precise estimation in plasma. Nonetheless, plasma catecholamines have proved valuable in the assessment of sympathoadrenal activity, and the usefulness and applicability of plasma catecholamine measurements is certain to increase with continued improvement in methodology and the greater accessability of reliable assay methods to increasing numbers of investigators.

8.3.2.2. Urinary Catecholamines

Measurements of urinary free catecholamine levels have several advantages over measurements of plasma catecholamine levels, as well as several important disadvantages. The concentration of free catecholamines in urine is such that accurate determination by classic chromatographic and fluorescent techniques is within the grasp of most laboratories. Quantitative separation of E and NE is relatively easy, and the concentration of both amines in timed urine collections of 1–2 hr can be measured accurately.[100] Furthermore, measurement of catecholamines in urine provides an integrated assessment of catecholamine production over discrete periods of time, thereby significantly reducing the sampling error inherent in the measurement of a substance with a short half-life in plasma. A disadvantage of urinary catecholamine determinations is the lack of precise data in man pertaining to the renal mechanisms involved in catecholamine excretion. Studies with the isolated perfused rat kidney[110] indicate net tubular secretion of both E and NE, and a linear relationship between catecholamine clearance and plasma catecholamine levels. Whether or not these findings are applicable to man remains to be seen, but, on the basis of these studies, it seems likely that urinary catecholamines do, in fact, accurately reflect catecholamine levels in plasma. The isolated perfused kidney also demonstrates significant metabolism of catecholamines, particularly via O-methylation. Clearly, metabolism of catecholamines by the kidney with the excretion of catecholamine metabolites in the urine is a potential variable that may decrease the reliability of measurements of urinary catecholamines. Of even greater significance, it seems likely that subtle alterations in renal function may alter urinary catecholamine excretion; it is not completely clear that normalizing catecholamine values for creatinine would overcome this difficulty, although factoring by creatinine should be carried out in physiological studies in order to correct for changes in GFR.

Another serious theoretical objection to the use of urinary catecholamines in the assessment of sympathoadrenal activity is often raised. When labeled catecholamines are infused into patients or experimental animals, free catecholamines in urine constitute a small percentage of the infused dose. Thus, it is argued that since free catecholamines comprise only about 10% of an infused dose of catecholamines, a small change in metabolic disposition could have a large effect on the ultimate free catecholamine excretion. Despite the validity of this objection, the percentage of an infused dose of catecholamine recovered as free catecholamine in the urine is relatively constant,[32] and capricious or systematic changes in catecholamine metabolism have not been demonstrated. It should be further emphasized that urinary NE excretion is subject to the same theoretical limitations outlined above for plasma NE, objections that depend on the relative instability of the pool of circulating NE and the fact that levels do not directly reflect turnover at the sympathetic nerve endings. An additional objection to measuring urine catecholamines rather than catecholamines in plasma is that determination of urinary catecholamines may miss a transient increase in catecholamine secretion; such a short burst could easily be missed in the relatively large background of a timed urine sample. It should be emphasized, however, that very frequent sampling of blood would be necessary to detect such a transient increase in plasma catecholamines.

8.3.3. Dopamine-β-Hydroxylase Activity in Plasma— A Measure of Sympathetic Activity?

8.3.3.1. The Enzyme Dopamine-β-Hydroxylase (DBH)

Dopamine-β-hydroxylase (DBH) is the enzyme that catalyzes the formation of NE from dopamine by hydroxylating the β-position on the side chain. It is present only in those tissues that synthesize and store NE and E, namely, the peripheral sympathetic nerve endings, the adrenal medulla, and the noradrenergic neurons of the CNS. It is a copper-containing enzyme of mol. wt. approximately 290,000.[111] Unlike the other enzymes involved in catecholamine biosynthesis, which are located free in the cytosol, DBH is localized in the subcellular particles that store catecholamines. Thus, the enzyme can be recovered from the chromaffin granules of the adrenal medulla and the granulated vesicles of the sympathetic nerve endings.[112,113] In the catecholamine storage particles, DBH exists in both a bound and a free form; the bound form appears to be a structural component of the storage particle itself, while the free form represents soluble enzyme protein that is located in the granule in conjunction with the other soluble granule constituents. The soluble particle constituents include, in addition to catecholamines and DBH, ATP and a soluble, specific protein named chromogranin[114] (Fig. 3).

8.3.3.1a. Release of DBH by Exocytosis. Work from a number of laboratories over the last ten years[114–116] has shown that release of catecholamines from the adrenal medulla and the sympathetic nerve endings occurs by the process of exocytosis. In response to acetylcholine liberated from the preganglionic splanchnic nerves that innervate the adrenal medulla, or in reponse to a propagated action potential in the sympathetic nerve endings, the catecholamine storage particles fuse with the cell membrane, and the entire soluble contents of the storage vesicle are released (see Fig. 3). The soluble particle contents are released in stoichiometric amounts, and the effluent of stimulated tissues contains these constituents in the same proportions as are present in the soluble contents of the storage particles.[113,117]

8.3.3.1b. Assay of DBH in Blood. The development of a sensitive assay for DBH allowed Weinshilboum and Axelrod to demonstrate measurable DBH activity in human serum.[118] There are several ways of assaying DBH in blood. The two commonly employed methods of measuring DBH activity in serum or plasma depend on the β-hydroxylation of tyramine, an artificial substrate added to plasma or serum in excess, with the formation of octopamine (Fig. 4). The original method of Axelrod is a radiometric enzymatic isotope derivative technique that utilizes purified phenylethanolamine-N-methyl transferase (Fig. 1) to measure the octopamine (see Fig. 4) formed from tyramine by transferring a labeled methyl group from S-adenosylmethionine to the N-methyl group of octopamine, and extracting the labeled product.

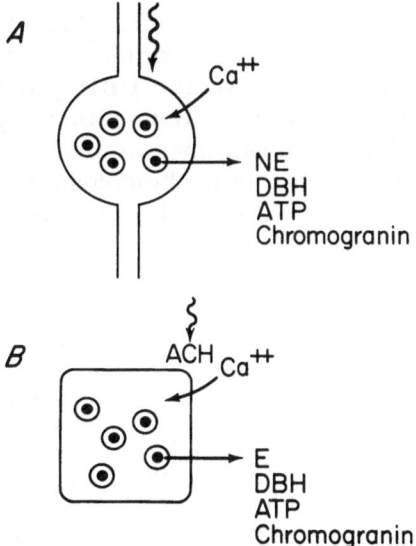

Fig. 3. Catecholamine release from the sympathetic nerve endings and adrenal medulla. Release of intragranular contents from (A) sympathetic nerve endings and (B) adrenal medullary chromaffin cell. The substituents are released in stoichiometric amounts, proportional to their concentration in the soluble portion of the storage particles.

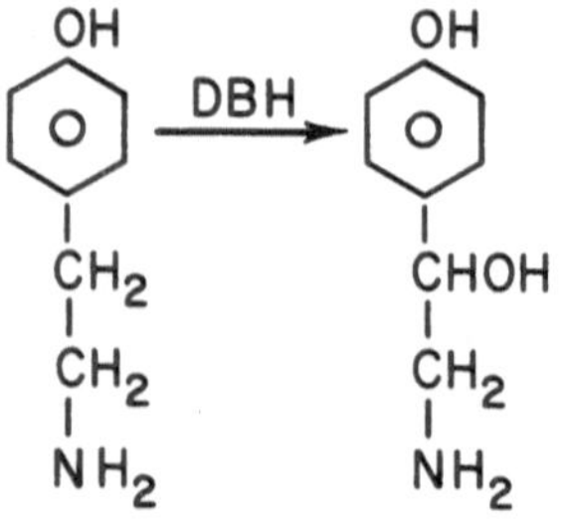

TYRAMINE   OCTOPAMINE

Fig. 4. Conversion of tyramine to octopamine by DBH. Assay of DBH activity in blood depends on the formation of octopamine from the artificial substrate tyramine. The octopamine formed can be measured by an isotope derivative technique utilizing phenylethanolamine-*N*-methyl transferase, or by a spectrophotometric technique after oxidation to *p*-hydroxybenzaldehyde.

This assay is cumbersome and subject to several theoretical[119] and methodological[120] problems; a simpler assay developed by Nagatsu and Udenfriend[119] also employs tyramine as an artificial substrate, but relies on the oxidation of the β-hydroxylated product (octopamine) to *p*-hydroxybenzaldehyde, which is determined spectrophotometrically. This assay is the one that has been most widely used in studies of DBH activity in blood in different pathophysiological states. In addition to assay of DBH activity in plasma, a radioimmunoassay for the DBH protein itself has been developed.[121,122] Although use of radioimmunoassay cast some initial doubts about the validity of using measurements of DBH activity in plasma,[123] more recent studies using homologous human DBH have shown a very close correlation between the measured enzyme protein by radioimmunoassay and the activity of DBH as measured by the spectrophotometric assay.[124]

The proportionate coupled release of DBH and catecholamines immediately raised hopes that the level of enzyme activity in blood might be a reasonable measure of sympathoadrenal activity. It was subsequently shown in a variety of studies in experimental animals that DBH in plasma originated in the sympathetic nerve endings, since adrenal demedullation had no appreciable affect on levels of the enzyme in plasma.[125] It was further shown that experimental maneuvers that increased sympathetic neuronal activity produced a significant increase in plasma DBH activity. For example, immobilization in rats, a maneuver known to increase NE turnover at the sympathetic nerve endings, resulted in a prompt and sustained increase in plasma DBH activity.[125] Stimulation of the splenic nerve of the cat caused release of both NE and DBH.[126] Studies with drugs supported the origin of DBH in sympathetic nerve endings. For example, treatment with 6-hydroxydopamine (an agent that destroys the sympathetic nerve endings) led to a significant reduction in plasma DBH activity.[127] Other agents, such as colchicine or vinblastine, that cause microtubular disaggregation and block the release of catecholamines in response to sympathetic nerve impulses decreased the release of DBH as well.[128] Calcium was shown to potentiate the release of both DBH and catecholamines in stimulated organ preparations *in vitro.*[111]

The initial studies in experimental animals thus supported the possible usefulness of measuring DBH activity in blood as a measure of sympathetic neuronal activity. This usefulness was further supported by the studies of Geffen and Rush,[121] which showed that DBH had a relatively long half-life in plasma, on the order of 3 hr, as compared with the very brief half-life of plasma catecholamines. DBH did not accumulate in adrenergically innervated tissues, suggesting that DBH is not subject to reuptake by the sympathetic nerve endings. All these studies indicated that measurement of DBH in blood might provide the elusive and long-sought measurement of sympathetic activity in man.

8.3.3.2. DBH Activity as a Measure of Sympathetic Activity

Unfortunately, the promise of DBH as an important measure of sympathetic activity has been largely unfulfilled. Although many of the studies in experimental animals quoted above showed concomitant alterations in plasma DBH activity and NE, the alterations in DBH levels were considerably smaller than corresponding alterations in NE release. Thus, in animals treated with 6-hydroxydopamine, despite impressive NE depletion from sympathetically innervated organs, plasma DBH fell only 25%[127]; similarly, in restraint or immobilization stress, plasma DBH levels increased only about 25%,[125] even though such maneuvers increase the turnover of NE at the sympathetic nerve endings manyfold. Furthermore, in isolated perfused organs, the release of NE is tightly coupled to sympathetic nerve stimulation, with almost no release during periods of nonstimulation. DBH, however, appears in the effluent or bath in relatively high concentrations in periods during which the nerves are not being stimulated, although stimulation does cause a further increase in DBH efflux.[128] Recent studies by Reid and Kopin[92,93] have shown that DBH levels in experimental animals reflect drug-induced changes in NE release rather poorly. Thus, phenoxybenzamine, an agent that markedly increases both NE turnover at the sympathetic nerve endings and plasma NE levels, had no effect on plasma DBH; on the other hand, ganglionic blockade, a maneuver that markedly diminished NE turnover, led to a prompt fall in plasma NE levels, but was without effect on plasma levels of

DBH. On the basis of these and other concomitant studies, Reid and Kopin[93] concluded that the level of DBH in blood reflects intraneuronal events other than release of NE by classic stimulus secretion coupling and exocytosis. It seems likely that much of plasma DBH activity results from the intraneuronal synthesis of the DBH enzyme and degradation of the intraneuronal storage vesicles of which DBH is a major component; only part of the DBH activity that reaches the plasma does so as a result of exocytosis, and therefore only a small proportion of the pool of circulating DBH reflects catecholamine release. These studies in experimental animals indicate that DBH may not be as sensitive an indicator of changes in sympathetic activity as previously thought.

Studies of DBH activity in man in general support the view that there is some correlation between DBH activity and sympathetic neuronal activity, but that the relationship is not direct. Thus, Wooten and Cardon[129] found that DBH activity increased significantly during exercise and during the cold pressor test, but the changes in DBH activity were small compared with the known changes in catecholamine metabolism that occur in these conditions. These authors were also unable to demonstrate any increase in DBH activity with tilting, a condition known to be associated with activation of the sympathetic nervous system. In a recent study,[94] plasma DBH levels correlated with plasma NE levels, and both were increased in response to maneuvers that activate the sympathetic nervous system, but the percentage change in plasma DBH activity was very much smaller than the change in plasma NE levels. Many of the reported studies of plasma DBH levels in humans have been done in patients with hypertension and hyperthyroidism; the results of studies in hyperthyroidism are described elsewhere (Section 8.4), but in general support the same conclusion. It is of additional interest that some patients appear to have a very low DBH level in their plasma, and evidence has been provided that a very low DBH level is inherited as an autosomal recessive trait.[130,131] Studies thus far, however, have not demonstrated any significant physiological correlates of this low DBH level.

In summary, it seems fair to say that plasma DBH levels do reflect sympathetic activity under certain conditions; there does seem to be, however, a large pool of DBH in plasma that gains access to the circulation by mechanisms other than exocytosis-induced release of catecholamines. Therefore, changes in DBH levels tend to be small compared with changes in plasma NE levels. It is also true that the normal range of DBH activity in human plasma is considerable[119]; studies involving sequential observations in a single subject are not affected by this variation, but studies of sympathetic activity involving mean values for groups of subjects compared one against the other are significantly limited by this factor. These disadvantages in DBH assay clearly offset the theoretical advantage resulting from the long plasma half-life of the enzyme and the absence of significant reuptake in the sympathetic nerve endings. It would seem from the available literature that plasma NE levels, despite their theoretical limitations, are a better indication of sympathetic neuronal activity than are plasma DBH levels. Pending the general availability of reliable methods for determining plasma catecholamine levels, however, DBH activity, which is relatively simple to assay, may provide some useful information about the functional state of the sympathetic nervous system.

8.4. Hyperthyroidism and the Sympathoadrenal System

Clinicians have puzzled over the role of the sympathoadrenal system in the pathogenesis of the clinical manifestations of hyperthyroidism for over 100 years. Infusions of catecholamines produce symptoms and signs similar to those observed in spontaneous hyperthyroidism: tachycardia, sweating, increased BMR, palpitations, tremor, and increase in cardiac contractility, all common manifestations of thyrotoxicosis, are reproduced by exogenous catecholamines or spontaneous activation of the sympathoadrenal system. Furthermore, some of the symptoms and signs of thyrotoxicosis are alleviated by adrenergic blocking agents that have no obvious effect on the production or metabolism of thyroid hormones. Therefore, physicians have long assumed that the hyperthyroid state either increases the activity of the sympathoadrenal system or increases the sensitivity of the cardiovascular system to the physiological effects of endogenous catecholamines. Neither of these presumed effects of hyperthyroidism has, however, been established; despite continued interest and investigation in this area. the participation of catecholamines in the clinical picture of thyrotoxicosis is not clearly established, and the relationship between the thyroid hormones and catecholamines, and between the sympathoadrenal system and clinical hyperthyroidism, remains uncertain.

Recent studies have clearly shown that the thyroid follicles are innervated with sympathetic nerve endings,[132-136] and catecholamines have been shown experimentally to increase the biosynthesis[132,137-139] and release of thyroid hormones[140-142] by a beta receptor mechanism.[143,144] There is no evidence, however, that the sympathetic nervous system is involved in the initiation or the maintenance of enhanced thyroid hormone output in hyperthyroidism. Most recent investigations have therefore centered around the effect of thyroid hormones on catecholamine metabolism and the effect of thyroid hormones on the sensitivity to catecholamines.

8.4.1. Effect of Thyroid Hormones on Catecholamine Biosynthesis, Metabolism, and Excretion

The effect of thyroid hormones on catecholamine metabolism in experimental animals and man has been well studied over the last ten years. There is uniform agreement that the sympathoadrenal system is not overactive in hyperthyroidism. Studies of NE biosynthesis and turnover in the hearts of experimental animals have clearly established that experimental hyperthyroidism is associated with normal or diminished sympathetic nervous activity,[145,146] and, conversely, that experimental thyroid deficiency is associated with a marked increase in sympathetic neuronal activity to the heart and other organs.[147,148] Urinary NE excretion is normal or low in patients with hyperthyroidism, and normal or increased in hypothyroid subjects.[149-151] The excretion of catecholamine metabolites (VMA and metanephrines) is not altered in hyperthyroidism.[150] Plasma NE levels are likewise low or normal in hyperthyroidism, and significantly increased in hypothyroidism.[152-154] Plasma DBH activity is decreased in hyperthyroidism,[155,156] and increased in hypothyroidism,[155] with normalization after treatment.[156] The urinary excretion of E is unchanged in hypo- or hyperthyroidism,[150,151] and plasma E levels are not significantly altered.[153] The clearance and secretion rates of E are not significantly altered in hyper- or hypothyroidism.[157]

The evidence thus clearly indicates that hyperthyroidism is not associated with increased endogenous production of catecholamines. Adrenal secretion of E is unaffected by thyroid status. The sympathetic nervous system is, if anything, suppressed by hyperthyroidism, while the hypothyroid state is clearly associated with increased sympathetic activity.

8.4.2. Effect of Thyroid Hormones on Sensitivity to Catecholamines

Catecholamine responses are generally held to be potentiated by thyroid hormone excess and diminished by thyroid hormone deficiency. Unfortunately, the literature in this area is complex and confusing. It seems clear that thyroid hormones have direct effects on the heart that resemble those of catecholamines; it appears that these effects may be additive with those of catecholamines; whether thyroid hormones enhance the responsiveness of the cardiovascular system to catecholamines remains uncertain. The evidence that catecholamines enhance certain metabolic and calorigenic effects of catecholamines appears to be on firmer ground.

8.4.2.1. Thyroid Hormones and the Cardiovascular Effects of Catecholamines

8.4.2.1a. Direct Effect of Thyroid Hormones on Cardiac Contractility and Heart Rate. Studies in a variety of experimental animals and man indicate that thyroid hormones increase cardiac contractility and heart rate. The cardiac effects of thyroid hormones, although they are similar to those of catecholamines, are not mediated by the sympathoadrenal system. That the positive chronotropic effect of thyroid is independent of catecholamines has been demonstrated in a number of ways. Explanted fragments of chick embryo cardiac muscle in tissue culture[158] and fetal mouse hearts maintained in organ culture[159] beat more rapidly when exposed to thyroid hormones under conditions in which the sympathetic innervation is not likely to be functional. Rats and mice with sympathetic nervous system and adrenal medulla completely ablated by a combination of chemical, immunological, and surgical techniques increase their heart rates when treated with T_4 or T_3 to the same extent as do animals with sympathetic nervous system intact.[160] Isolated rat hearts beat more rapidly when exposed to varying doses of thyroid hormones *in vitro.*[161] Studies with autonomic blocking agents in both animals[162] and patients[163] have also shown a direct effect of thyroid hormone on heart rate independent of autonomic influences.

Similarly, thyroid hormones have been shown to enhance myocardial contractility directly, without the intervention of the sympathetic nervous system, in both isolated cat papillary muscles[164] and intact dogs.[165] Studies with β-blockers in hyperthyroid patients have also indicated increased cardiac contractility independent of adrenergic activity.[166] Interestingly enough, though the direct effects of thyroid hormones on the heart resemble those of catecholamines, the effect of thyroid hormones on the peripheral vasculature is quite different; in hyperthyroidism, peripheral vasodilation occurs, with a marked lowering of the total peripheral resistance,[167] although the vasodilation may be secondary to changes in tissue metabolism.

The mode of action of thyroid hormone in increasing heart rate and myocardial contractility is uncertain. It has been demonstrated that thyroid hormones activate adenylate cyclase when added *in vitro* to homogenates of cat heart; cyclase activation by thyroid hormones in this *in vitro* system is not blocked by β-blockers, and is additive with the activation produced by NE.[168] The importance of myocardial adenylate cyclase as a mediator of the effects of thyroid hormone on heart rate and contractility is, however, seriously in question. The hearts of animals made hyperthyroid by exogenous thyroxine do not differ from those of euthyroid controls in adenylate cyclase activity or in the activation of adenylate cyclase by NE[169–171]; the dose–response curve for cardiac contractility and adenylate cyclase activation is identical in both hyperthyroid and euthyroid animals.[170] Furthermore, hearts of rats pretreated with triiodothyronine do not have increased levels of cAMP,[171] and respond normally to catecholamines with respect to both contractility and the accumulation of cAMP.[172] Thus, there is very little evidence that adenylate cyclase activation mediates the increase in cardiac contractility or heart rate induced by thyroid hormones.

8.4.2.1b. Sensitivity of the Cardiovascular System to Catecholamines in Relation to Thyroid Status—Studies in Experimental Animals. Many studies over the last 50 years have been said to show an increase in the sensitivity of the heart and vasculature to catecholamines in the presence of thyroid hormone excess.[173] In general, these investigations have shown that the heart rate response to catecholamines is more marked in hyperthyroid than in normal animals.[174–178] Other studies have shown that tolerance to the toxic effects of catecholamines is decreased by thyroid hormone administration and increased by antithyroid drugs.[179,180] It is doubtful, however, that these studies have adequately confronted the question of sensitivity to catecholamines. A change in sensitivity should be associated with a shift to the left in the dose–response relationship, and with a significant decrease in either the threshold concentration or the concentration necessary to produce half-maximal activity.[181] The oft-quoted studies do not fulfill these criteria. Several recent studies, however, designed specifically to answer the question of sensitivity, have provided evidence that hyperthyroidism in the experimental animal does not alter the responsiveness of the cardiovascular system to catecholamines.[162,182–185] These studies have been performed in rats, rabbits, and dogs; taken as a group, they provide convincing evidence that experimental hyperthyroidism does not alter the sensitivity of the cardiovascular system to infused catecholamines or sympathetic nerve stimulation. In these studies, dose–response relationships for catecholamine-induced changes in heart rate, blood pressure, and vascular or cardiac contractility were examined; there was no significant displacement of the dose–response curve in thyroid hormone–treated animals. In one of the studies,[185] denervation with 6-hydroxy-dopamine clearly produced the expected shift in the dose–response relationship toward increased sensitivity to catecholamines, while thyroxine was without effect on the dose–response curve.

    Two recent studies have, however, demonstrated a significant shift in the dose–response curve in relation to a change in thyroid status.[186,187] Isolated aortic rings from hyperthyroid rats were shown to develop a greater isometric tension at a given NE concentration than did rings from normal rats, while the converse was true in aortic rings from hypothyroid animals.[186] Similarly, the isolated fetal mouse heart in organ culture has been demonstrated to beat faster at a given NE concentration after incubation *in vitro* with triiodothyronine.[187] Furthermore, increased binding of ^{3}H-NE to a subcellular particulate fraction of rat heart thought to contain the β-adrenergic receptor has been demonstrated in hearts from hyperthyroid animals.[188] This study provides a possible mechanism for increased sensitivity to catecholamines in hyperthyroidism. However, as described above, the majority of recent studies have not found a significant change in the dose–response relationship between catecholamines and cardiovascular activation as a function of either thyroid hormone excess or deficiency. The reason for conflicting results is not clear, although differences in experimental techniques, which are difficult to evaluate at a distance, probably contribute to the confusion.

Other studies that purport to demonstrate an effect of thyroid hormone on sensitivity to catecholamines can be questioned with regard to the specificity of the effect observed.[189] In a study of several isolated tissues from rats and guinea pigs, thyroxine pretreatment was noted to increase the sensitivity of the isolated perfused heart to catecholamines; while NE and E produced a greater rise in heart rate in thyroxine-pretreated animals than in normal controls, acetylcholine produced a significantly greater decrease.[189] In the same study, the contractility of isolated aortic strips was studied, and thyroxine pretreatment was found to decrease contractility in response to NE and E, as well as to histamine and 5-HT. It thus appears possible that some of the reported effects of thyroxine on catecholamine sensitivity may be nonspecific, rather than selective.

It is worth noting one additional area that needs further study. An interesting body of literature is developing that suggests hypothyroidism is associated with a change in the normal balance of alpha and beta receptors.[190] Thus, rat atria, rabbit aorta, and rat tail artery from hypothyroid animals respond with an increase in sensitivity to alpha receptor agonists, and with a decrease in responsiveness to beta receptor stimulation.[190–193] It has been postulated that in hypothyroidism, the balance of alpha and beta receptors in different tissues may change in favor of the alpha receptor, and that this interconversion may be a thyroid-induced allosteric change in a single adrenergic receptor.[190] This hypothesis is substantiated by the fact that atria from hypothyroid rats have been demonstrated to bind more labeled phenoxybenzamine than do atria from euthyroid control animals,[190] suggesting an increase in the number of alpha receptors. The converse, i.e., augmentation or recruitment of beta receptors in the presence of hyperthyroidism, has apparently not been demonstrated. Augmentation in the number of beta receptors by recruitment of alpha receptors or undifferentiated adrenergic receptors in the presence of increased thyroid hormone should result in enhanced β-adrenergic sensitivity in the presence of hyperthyroidism; as indicated above, such enhanced sensitivity has not been uniformly or reproducibly demonstrated. Nonetheless, this intriguing hypothesis deserves further work, and may explain some of the observed changes in sensitivity to catecholamines in hypo- and hyperthyroid states.

In summary, while the studies in experimental animals do not exclude the possibility of an effect of thyroid hormone on sensitivity to catecholamines, the available evidence favors the conclusion that experimental hyperthyroidism is not associated with enhanced reactivity of the heart and vasculature to catecholamines. It should be noted, moreover, that even if increased sensitivity to catecholamines resulted in enhanced adrenergic responses, the latter should be transient rather than sustained. Reflex suppression of the sympathoadrenal outflow would be the expected result of enhanced adrenergic responses, unless other, undefined factors related to the hyperthyroid state alter the suppressibility of the sympathoadrenal system. The possibility of an effect of thyroid hormones to inhibit an appropriate reduction in central sympathetic outflow needs to be considered.

8.4.2.1c. Cardiovascular Responses to Catecholamines in Thyrotoxic Patients. Several widely quoted studies in patients have purported to show an enhanced effect of catecholamines on heart rate and blood pressure in the presence of hyperthyroidism,[194–196] with restoration of normal responsiveness after treatment.[195] More recent studies, however, both in normal persons made hyperthyroid with triiodothyronine and in patients with spontaneous hyperthyroidism before and after treatment,[197,198] have not confirmed these earlier works: a variety of hemodynamic responses to varying doses of both E and NE were noted to be similar in the euthyroid and hyperthyroid state. The reason for the differences between the early[194–196] and more recent studies[197,198] is not clear, and the question of increased cardiovascular responsiveness in hyperthyroid patients is still unanswered.

8.4.2.2. Metabolic and Calorigenic Effects of Catecholamines in Relation to Thyroid Status

The metabolic effects of catecholamines, in distinction to the cardiovascular effects, appear to vary with the level of thyroid hormone.[199]

There is sound evidence that thyroid hormones and catecholamines are synergistic in their effects on lipolysis, glycogenolysis in heart, and non-shivering thermogenesis. Thus, catecholamine-stimulated lipolysis is enhanced *in vitro* in fat pads of hyperthyroid animals.[200] These studies clearly show a leftward displacement of the dose–response relationship between catecholamines and lipolysis in thyroid-treated animals. Lipolysis induced by E is decreased in isolated fat cells from hypothyroid rats,[201] and markedly diminished in fat cells of hypothyroid patients.[202] Adenylate cyclase and cAMP appear to be involved in catecholamine-stimulated lipolysis, and increased adenylate cyclase levels in the adipose tissue of thyroid-pretreated rats has been reported,[203] but the precise effect of thyroid hormone on this system is not known. Similarly, catecholamines are necessary for the normal activation of cardiac phosphorylase A by thyroid hormones,[160,204] and thyroid pretreatment potentiates catechola-mine activation of this enzyme.[205] The role of adenylate cyclase in this system is uncertain.[206] Recent studies in hyperthyroid patients indicate that infusions of E cause a greater rise in urinary and plasma cAMP levels than in euthyroid controls, and that this epinephrine-induced cAMP rise is blunted by propranolol.[207,208] Hypothyroid patients, by contrast, show no rise in plasma cAMP in response to E. The origin of the cAMP appearing in the urine and plasma in these studies is not known. This finding is not specific for E, since both glucagon and parathormone induce a greater rise in plasma cAMP in hyperthyroid patients than in euthyroid or hypothyroid subjects.[208] Further studies are required to determine the significance of these changes in plasma cAMP.

Finally, a substantial body of evidence indicates that cold acclimatiza-tion and the generation of heat from nonshivering thermogenesis involves an interaction of thyroid hormones and catecholamines.[209–211] For example, in the newborn mouse, thyroxine pretreatment is needed for a full calorigenic effect of NE.[212,213] In adult rats, pretreatment with both thyroxine and catecholamines is necessary if normal animals are to approach cold-acclimatized animals in their response to cold stress.[214]

Synergism between catecholamines and thyroid hormones may thus explain, in part, the increased free fatty acid turnover, and increased heat production characteristic of the hyperthyroid state.

8.4.3. Adrenergic Blocking Agents in the Treatment of Hyperthyroidism

8.4.3.1. The Choice of an Antiadrenergic Agent

Reserpine, guanethidine, and propranolol have all been shown to block some of the manifestations of thyrotoxicosis, and these agents have proved useful in the management of certain patients with hyperthyroidism. The mechanism of action of these antiadrenergic agents is different: reserpine depletes catecholamines in the CNS and peripheral sympathetic nerve endings, thereby reducing both central sympathetic outflow and release of neurotransmitter from the peripheral nerve endings; guanethidine is a neuron-blocking agent that prevents the release of NE from the peripheral sympathetic nerve endings without any effect on the CNS; propranolol selectively blocks the beta receptors in peripheral tissues and the CNS. Although propranolol possesses, in addition to its β-blocking properties, a significant membrane-stabilizing effect similar to that of local anesthetic agents, it is clear that the beneficial effects of propranolol in hyperthyroidism are due predominatly to its β-blocking properties, since (1) the d-isomer of propranolol, which is without β-blocking effect (but which possesses the membrane-stabilizing properties), is less effective than propanolol in reducing the sympathomimetic features of hyperthyroidism[215]; and (2) other β-blocking agents (which have no membrane stabilizing effect) are as effective as propranolol.[166]

Propranolol is clearly the adrenergic blocking agent of choice in the treatment of hyperthyroidism. Although reserpine is of established clinical benefit in the treatment of severe thyrotoxicosis or thyroid storm,[216] the usefulness of this agent is limited by severe side effects (mental depression, gastrointestinal hemorrhage), pronounced sedation, slow onset, and long duration of action. It is still used in those cases in which the sedative effect is desirable, as when marked agitation accompanies severe thyrotoxicosis. Guanethidine has demonstrated effectiveness in the treatment of patients with moderate to severe thyrotoxicosis,[216-218] but its clinical usefulness is limited by the slow onset and long duration of its actions and the side effects associated with marked sympathetic blockade, particularly orthostatic hypotension. Propranolol has a relatively rapid onset and short duration of action, and a low incidence of side effects. It is the agent that has been used most extensively in the symptomatic modification of hyperthyroidism, and is the drug of first choice when the clinical situation requires the use of an antiadrenergic agent.[219-224] The major side effects of propranolol, when it is used in the doses required for severe thyrotoxicosis or thyroid storm, include: exacerabation of heart failure, due to the negative inotropic effect resulting from the removal of sympathetic reinforcement; bronchospasm in asthmatic patients or patients with chronic lung disease; and hypoglycemic reactions in insulin-requiring diabetics. These potential adverse reactions should be anticipated in predisposed subjects.

Some workers have cautioned that the reduction of cardiac output following adrenergic blockade in hyperthyroidism may be associated with a significant decrease in tissue perfusion and the attendant risk of tissue anoxia.[166] The increase in cardiac output in hyperthyroidism, however, is far in excess of the increase in O_2 consumption,[167] and untoward effects on tissue perfusion have rarely been noted clinically.

8.4.3.2. Effects of Adrenergic Blocking Agents in Hyperthyroidism

The effects of adrenergic blocking agents on the clinical and hemodynamic manifestations of spontaneous and experimentally induced thyrotoxicosis have been extensively studied (Table III). There is general agreement that adrenergic blockade does not alter thyroid function tests, as reflected in the plasma level of thyroid hormones or the thyroid uptake of[131]I. The BMR is often reduced by adrenergic blockade, although not to normal levels.[217,225] Oxygen consumption and weight loss are not returned to normal, although improvement has been noted in some studies.[222,224-227] Improvement in negative nitrogen balance (although not to normal levels) has recently been reported[227]; the increased loss of urinary calcium, phosphorus, and hydroxyproline in hyperthyroidism is not, however, affected by adrenergic blockade,[227] although in 2 cases, propranolol administration reversed hypercalcemia by a mechanism independent of PTH.[228] Tremor, hyperreflexia, widened palpebral fissure, and excessive sweating are improved significantly by adrenergic blocking

Table III.   Effects of Adrenergic Blockade in Hyperthyroidism

Predictability of effect	Symptom	Sign or laboratory
Beneficial effect usually achieved	Pulse Tremor Nervousness Sweating	Palpitation Pulse pressure Hyperreflexia Widened palpebral fissure Urinary nitrogen loss[a] Elevated serum calcium[a]
Less regularly beneficial or partial response only	Heat intolerance	Myocardial contractility Weight loss Oxygen consumption BMR Skin temperature
No effect	—	Calcium excretion[a] Hydroxyproline excretion[a] Plasma T_4 ^{131}I uptake

[a]Recently reported; needs confirmation.

agents, but skin temperature and heat intolerance are less regularly improved.[220,222,224,229,230]

The hemodynamic effects of adrenergic blockade in thyrotoxicosis have been well studied,[166,215,231-234] and most studies—but not all[231,232]—show a significant decrease in heart rate, pulse pressure, systolic blood pressure, and cardiac output with prolongation of the circulation time. The heightened myocardial contractility of hyperthyroidism is not restored to normal.[166,234]

8.4.3.3. Clinical Usefulness of Adrenergic Blocking Agents in Thyrotoxicosis

Because adrenergic blocking agents control some of the manifestations of thyrotoxicosis, they have been used in a number of circumstances in the management of patients with hyperthyroidism. It is important to emphasize that the use of adrenergic blocking agents in the treatment of thyrotoxicosis is clearly secondary to the usual forms of treatment that diminish thyroid hormone production. Adrenergic blocking agents do not modify the underlying disease process; they produce only symptomatic improvement, and should be regarded as adjuncts to the conventional forms of definitive treatment (i.e., either thyroid ablation by radioactive iodine or surgery or a prolonged course of a thionamide). Adrenergic blocking agents should not be substituted for thionamides as a form of medical treatment, since symptomatic control is incomplete with adrenergic blockade alone,[222] and the metabolic parameters of the disease are not corrected,[227] with potential long-term detriment. Despite the caveats, adrenergic blocking agents have been widely used in a number of clinical situations, and have significantly improved the management of the thyrotoxic patient,[235] but always as an adjunct to some form of definitive treatment. Experience with adrenergic blocking agents has been accumulated in the following clinical situations.

a. In *thyroid storm* or *severe thyrotoxicosis*,[218,221,223] the clinical benefit from adrenergic blocking agents is often striking and occasionally lifesaving. Adrenergic blocking agents may be expected to control the tachycardia (sinus or supraventricular), decrease pulse pressure, prolong circulation time, and increase cardiac output; congestive heart failure or pulmonary edema may actually be improved, despite the negative inotropic effect, because of the reduction in pulse rate and reduction in the high output state.

Reserpine,[216] guanethidine,[218] and propranolol[221,223] have demonstrated efficacy in severe thyrotoxicosis. Reserpine, in doses of 2–5 mg i.m. every 4–6 hr; guanethidine, 50–150 mg p.o./day; or propranolol, 40–80 mg p.o. every 6 hr, or 1 mg i.v. p.r.n., all produce striking improvement in the patient with severe thyrotoxicosis or thyroid storm. Propranolol is generally the most useful agent because of its rapid onset and short duration of action. The dose of propranolol should be titrated to control the tachycardia and the manifestations of hyperdynamic circulation. Reserpine should be reserved for those patients in whom sedation is desirable, and guanethidine for those in whom a long duration of action is required. The adrenergic blocking drugs will buy time while the other measures aimed specifically at reducing serum thyroid hormone levels become effective.

   b. In patients with *mild to moderate thyrotoxicosis,* in whom the tachycardia, palpitations, heat intolerance, sweating, nervousness, and irritability are troublesome, propranolol may be of distinct clinical benefit.[220] Patients in this category do not warrant the use of reserpine or guanethidine. Many patients will respond to a dose of propranolol as low as 10 mg q.i.d.; the dose can be titrated upward as needed. The propranolol may be continued until the effects of the definitive therapy have resulted in reduction of the circulating level of thyroid hormone. Thus, in patients being treated primarily with a thionamide, propranolol may be continued for the first 4–6 weeks of treatment, and then gradually reduced as the euthyroid state is achieved. In patients treated with ^{131}I, propranolol, either alone or in combination with inorganic iodide, may maintain the hyperthyroid patient in a reasonable clinical state while awaiting the full effects of ^{131}I treatment to develop.[236]

   c. In patients *incompletely prepared for surgery or* [131]*I therapy,* or who are *allergic to thionamides,* propranolol is an important adjunct of medical management. Hyperthyroid patients who require emergency surgery and who are still thyrotoxic may be managed through the operative period by a regimen of propranolol and Lugol's solution.[237,238] Similarly, patients who require ^{131}I treatment at a time when they are still thyrotoxic may be treated with propranolol; this treatment reduces the symptoms that may be associated with any radiation thyroiditis that accompanies the ^{131}I treatment. In patients with cardiac disease, treatment with propranolol is an especially important adjunct around the time of administration of ^{131}I, since these patients are likely to be more sensitive to the release of thyroid hormones, and are at greater risk of suffering an attack of coronary insufficiency or developing an arrhythmia.

   d. In *pregnant women* who develop hyperthyroidism, the use of propranolol has been tentatively suggested. In a recently reported series,[239] 4 thyrotoxic pregnant women were treated with doses of propranolol between 80 and 240 mg/day. The hyperthyroidism was well controlled in all, and no adverse effects on either the course of labor or the fetus were noted. Before propranolol can be recommended as routine treatment in pregnant women with hyperthyroidism, however, further studies are necessary to confirm that propranolol does not interfere with normal labor and delivery, and has no adverse effects on the fetus. Propranolol may, however, be an important adjunct in the treatment of hyperthyroidism in pregnancy in the future, if its safety can be confirmed.

8.4.3.4. An Open Question: Why Are Adrenergic Blocking Agents Efficacious in the Symptomatic Treatment of Hyperthyroidism?

Since catecholamine production is not increased in hyperthyroidism, and since it is not likely that hyperthyroidism significantly enhances the effects of catecholamines on peripheral tissues, it is not at all clear why adrenergic blockade results in suppression of some of the manifestations of the hyperthyroid state. Indeed, it is not possible to answer this question with certainty at present. It seems likely, that in hyperthyroidism, the effects of catecholamines and thyroid hormones are additive; both increase heart rate, enhance myocardial contractility, stimulate lipolysis, and induce nonshivering thermogenesis. It is possible that the level of sympathoadrenal activity in hyperthyroidism, although clearly within the normal range, is inappropriately high, given the circulatory and metabolic state of the hyperthyroid individual. This view implies a failure of the sympathoadrenal system to suppress normally in hyperthyroidism. It remains to be demonstrated, however, that supressibility of the sympathoadrenal system is actually impaired in hyperthyroidism.

References

1. Winkler, H., and Smith, A. D., 1972, Pheochromocytoma and other catecholamine producing tumors, *in: Catecholamines, Handbook of Experimental Pharmacology* (H. Blaschko and E. Muscholl, eds.), pp. 900–933, Springer-Verlag, Berlin.
2. Carman, C. T., and Brashear, R. E., 1960, Pheochromocytoma as an inherited abnormality, *N. Engl. J. Med.* **263:**419–423.
3. Hermann, H., and Mornex, R., 1964, *Human Tumors Secreting Catecholamines*, The Macmillan Co., New York.
4. Steiner, A. L., Goodman, A. D., and Powers, S. R., 1968, Study of a kindred with pheochromocytoma, medullary thyroid carcinoma, hyperparathyroidism and Cushing's disease: Multiple endocrine neoplasia, type 2, *Medicine* **47:**371–409.
5. Ljungberg, O., 1972, On medullary carcinoma of the thyroid, *Acta Pathol. Microbiol. Scand. Sect. A Suppl.* **231:**1–56.
6. Melvin, K. E. W., Tashjian, A. H., Jr., and Miller, H. H., 1972, Studies in familial (medullary) thyroid carcinoma, *Recent Prog. Horm. Res.* **28:**399–470.

7. Hamilton. B. P. M., Landsberg, L., Levine, R. J., and Tashjian, A. H., Jr., 1973, Sipple's syndrome: Results of screening a large family, *Clin. Res.* **21:**979.
8. Wermer, P., 1954, Genetic aspects of adenomatosis of endocrine glands, *Amer. J. Med.* **16:**363–371.
9. Wermer, P., 1963, Endocrine adenomatosis and peptic ulcer in a large kindred, *Amer. J. Med.* **35:**205–212.
10. Ballard, H. S., Frame, B., and Hartsock, R. J., 1964, Familial multiple-endocrine adenoma–peptic ulcer complex, *Medicine* **43:**481–516.
11. Williams, E. D., and Celestin, L. R., 1962, The association of bronchial carcinoid and pluriglandular adenomatosis, *Thorax* **17:**120–127.
12. Snyder, N., III, Scurry, M. T., and Deiss, W. P., Jr., 1972, Five families with multiple endocrine adenomatosis, *Ann. Intern. Med.* **76:**53–58.
13. Synder, N., Scurry, M., and Hughes, W., 1974, Hypergastrinemia in familial multiple endocrine adenomatosis, *Ann. Intern. Med.* **80:**321–325.
14. Samaan, N. A., Hickey, R. C., Bedner, T. D., and Ibanez, M. L., 1975, Hyperparathyroidism and carcinoid tumor, *Ann. Intern. Med.* **82:**205–207.
15. Das Gupta, T. K., and Brasfield, R. D., 1971, Von Recklinghausen's disease, *CA* **21:**174–183.
16. Glushien, A. S., Mansuy, M. M., and Littman, D. S., 1953, Pheochromocytoma: Its relationship to the neurocutaneous syndromes, *Amer. J. Med.* **14:**318–327.
17. Sipple, J. H., 1961, The association of pheochromocytoma with carcinoma of the thyroid gland, *Amer. J. Med.* **31:**163–166.
18. Cushman, P., Jr., 1962, Familial endocrine tumors: Report of two unrelated kindred affected with pheochromocytomas, one also with multiple thyroid carcinomas, *Amer. J. Med.* **32:**352–360.
19. Nourok, D. S., 1964, Familial pheochromocytoma and thyroid carcinoma, *Ann. Intern. Med.* **60:**1028–1040.
20. Schimke, R. N., and Hartmann, W. H., 1965, Familial amyloid-producing medullary thyroid carcinoma and pheochromocytoma, *Ann. Intern. Med.* **63:**1027–1039.
21. Sapira, J. D., Altman, M., Vandyk, K., and Shapiro, A. P., 1965, Bilateral adrenal pheochromocytoma and medullary thyroid carcinoma, *N. Engl. J. Med.* **273:**140–143.
22. Williams, E. D., Brown, C. L., and Doniach, I., 1966, Pathological and clinical findings in a series of 67 cases of medullary carcinoma of the thyroid, *J. Clin. Pathol.* **19:**103–113.
23. Manning, P. C., Jr., Molnar, G. D., Black, B. M., Priestly, J. T., and Woolner, L. B., 1963, Pheochromocytoma, hyperparathyroidism, and thyroid carcinoma occurring coincidentally: Report of case, *N. Engl. J. Med.* **268:**68–72.
24. Sarosi, G., and Doe, R. P., 1968, Familial occurence of parathyroid adenomas, pheochromocytoma, and medullary carcinoma of the thyroid with amyloid stroma (Sipple's syndrome), *Ann. Intern. Med.* **68:**1305–1309.
25. Williams, E. D., 1966, Histogenesis of medullary carcinoma of the thyroid, *J. Clin. Pathol.* **19:**114–118.
26. Tashjian, A. H., Jr., and Melvin, K. E. W., 1968, Medullary carcinoma of the thyroid gland: Studies of thyrocalcitonin in plasma and tumor extracts, *N. Engl. J. Med.* **279:**279–283.
27. Dubé, W. J., Bell, G. O., and Aliapoulios, M. A., 1969, Thyrocalcitonin activity in metastatic medullary thyroid carcinoma: Further evidence of its parafollicular cell origin, *Arch. Intern. Med.* **123:**423–427.

28. Tashjian, A. H., Jr., Howland, B. G., Melvin, K. E. W., and Stratton Hill, C., Jr., 1970, Immunoassay of human calcitonin: Clinical measurement, relationship to serum calcium and studies in patients with medullary carcinoma, *N. Engl. J. Med.* **283:**890–895.
29. Melvin, K. E. W., Miller, H. H., and Tashjian, A. H., Jr., 1971, Early diagnosis of medullary carcinoma of the thyroid gland by means of calcitonin assay, *N. Engl. J. Med.* **285:**1115–1120.
30. Jackson, C. E., Tashjian, A. H., Jr., and Block, M. A., 1973, Detection of medullary thyroid cancer by calcitonin assay in families, *Ann. Intern. Med.* **78:**845–852.
31. Goltzman, D., Potts, J. T., Jr., Ridgway, E. C., and Maloof, F., 1974, Calcitonin as a tumor marker: Use of the radioimmunoassay for calcitonin in the postoperative evaluation of patients with medullary thyroid carcinoma, *N. Engl. J. Med.* **290:**1035–1039.
32. Levine, R. J., and Landsberg, L., 1974, Catecholamines and the adrenal medulla, in: *Duncan's Diseases of Metabolism* (P. K. Bondy and L. E. Rosenberg, eds.), pp. 1181–1224, W. B. Saunders Co., Philadelphia.
33. Carney, J. A., Sizemore, G. W., Tyce, G. M., 1975, Bilateral adrenal medullary hyperplasia in multiple endocrine neoplasia, type 2: The precursor of bilateral pheochromocytoma, *Mayo Clin. Proc.* **50:**3–10.
34. Marks, A. D., and Channick, B. J., 1974, Extra-adrenal pheochromocytoma and medullary thyroid carcinoma with pheochromocytoma, *Arch. Intern. Med.* **134:**1106–1109.
35. Roth, R. H. Stjänne, L., Levine, R. J., and Giarman, N. J., 1968, Abnormal regulation of catecholamine synthesis in pheochromocytoma, *J. Lab. Clin. Med.* **72:**397–403.
36. Nagatsu, T., Yamamoto, T., and Nagatsu, I., 1970, Partial separation and properties of tyrosine hydroxylase from the human pheochromocytoma: Effect of norepinephrine, *Biochim. Biophys. Acta* **198:**210–218.
37. Waymire, J. C., Weiner, N., Schneider, F. H., Goldstein, M., and Freedman, L. S., 1972, Tyrosine hydroxylase in human adrenal and pheochromocytoma: Localization, kinetics, and catecholamine inhibition, *J. Clin. Invest.* **51:**1798–1804.
38. Engelman, K., and Sjoerdsma, A., 1971, The adrenal medulla: Catecholamines and pheochromocytoma, in: *Clinician—1*, pp. 111–125, Medcom, New York.
39. Hamilton, B. P. M., Landsberg, L., and Levine, R. J., 1974, Sipple's syndrome: Familial medullary carcinoma of the thyroid, hyperparathyroidism and epinephrine-secreting pheochromocytoma, *Endocrinology Suppl.:* A-244.
40. Chong, G. C., Beahrs, O. H., Sizemore, G. W., and Woolner, L. H., 1975, Medullary carcinoma of the thyroid gland, *Cancer* **35:**695–704.
41. Khairi, M. R. A., Dexter, R. N., Burzynski, N. J., and Johnston, C. C., 1975, Mucosal neuroma, pheochromocytoma and medullary thyroid carcinoma: Multiple endocrine neoplasia type 3, *Medicine* **54:**89–112.
42. Cervi-Skinner, S. J., 1973, Case records of the Massachusetts General Hospital, *N. Engl. J. Med.* **289:**472–479.
43. Sjoerdsma, A., Engelman, K., Waldmann, T. A., Cooperman, L. H., and Hammond, W. G., 1966, Pheochromocytoma: Current concepts of diagnosis and treatment, *Ann. Intern. Med.* **65:**1302–1326.
44. Engelman, K., and Hammond, W. G., 1968, Adrenaline production by an intrathoracic pheochromocytoma, *Lancet* **1:**609–611.

45. Sheps, S. G., and Maher, F. T., 1968, Histamine and glucagon tests in diagnosis of pheochromocytoma, *J. Amer. Med. Assoc.* **205:**895–899.
46. Levey, G. S. Weiss, S. R., and Ruiz, E., 1975, Characterization of the glucagon receptor in a pheochromocytoma, *J. Clin. Endocrinol. Metab.* **40:**720–723.
47. Siqueira-Filho, A. G., Sheps, S. G., Mahler, F. T., Jiang, N. S., and Elveback, L. R., 1975, Glucagon-blood catecholamine test: Use in isolated and familial pheochromocytoma, *Arch. Intern. Med.* **135:**1227–1231.
48. Hill, C. S., Jr., Ibanez, M. L., Samaan, N. A., Ahearn, M. J., and Clark, R. L., 1973, Medullary (solid) carcinoma of the thyroid gland: An analysis of the M. D. Anderson Hospital experience with patients with the tumor, its special features, and its histogenesis, *Medicine* **52:**141–171.
49. Hazard, J. B., Hawk, W. A., and Crile, G., 1959, Medullary (solid) carcinoma of the thyroid—A Clinicopathologic entity, *J. Clin. Endocrinol.* **19:**152–161.
50. Wolfe, H. J., Melvin, K. E. W., Cervi-Skinner, S. J., Al Saadi, A. A., Juliar, J. F., Jackson, C. E., and Tashjian, A. H., Jr., 1973, C-Cell hyperplasia preceding medullary thyroid carcinoma, *N. Engl. J. Med.* **289:**437–441.
51. Wolfe, H. J., DeLellis, R. A., Voelkel, E. F., and Tashjian, A. H., Jr., 1975, Distribution of calcitonin-containing cells in the normal neonatal human thyroid gland: A correlation of morphology with peptide content, *J. Clin. Endocrinol. Metab.* **41:**1076–1081.
52. Baylin, S. B., Beaven, N. A., Buja, L. M., and Keiser, H. R., 1972, Histaminase activity: A biochemical marker for medullary carcinoma of the thyroid, *Amer. J. Med.* **53:**723–733.
53. Williams, E. D., Karim, S. M. M., and Sandler, M., 1968, Prostaglandin secretion by medullary carcinoma of the thyroid, *Lancet* **1:**22–23.
54. Moertel, C. G., Beahrs, O. H., Woolner, L. B., and Tyce, G. M., 1965, "Malignant carcinoid syndrome" associated with non-carcinoid tumors, *N. Engl. J. Med.* **273:**244–248.
55. Donahower, G. F., Schumacher, O. P., and Hazard, J. B., 1968, Medullary carcinoma of the thyroid—A cause of Cushing's syndrome: Report of two cases, *J. Clin. Res.* **28:**1199–1204.
56. Melvin, K. E. W., Tashjian, A. H., Jr., Cassidy, C. E., and Givens, J. R., 1970, Cushing's syndrome caused by ACTH- and calcitonin-secreting medullary carcinoma of the thyroid, *Metabolism* **19:**831–838.
57. Hennessy, J. F., Wells, S. A., Jr., Ontjes, D. A., and Cooper, C. W., 1974, A comparison of pentagastrin injection and calcium infusion as provocative agents for the detection of medullary carcinoma of the thyroid, *J. Clin. Endocrinol. Metab.* **39:**487–495.
58. Sizemore, G. W., and Go, V. L. W., 1975, Stimulation tests for diagnosis of medullary thyroid carcinoma, *Mayo Clin. Proc.* **50:**53–56.
59. Deftos, L. J., Goodman, A. D., Engelman, K., and Potts, J. T., Jr., 1971, Suppression and stimulation of calcitonin secretion in medullary thyroid carcinoma, *Metabolism* **20:**428–431.
60. Wells, S. A., Jr., Cooper, C. W., and Ontjes, D. A., 1975, Stimulation of thyrocalcitonin secretion by ethanol in patients with medullary thyroid carcinoma—an effect apparently not mediated by gastrin, *Metabolism* **24:**1215–1219.
61. Anast, C., David, L., Winnacker, J., Glass, R., Baskin, W., Brubaker, L., and Burns, T., 1975, Serum calcitonin–lowering effect of magnesium in patients with medullary carcinoma of the thyroid, *J. Clin. Invest.* **56:**1615–1621.

62. Deftos, L. J., and Parthemore, J. G., 1974, Secretion of parathyroid hormone in patients with medullary thyroid carcinoma, *J. Clin. Invest.* **54:**416–420.
63. Indech, M., and Jowsey, J., 1971, Secondary hyperparathyroidism produced in kittens repeatedly given porcine calcitonin, *Endocrinology* **88:**1489–1496.
64. Keiser, H. R., Beaven, M. A., Doppman, J., Wells, S., Jr., and Buja, L. M., 1973, Sipple's syndrome: Medullary thyroid carcinoma, pheochromocytoma, and parathyroid disease, *Ann. Intern. Med.* **78:**561–579.
65. Ross, E. J., Prichard, B. N. C., Kaufman, L., Robertson, A. I. G., and Harries, B. J., 1967, Preoperative and operative management of patients with phaeochromocytoma, *Br. Med. J.* **1:**191–198.
66. Ross, E. J., 1967, Safer surgery for patients with pheochromocytomas, *Amer. Heart J.* **74:**443–445.
67. Gloltzman, D., 1975, Case records of the Massachusetts General Hospital, *N. Engl. J. Med.* **293:**1085–1092.
68. Williams, E. D., and Pollock, D. J., 1966, Multiple mucosal neuromata with endocrine tumours: A syndrome allied to von Recklinghausen's disease, *J. Pathol. Bacteriol.* **91:**71–80.
69. Schimke, R. N., Hartmann, W. H., Prout, T. E., Rimoin, D. L., 1968, Syndrome of bilateral pheochromocytoma, medullary thyroid carcinoma and multiple neuromas: A possible regulatory defect in the differentiation of chromaffin tissue, *N. Engl. J. Med.* **279:**1–7.
70. Gorlin, R. J., Sedano, H. O., Vickers, R. A., and Cervenka, J., 1968, Multiple mucosal neuromas, pheochromocytoma and medullary carcinoma of the thyroid—A syndrome, *Cancer* **22:**293–299.
71. Block, M. B., Roberts, J. P., Kadair, R. G., Seyfer, A. E., Hull, S. F., and Nofeldt, F. D., 1975, Multiple endocrine adenomatosis type 11b: Diagnosis and treatment, *J. Amer. Med. Assoc.* **234:**710–714.
72. Pearse, A. G. E., 1969, The cytochemistry and ultrastructure of polypeptide hormone–producing cells of the APUD series and the embryologic, physiologic and pathologic implications of the concept, *J. Histochem. Cytochem.* **17:**303–313.
73. Pearse, A. G. E., 1974, The APUD cell concept and its implications in pathology, *Pathol. Annu.* **9:**27–42.
74. Pearse, A. G. E., and Polak, J. M., 1971, Neural crest origin of the endocrine polypeptide (APUD) cells of the gastrointestinal tract and pancreas, *Gut* **12:**783–788.
75. Pearse, A. G. E., Polak, J. M., and Heath, C. M., 1973, Development, differentiation and derivation of the endocrine polypeptide cells of the mouse pancreas: Immunofluorescence, cytochemical and ultrastructural studies, *Diabetologia* **9:**120–129.
76. Owman, C., Hakanson, R., and Sundler, F., 1973, Occurrence and function of amines in endocrine cells producing polypeptide hormones, *Fed. Proc. Fed. Amer. Soc. Exp. Biol.* **32:**1785–1791.
77. Tishler, A. S., and Greene, L. A., 1975, Nerve growth factor–induced process formation by cultured rat pheochromocytoma cells, *Nature* **258:**341, 342.
78. Greene, L. A., and Tishler, A. S., 1976, Establishment of a noradrenergic clonal line of rat adrenal pheochromocytoma cells which respond to nerve growth factor, *Proc. Nat. Acad. Sci. U.S.A.* **73:**2424–2428.
79. Biales, B., Dichter, M., and Tischler, A., 1975, Electrical excitability of cultured adrenal medulla, *Neurosci. Abstr.* **1:**460.
80. Tischler, A. S., Dichter, M., Biales, B., and Posner, M., 1975, The neural

properties of pheochromocytoma cells in culture—Preliminary observations, *Lab. Invest.* **32**:21–22.

81. Tischler, A. S. Dichter, M. A., Biales, B., DeLellis, R. A., and Wolfe, H., 1976, Neural properties of cultured human endocrine tumors of neural crest origin, *Science* **192**:902–904.

82. Levi-Montalcini, R., and Angeletti, P. U., 1968, Nerve growth factor, *Physiol. Rev.* **48**:534–569.

83. Hogue-Angeletti, R. A., Bradshaw, R. A., and Frazier, W. A., 1975, Nerve growth factor: Structure and mechanism of action, *Adv. Metab. Disord.* **8**:285–299.

84. Banerjee, S. P., Cuatrecasas, P., and Snyder, S. H., 1975, Nerve factor receptor binding: Influence of enzymes, ions, and protein reagents, *J. Biol. Chem.* **250**:1427–1433.

85. Bigazzi, M. Revoltella, R., and Casciano, S., 1975, High level of nerve growth factor (NGF) in the serum of a patient with medullary carcinoma of the thyroid gland, *Excerpta Med. Int. Cong. Ser.* 361, p. 92.

86. Vance, J. E., Stoll, R. W., Kitabchi, A. E., Buchanan, K. D., Hollander, D., Williams, R. H., 1972, Familial nesidioblastosis as the predominant manifestation of multiple endocrine adenomatosis, *Amer. J. Med.* **52**:211–227.

87. Paloyan, E., Lawrence, A. M., Straus, F. H., II, Paloyan, D., Harper, P. V., and Cummings, D., 1967, Alpha cell hyperplasia in calcific pancreatitis associated with hyperparathyroidism, *J. Amer. Med Assoc.* **200**:757–761.

88. Iversen, L. L., 1973, Catecholamine uptake processes, *Br. Med. Bull.* **29**:130–135.

89. Bhagat, B., and Zeidman, H., 1970, Increased retention of norepinephrine-^{3}H in vas deferens during nerve stimulation, *Amer. J. Physiol.* **219**:691–696.

90. Rosell, S., Kopin, I. J., and Axelrod, J., 1963, Fate of H^3-noradrenaline in skeletal muscle before and following sympathetic stimulation, *Amer. J. Physiol.* **205**:317–321.

91. Yamaguchi, N., deChamplain, J., and Nadeau, R., 1975, Correlation between the response of the heart to sympathetic stimulation and the release of endogenous catecholamines into the coronary sinus of the dog, *Circ. Res.* **36**:662–668.

92. Reid, J. L., and Kopin, I. J., 1974, Significance of plasma dopamine beta-hydroxylase activity as an index of sympathetic neuronal function, *Proc. Nat. Acad. Sci. U.S.A.* **71**:4392–4394.

93. Reid, J. L., and Kopin, I. J., 1975, The effects of ganglionic blockade, resperine and vinblastine on plasma catecholamines and dopamine beta-hydroxylase in the rat, *J. Pharmacol. Exp. Ther.* **193**:748–756.

94. Ziegler, M. G., Lake, C. R., and Kopin, I. J., 1976, Deficient sympathetic nervous response in familial dysantonomia, *N. Engl. J. Med.* **294**:630–633.

95. Landsberg, L., and Axelrod, J., 1968, Influence of pituitary, thyroid, and adrenal hormones on norepinephrine turnover and metabolism in the rat heart, *Circ. Res.* **22**:559–571.

96. Taubin, H. L., Djahanguiri, B., and Landsberg, L., 1972, Norepinephrine concentraiton and turnover in different regions of the gastrointestinal tract of the rat. An approach to the evaluation of sympathetic activity in the gut, *Gut* **13**:790–795.

97. Young, J. B., Landsberg, L., and Arky, R., 1976, Pancreatic norepinephrine (NE) turnover in the rat: A method for assessing the sympathetic regulation of the endocrine pancreas, *Diabetes*(Suppl. 1) **25**:391.

98. Engelman, K., Portnoy, B., and Lovenberg, W., 1968, A sensitive and

specific double-isotope derivative method for the determination of catecholamines in biological specimens, *Amer. J. Med. Sci.* **255**:259–268.

99. Christensen, N. J., 1973, Plasma noradrenaline and adrenaline in patients with thyrotoxicosis and myxoedema, *Clin. Sci. Mol. Med.* **45**:163–171.

100. Danon, A., and Sapira, J. D., 1972, Binding of catecholamines to human serum albumin, *J. Pharmacol. Exp. Ther.* **182**:295–302.

101. Collier, J. G., 1972, New dialysis technique for the continuous measurement of the concentration of vaso-active hormones, *Br. J. Pharmacol.* **44**:383P.

102. May, P., Sanders, F. J., and Donabedian, R. K., 1974, Binding of catechol derivatives to human serum proteins, *Experientia* **30**:304–305.

103. Powis, G., 1975, The binding of catecholamines to human serum proteins, *Biochem. Pharmacol.* **24**:707–712.

104. Jiang, N. S., Machacek, D., and Wadel, O. P., 1976, Further study on the two-column plasma catecholamine assay, *Mayo Clin. Proc.* **51**:112–116.

105. Friedman, M., Byers, S. O., Diamant, J., and Rosenman, R. H., 1975, Plasma catecholamine response of coronary-prone subjects (type A) to a specific challenge, *Metabolism* **24**:205–210.

106. Saelens, J. K., Schoen, M. S., and Koracsics, G. B., 1967, An enzyme assay for norepinephrine in brain tissue, *Biochem. Pharmacol.* **16**:1043–1049.

107. Whitby, L. G., Axelrod, J., and Weil-Malherbe, H., 1961, The fate of ^{3}H-norepinephrine in animals, *J. Pharmacol. Exp. Ther.* **132**:193–201.

108. Landsberg, L., 1976, Extraneuronal uptake and metabolism of [^{3}H]-L-norepinephrine by the rat duodenal mucosa, *Biochem. Pharmacol.* **25**:729–731.

109. Young, J. B., Landsberg, L., and Knopp, R. H., 1976, Effect of intravenous glucagon on urinary catecholamine excretion in normal man, *Metabolism* **25**:233–237.

110. Silva, P., Besarab, A., and Landsberg, L., 1976, Catecholamine clearance by the isolated perfused rat kidney: Preferential excretion and metabolism of epinephrine, *Clin Res.* **24**:258A.

111. Axelrod, J., 1972, Dopamine-beta-hydroxylase: Regulation of its synthesis and release from nerve terminals, *Pharmacol. Rev.* **24**:233–243.

112. Potter, L. T., and Axelrod, J., 1963, Properties of norepinephrine storage particles of the rat heart, *J. Pharmacol. Exp. Ther.* **142**:299–305.

113. Viveros, O. H., Argueros, L., and Kirshner, N., 1968, Release of catecholamines and dopamine-beta-hydroxylase from the adrenal medulla, *Life Sci.* **7**:609–618.

114. Smith, A. D., and Winkler, H., 1972, Fundamental mechanisms in the release of catecholamines, *in: Catecholamines, Handbook of Experimental Pharmacology* (H. Blaschko and E. Muscholl, eds.), pp. 538–617, Springer-Verlag, Berlin.

115. Douglas, W. W., 1968, Stimulus–secretion coupling: The concept and clues from chromaffin and other cells, *Br. J. Pharmacol.* **34**:451–474.

116. Kirshner, N., and Viveros, O. H., 1972, The secretory cycle in the adrenal medulla, *Pharmacol. Rev.* **24**:385–398.

117. Weinshilboum, R. M., Thoa, N. B., Johnson, D. G., Kopin, I. J., and Axelrod, J., 1971, Proportional release of norepinephrine and dopamine-beta-hydroxylase from sympathetic nerves, *Science* **174**:1349–1351.

118. Weinshilboum, R., and Axelrod, J., 1971, Serum dopamine-beta-hydroxylase activity, *Circ. Res.* **28**:307–315.

119. Nagatsu, T., and Udenfriend, S., 1972, Photometric assay of dopamine-beta-hydroxylase activity in human blood, *Clin. Chem.* **18**:980–983.

120. Laduron, P., 1975, Scope and limitation in dopamine-beta-hydroxylase measurement, *Biochem. Pharmacol.* **24:**557–562.
121. Rush, R. A., and Geffen, L. B., 1972, Radioimmunoassay and clearance of circulating dopamine-beta-hydroxylase, *Circ. Res.* **31:**444–452.
122. Rush, R. A., Kindler, S. H., and Udenfriend, S., 1975, Solid-phase radioimmunoassay on polystyrene beads and its application to dopamine-beta-hydroxylase, *Clin. Chem.* **21:**148–150.
123. Rush, R. A., Thomas, P. E., Nagatsu, T., and Udenfriend, S., 1974, Comparison of human serum dopamine-beta-hydroxylase levels by radioimmunoassay and enzymatic assay, *Proc. Nat. Acad. Sci. U.S.A.* **71:**872–874.
124. Rush, R. A., Thomas, P. E., and Udenfriend, S., 1975, Measurement of human dopamine-beta-hydroxylase in serum by homologous radioimmunoassay, *Proc. Nat. Acad. Sci. U.S.A.* **72:**750–752.
125. Weinshilboum, R. M., Kvetnansky, R., Axelrod, J., and Kopin, I. J., 1971, Elevation of serum dopamine-beta-hydroxylase activity with forced immobilization, *Nature* **230:**287–288.
126. Gerwirtz, G. P., and Kopin, I. J., 1970, Release of dopamine-beta-hydroxylase with norepinephrine during rat splenic nerve stimulation, *Nature* **227:**406–407.
127. Weinshilboum, R. M., and Axelrod, J., 1971, Serum dopamine-beta-hydroxylase: Decrease after chemical sympathectomy, *Science* **173:**931–934.
128. Thoa, N. B., Wooten, F., Axelrod, J., and Kopin, I. J., 1972, Inhibition of release of dopamine-beta-hydroxylase and norepinephrine from sympathetic nerves by colchicine, vinblastine, or cyctochalasin-B, *Proc. Nat. Acad. Sci. U.S.A.* **69:**520–522.
129. Wooten, G. F., and Cardon, P. V., 1973, Plasma dopamine-beta-hydroxylase activity: Elevation in man during cold pressor test and exercise, *Arch. Neurol.* **28:**103–106.
130. Weinshilboum, R. M., and Axelrod, J., 1971, Reduced plasma dopamine-beta-hydroxylase activity in familial dysantonomia, *N. Engl. J. Med.* **285:**938–942.
131. Weinshilboum, R. M., Schrott, H. G., Raymond, F. A., Weidman, W. H., and Elveback, L. R., 1975, Inheritance of very low serum dopamine-beta-hydroxylase activity, *Amer. J. Hum. Genet.* **27:**573–585.
132. Melander, A., Sundler, F., and Westgren, U., 1973, Intrathyroidal amines and the synethesis of thyroid hormone, *Endocrinology* **93:**193–200.
133. Melander, A., Ericson, L. E., Sundler, F., and Ingbar, S. H., 1974, Sympathetic innervation of the mouse thyroid and its significance in thyroid hormone secretion, *Endocrinology* **94:**959–966.
134. Melander, A., Ericson, L. E., Ljunggren, J.-G., Norberg, K.-A., Persson, B., Sundler, F., Tibblin, S., and Westgren, U., 1974, Sympathetic innervation of the normal human thyroid., *J. Clin. Endocrinol. Metab.* **39:**713–718.
135. Tice, L. W., and Creveling, C. R., 1975, Electron microscopic identification of adrenergic nerve endings on thyroid epithelial cells, *Endocrinology* **97:**1123–1129.
136. Melander, A., Sundler, F., and Westgren, U., 1975, Sympathetic innervation of the thyroid: Variation with species and with age, *Endocrinology* **96:**102–106.
137. Maayan, M. L., and Ingbar, S. H., 1970, Effect of epinephrine on iodine and intermediary metabolism in isolated thyroid cells, *Endocrinology* **87:**588–595.
138. Ahn, C. S., 1971, Glycogen metabolism of the thyroid, *Endocrinology* **88:**1341–1348.

139. Maayan, M. L., Shapiro, R., and Ingbar, S. H., 1973, Epinephrine precursors: Effects on the iodine and intermediary metabolism of isolated calf thyroid cells, *Endocrinology* **92:**912–916.
140. Ericson, L. E., Melander, A., Owman, C., and Sundler, F., 1970, Endocytosis of thyroglobulin and release of thyroid hormone in mice by catecholamines and 5-hydroxytryptamine, *Endocrinology* **87:**915–923.
141. Melander, A., Nelsson, E., and Sundler, F., 1972, Sympathetic activation of thyroid hormone secretion in mice, *Endocrinology* **90:**194–199.
142. Coleoni, A. H., 1972, Effects of the administration of catecholamine-depleting drugs on the thyroid function of the rat, *Pharmacology* **8:**300–310.
143. Marshall, N. J., Von Borcke, S., and Malan, P. G., 1975, Studies on isoproterenol stimulation of adenyl cyclase in membrane preparations from the bovine thyroid, *Endocrinology* **96:**1520–1524.
144. Melander, A., Ranklev, E., Sundler, F., and Westgren, U., 1975, Beta$_2$-adrenergic stimulation of thyroid hormone secretion, *Endocrinology* **97:**332–336.
145. Beley, A., Rochette, L., and Bralet, J., 1973, Influence du traitement par la thyroxine et le propylthiouracile sur le taux de renouvellement de la noradrenaline dans huit organes peripheriques du rat, *Arch. Int. Physiol. Biochim.* **81:**287–298.
146. Prange, A. J., Jr., Meek, J. L., and Lipton, M. A., 1970, Catecholamines: Diminished rate of synthesis in rat brain and heart after thyroxine pretreatment, *Life Sci.* **9:**901–907.
147. Landsberg, L., and Axelrod, J., 1968, Influence of pituitary, thyroid, and adrenal hormones on norepinephrine turnover and metabolism in the rat heart, *Circ. Res.* **22:**559–571.
148. Landsberg, L., DeChamplain, J., and Axelrod, J., 1969, Increased biosynthesis of cardiac norepinephrine after hypophysectomy, *J. Pharmacol. Exp. Ther.* **165:**102–107.
149. Kuschke, H. J., Wernze, H., and Becker, G., 1960, Sympatho-adrenal activity in thyrotoxicosis, *Br. Med. J.* **2:**1656.
150. Wiswell, J. G., Hurwitz, G. E., Corohno, V., Bing, O. H. L., and Child, D. L., 1963, Urinary catecholamines and their metabolites in hyperthyroidism and hypothyroidism, *J. Clin. Endocrinol. Metab.* **23:**1102–1106.
151. Bayliss, R. I. S., and Edwards, O. M., 1971, Urinary excretion of free catecholamines in Graves' disease, *Endocrinology* **49:**167–173.
152. Christensen, N. J., 1972, Increased levels of plasma noradrenaline in hypothyroidism, *J. Clin. Endocrinol. Metab.* **35:**359–363.
153. Christensen, N. J., 1973, Plasma noradrenaline and adrenaline in patients with thyrotoxicosis and myxoedema, *Clin. Sci. Mol. Med.* **45:**163–171.
154. Stoffer, S. S., Jiang, N.-S., Gorman, C. A., and Pikler, G. M., 1973, Plasma catecholamines in hypothyroidism and hyperthyroidism, *J. Clin. Endocrinol. Metab.* **36:**587–589.
155. Nishizawa, Y., Hamada, N., Fujii, S., Morii, H., Okuda, K., and Wada, M., 1974, Serum dopamine-beta-hydroxylase activity in thyroid disorders, *J. Clin. Endocrinol. Metab.* **39:**599–602.
156. Noth, R. H., and Spaulding, S. W., 1974, Decreased serum dopamine-beta-hydroxylase in hyperthyroidism, *J. Clin. Endocrinol. Metab.* **39:**614–617.
157. Coulombe, P., Dussault, J. H., Letarte, J., and Simard, S. J., 1976, Catecholamine metabolism in thyroid diseases. I. Epinephrine secretion rate in hyperthyroidism and hypothyroidism, *J. Clin. Endocrinol. Metab.* **42:**125–131.

158. Markowitz, C., and Yater, W. M., 1932, Response of explanted cardiac muscle to thyroxine, *Amer. J. Physiol.* **100:**162–166.
159. Wildenthal, K., 1971, Responses to cardioactive drugs of fetal mouse hearts maintained in organ culture, *Amer. J. Physiol.* **221:**238–241.
160. Nemecek, G. M., and Hess, M. E., 1974, Cardiovascular and metabolic responses to thyroid hormones in animals after sympathectomy or treatment with nerve growth factor, *Neuropharmacology* **13:**317–332.
161. Thier, M. D., Gravenstein, J. S., and Hoffman, R. G., 1962, Thyroxin, reserpine, epinephrine and temperature on atrial rate, *J. Pharmacol. Exp. Ther.* **136:**133–141.
162. Cairoli, V. J., and Crout, J. R., 1967, Role of the autonomic nervous system in the resting tachycardia of experimental hyperthyroidism, *J. Pharmacol. Exp. Ther.* **158:**55–65.
163. McDevitt, D. G., Shanks, R. G., Hadden, D. R., Montgomery, D. A. D., and Weaver, J. A., 1968, The role of the thyroid in the control of heart-rate, *Lancet* **1:**998–1000.
164. Buccino, R. A., Spann, J. F., Jr., Pool, P. E., Sonnenblick, E. H., and Braunwald, E., 1967, Influence of the thyroid state on the intrinsic contractile properties and energy stores of the myocardium, *J. Clin. Invest.* **46:**1669–1682.
165. Taylor, R. R., Covell, J. W., and Ross, J., Jr., 1969, Influence of the thyroid state on left ventricular tension–velocity relations in the intact, sedated dog, *J. Clin. Invest.* **48:**775–784.
166. Grossman, W., Robin, N. I., Johnson, L. W., Brooks, H. L., Selenkow, H. A., and Dexter, L., 1971, The enhanced myocardial contractility of thyrotoxicosis: Role of the beta adrenergic receptor, *Ann. Intern. Med.* **74:**869–874.
167. DeGroot, L. J., and Leonard, J. J., 1970, Hyperthyroidism as a high cardiac output state, *Amer. Heart J.* **79:**265–275.
168. Levey, G. S., and Epstein, S. E., 1969, Myocardial adenyl cyclase: Activation by thyroid hormones and evidence for two adenyl cyclase systems, *J. Clin. Invest.* **48:**1663–1669.
169. Sobel, B. E., Dempsey, P. J., and Cooper, T., 1969, Normal myocardial adenyl cyclase activity in hyperthyroid cats, *Proc. Soc. Exp. Biol. Med.* **132:**6–9.
170. Levey, G. S., Skelton, C. L., and Epstein, S. E., 1969, Influence of hyperthyroidism on the effects of norepinephrine on myocardial adenyl cyclase activity and contractile state, *Endocrinology* **85:**1004–1009.
171. McNeill, J. H., Muschek, L. D., and Brody, T. M., 1969, The effect of triiodothyronine on cyclic AMP, phosphorylase, and adenyl cyclase in rat heart, *Can. J. Physiol. Pharmacol.* **47:**913–916.
172. Young, B. A., and McNeill, J. H., 1974, The effect of noradrenaline and tyramine on cardiac contractility, cyclic AMP, and phosphorylase α in normal and hyperthyroid rats, *Can. J. Physiol. Pharmacol.* **52:**375–383.
173. Waldstein, S. S., 1966, Thyroid–catecholamine interrelations, *Annu. Rev. Med.* **17:**123–132.
174. Sawyer, M. E. M., and Brown, M. G., 1935, The effect of thyroidectomy and thyroxine on the response of the denervated heart to injected and secreted adrenine, *Amer. J. Physiol.* **110:**620–635.
175. McDonald, C. H., Shepeard, W. L., Green, M. F., and DeGroat, A. F., 1935, Response of the hyperthyroid heart to epinephrine, *Amer. J. Physiol.* **112:**227–230.

176. Brewster, W. R., Jr., Isaacs, J. P., Osgood, P. F., and King, T. L., 1956, The hemodynamic and metabolic interrelationships in the activity of epinephrine, norepinephrine and the thyroid hormones, *Circulation* **13**:1–20.

177. Thier, M. D., Gravenstein, J. S., and Hoffmann, R. G., 1962, Thyroxin, reserpine, epinephrine and temperature on atrial rate, *J. Pharmacol. Exp. Ther.* **136**:133–141.

178. Cravey, G. M., and Gravenstein, J. S., 1965, The effect of thyroxin, corticosteroids, and epinephrine on atrial rate, *J. Pharmacol. Exp. Ther.* **148**:75–79.

179. Rosenblum, H., Hahn, R. G., and Levine, S. A., 1933, Epinephrine: Its effect on the cardiac mechanism in experimental hyperthyroidism and hypothyroidism, *Arch. Intern. Med.* **51**:279–289.

180. Raab, W., 1944, Epinephrine tolerance of the heart altered by thyroxine and thiouracil, *J. Pharmacol. Exp. Ther.* **82**:330–338.

181. Levey, G. S., 1971, Catecholamine sensitivity, thyroid hormone and the heart, *Amer. J. Med.* **50**:413–420.

182. Margolius, H. S., and Gaffney, T. E., 1965, The effects of injected norepinephrine and sympathetic nerve stimulation in hypothyroid and hyperthyroid dogs, *J. Pharmacol. Exp. Ther.* **149**:329–335.

183. Van der Schoot, J. B., and Moran, N. C., 1965, An experimental evaluation of the reputed influence of thyroxine on the cardiovascular effects of catecholamines, *J. Pharmacol. Exp. Ther.* **149**:336–345.

184. Anton, A. H., and Gravenstein, J. S., 1970, Studies on thyroid–catecholamine interactions in the isolated rabbit heart, *Eur. J. Pharmacol.* **10**:311–318.

185. Brus, R., Hess, M. E., and Jacobowitz, D., 1970, Effect of 6-hydroxydopamine and thyroxine on chronotropic response to norepinephrine, *Eur. J. Pharmacol.* **10**:323–327.

186. Field, F. P., Janis, R. A., and Triggle, D. J., 1973, Relationship between aortic reactivity and blood pressure of renal hypertensive, hyperthyroid, and hypothyroid rats, *Can. J. Physiol. Pharmacol.* **51**:344–353.

187. Wildenthal, K., 1972, Studies of isolated fetal mouse hearts in organ culture: Evidence for a direct effect of triiodothyronine in enhancing cardiac responsiveness to norepinephrine, *J. Clin. Invest.* **51**:2702–2709.

188. Will-Shahab, L., and Wollenberger, A., 1974, Influence of thyroid state on the binding of noradrenaline to a cardiac subcellular fraction containing the beta-adrenoreceptor, *Acta Biol. Med. Ger.* **32**:K1–K8.

189. Coville, P. F., and Telford, J. M., 1970, Influence of thyroid hormones on the sensitivity of cardiac and smooth muscle to biogenic amines and other drugs, *Br. J. Pharmacol.* **39**:49–68.

190. Kunos, G., Vermes-Kunos, I., and Nickerson, M., 1974, Effects of thyroid state on adrenoreceptor properties, *Nature* **250**:779–781.

191. Nakashima, M., Maeda, K., Sekiya, A., and Hagino, Y., 1971, Effect of hypothyroid status on myocardial responses to sympathomimetic drugs, *Jpn. J. Pharmacol.* **21**:819–825.

192. Rosenqvist, Y., and Boreus, L. O., 1972, Enhancement of the alpha adrenergic response in aorta from hypothyroid rabbits, *Life Sci.* **11**:595–604.

193. Fregly, M. J., Nelson, E. L., Jr., Resch, G. E., Field, E. P., and Luthuer, L. O., 1975, Reduced beta-adrenergic responsiveness in hypothyroid rats, *Amer. J. Physiol.* **229**:916–924.

194. Goetsch, E., 1918, Newer methods in the diagnosis of thyroid disorders: Pathological and clinical, *N. Y. State J. Med.* **18**:259–267.

195. Schneckloth, R. E., Kurland, G. S., and Freedberg, A. S., 1953, Effect of

variation in thyroid function on the pressor response to norepinephrine in man, *Metabolism* **2**:546–555.

196. Murray, J. F., and Kelley, J. J., Jr., 1959, The relation of thyroidal hormone level to epinephrine response: A diagnostic test for hyperthyroidism, *Ann. Intern. Med.* **51**:309–321.

197. Aoki, V. S., Wilson, W. R., Theilen, E. O., Lukensmeyer, W. W., and Leaverton, P. E., 1967, The effects of triiodothyronine on hemodynamic responses to epinephrine and norepinephrine in man, *J. Pharmacol. Exper. Ther.* **157**:62–68.

198. Aoki, V. S., Wilson, W. R., and Theilen, E. O., 1972, Studies of the reputed augmentation of the cardiovascular effects of catecholamines in patients with spontaneous hyperthyroidism, *J. Pharmacol. Exp. Ther.* **181**:362–368.

199. Bray, G. A., 1966, Studies on the sensitivity to catecholamines after thyroidectomy, *Endocrinology* **79**:554–564.

200. Brodie, B. B., Davies, J. I., Hynie, S., Krinshna, G., and Weiss, B., 1966, Interrelationships of catecholamines with other endocrine systems, *Pharmacol. Rev.* **18**:273–289.

201. Ichikawa, A., Matsumoto, H., Sakato, N., and Tomita, K., 1971, Effect of thyroid hormones on epinephrine-induced lipolysis in adipose tissue of rats, *J. Biochem. (Tokyo)* **69**:1055–1064.

202. Rosenquist, U., 1972, Adrenergic receptor response in hypothyroidism. An *in vitro* study on human adipose tissue and rabbit aorta, *Acta Physiol. Scand. Suppl.* **532**:1–28.

203. Krishna, G., Hynie, S., and Brodie, B. B., 1968, Effects of thyroid hormones on adenyl cyclase in adipose tissue and on free fatty acid mobilization, *Proc. Nat. Acad. Sci. U.S.A.* **59**:884–889.

204. Hess, M. E., and Shanfeld, J., 1965, Cardiovascular and metabolic interrelationships between thyroxine and the sympathetic nervous system, *J. Pharmacol. Exp. Ther.* **148**:290–297.

205. McNeill, J. N., and Brody, T. M., 1968, The effect of triiodothyronine pretreatment on amine-induced rat cardiac phosphorylase activation, *J. Pharmacol. Exp. Ther.* **161**:40–46.

206. Frazer, A., Hess, M. E., and Shanfeld, J., 1969, The effects of thyroxine on rat heart adenosine 3′,5′-monophosphate, phosphorylase "b" kinase and phosphorylase "a" activity, *J. Pharmacol. Exp. Ther.* **170**:10–16.

207. Guttler, R. B., Shaw, J. W., Otis, C. L., and Nicoloff, J. T., 1975, Epinephrine-induced alterations in urinary cyclic AMP in hyper- and hypothyroidism, *J. Clin. Endocrinol. Metab.* **41**:707–711.

208. Guttler, R. B., Otis, C. L., Shaw, J. W., Warren, D. W., and Nicoloff, J. T., 1975, The effect of thyroid hormone on adenyl cyclase (AC)—A potential site for thyroid hormone action, *Proceedings of the International Conference on Thyroid Hormone Metabolism*, Glasgow, Scotland, August 7–9, *Excerpta Med. Int. Congr. Ser.*

209. Gale, C. C., 1973, Neuroendocrine aspects of thermoregulation, *Annu. Rev. Physiol.* **35**:391–430.

210. Jansky, L., 1973, Non-shivering thermogenesis and its thermoregulatory significance, *Biol. Rev.* **48**:85–132.

211. Sellers, E. A., Flattery, K. V., Shum, A., and Johnson, G. E., 1971, Thyroid status in relation to catecholamines in cold and warm environment, *Can. J. Physiol. Pharmacol.* **49**:268–275.

212. Steele, R. E., and Wekstein, D. R., 1973, Effects of thyroxine on calorigenic

response of the newborn rat to norepinephrine, *Amer. J. Physiol.* **224**:979–984.

213. Kaciuba-Uscilko, H., 1971, The effect of previous thyroxine administration on the metabolic response to adrenaline in new-born pigs, *Biol. Neonate* **19**:220–226.

214. Leblanc, J., and Villemarie, A., 1970, Thyroxine and noradrenaline on noradrenaline sensitivity, cold resistance, and brown fat, *Amer. J. Physiol.* **218**:1742–1745.

215. Howitt, G., Rowlands, D. J., Leung, D. Y. T., and Logan, W. F. W. E., 1968, Myocardial contractility, and the effects of beta-adrenergic blockade in hypothyroidism and hyperthyroidism, *Clin. Sci.* **34**:485–495.

216. Canary, J. J., Schaaf, M., Duffy, B. J., Jr., and Kyle, L. H., 1957, Effects of oral and intramuscular administration of reserpine in thyrotoxicosis, *N. Engl. J. Med.* **257**:435–442.

217. Gaffney, T. E., Braunwald, E., and Kahler, R. L., 1961, Effect of guanethidine on tri-iodothyronine-induced hyperthyroidism in man, *N. Engl. J. Med.* **265**:16–20.

218. Mazzaferri, E. L., and Skillman, T. G., 1969, Thyroid storm: A review of 22 episodes with special emphasis on the use of guanethidine, *Arch. Intern. Med.* **124**:684–690.

219. Hadden, D. R., Montgomery, D. A. D., Shanks, R. G., and Weaver, J. A., 1968, Propranolol and iodine-131 in the management of thyrotoxicosis, *Lancet* **2**:852–854.

220. Shanks, R. G., Hadden, D. R., Lowe, D. C., McDevitt, D. G., and Montgomery, D. A. D., 1969, Controlled trial of propranolol in thyrotoxicosis, *Lancet* **1**:993, 994.

221. Das, G., and Krieger, M., 1969, Treatment of thyrotoxic storm with intravenous administration of propranolol, *Ann. Intern. Med.* **70**:985–988.

222. McLarty, D. G., Brownlie, B. E. W., Alexander, W. D., Papapetrow, P. D., and Horton, P., 1973, Remission of thyrotoxicosis during treatment with propranolol, *Br. Med. J.* **2**:332–334.

223. Mackin, J. F., Canary, J. J., and Pittman, C. S., 1974, Thyroid storm and its management, *N. Engl. J. Med.* **291**:1396–1398.

224. Mazzaferri, E. L., Reynolds, J. C., Young, R. L., Lt. Col., Thomas, C. N., Lt. Col., and Parisi, A. F., 1976, Propranolol as primary therapy for thyrotoxicosis, *Arch. Intern. Med.* **136**:50–56.

225. Lee, W. Y., Bronsky, D., and Waldstein, S. S., 1962, Studies of thyroid and sympathetic nervous system interrelationships. II. Effects of guanethidine on manifestations of hyperthyroidism, *J. Clin. Endocrinol. Metab.* **22**:879–885.

226. Stout, B. D., Wiener, L., and Cox, J. W., 1969, Combined alpha and beta sympathetic blockade in hyperthyroidism, *Ann. Intern. Med.* **70**:963–970.

227. Georges, L. P., Santangels, R. P., Macklin, J. F., and Carnary, J. J., Metabolic effects of propranolol in thyrotoxicosis. I. Nitrogen, calcium, and hydroxyproline, *Metabolism* **1**:11–21.

228. Rude, R. K., Oldham, S. B., Singer, F. R., and Nicoloff, J. T., 1976, Treatment of thyrotoxic hypercalcemia with propranolol, *N. Engl. J. Med.* **294**:431–433.

229. Allen, J. A., Lowe, D. C., Roddie, I. C., and Wallace, W. F. M., 1973, Studies on sweating in clinical and experimental thyrotoxicosis, *Clin. Sci. Mol. Med.* **45**:765–773.

230. Grossman, W., Robin, N. I., Johnson, L. W., Brooks, H., Selenkow, H. A., and Dexter, L., 1971, Effects of beta blockade on the peripheral manifestations of thyrotoxicosis, *Ann. Intern. Med.* **74:**875–879.

231. Wilson, W. R., Theilen, E. O., and Fletcher, F. W., 1964, Pharmacodynamic effects of beta-adrenergic receptor blockade in patients with hyperthyroidism, *J. Clin. Invest.* **43:**1697–1703.

232. Wilson, W. R., Theilen, E. O., Hege, J. H., and Valenca, M. R., 1966, Effects of beta-adrenergic receptor blockade in normal subjects before, during, and after triiodothyronine-induced hypermetabolism, *J. Clin. Invest.* **45:**1159–1169.

233. Wiener, L., Stout, B. D., and Cox, J. W., 1969, Influence of beta sympathetic blockade (propranolol) on the hemodynamics of hyperthyroidism, *Amer. J. Med.* **46:**227–233.

234. Pietras, R. J., Real, M. D., Poticha, G. S., Bronsky, D., and Waldstein, S. S., 1972, Cardiovascular response in hyperthyroidism: Influence of androgenic-receptor blockade, *Arch. Intern. Med.* **129:**426–429.

235. Riddle, M. C., and Schwartz, T. B., 1970, New tactics for hyperthyroidism: Sympathetic blockade, *Ann. Intern. Med.* **72:**749, 750.

236. Sterling, K., and Hoffenberg, R., 1971, Beta blocking agents and antithyroid drugs as adjuncts to radioiodine therapy, *Semin. Nucl. Med.* **1:**422–431.

237. Pimstone, B., and Joffe, B., 1970, The use and abuse of beta-adrenergic blockade in the surgery of hyperthyroidism, *S. Afr. Med. J.* **44:**1059–1061.

238. Cook, D. R., and Chodoff, P., 1970, Anesthetic management of an incompletely controlled hyperthyroid patient for thyroidectomy, *Anesthesiology* **33:**562–564.

239. Langer, A., Hung, C. T., McA'nulty, J. A., Harrigan, J. T., and Washington, E., 1974, Adrenergic blockade: A new approach to hyperthyroidism during pregnancy, *Obstet. Gynecol.* **44:**181–186.

9

Calcitonin

Louis V. Avioli

9.1. Introduction

Today, when one is asked to enumerate those hormones that play an integral role in maintaining the "internal milieu" with respect to calcium and inorganic phosphate, the response is universally "parathyroid hormone, calcitonin, and vitamin D." The parathyroid glands were first recognized in a dissection of an Indian rhinoceros by Sir Richard Owen in 1852, and for years were considered the sole guardian of mineral and skeletal homeostasis. During the past 25 years, considerable knowledge has accumulated with regard to the nature of the secreted hormone, factors that control or modulate parathyroid hormone synthesis and release, and the target organ response or responses to hormonal stimulation.[1-11] In contrast, only within the last decade have rapid advances in

LOUIS V. AVIOLI • Department of Medicine, Washington University School of Medicine, St. Louis, Missouri 63110.

our knowledge of the enzymatic, ionic, and hormonal control of vitamin D metabolism been made, and the nature of the target organ response to its hydroxylated metabolites defined.[12] Integrated feedback control circuits that regulate parathyroid hormone and vitamin D metabolism have been documented and the interactions of these hormones on bone, intestine, and kidney reevaluated.

In a comparable fashion, since a "hypocalcemic substance" (i.e., calcitonin) was first demonstrated in extracts of rat thyroids by Hirsch and collegues in 1963,[13] its role in maintaining mineral homeostasis has undergone extensive analyses within the last decade. Mechanisms that regualte the secretion and biological activity of calcitonin have been explored both in a variety of lower animal species and in patients with medullary carcinoma, and the sequence for the 32-amino acid calcitonin peptide isolated from human, bovine, ovine, salmon, and porcine thyroid glands has been defined.[14,15] Despite these many contributions, which stem primarily from a combination of *in vitro* experiments on thyroid or ultimobranchial tissue, *in situ* perfusions of the thyroid gland of pigs, goats, cows, and dogs, and *in vivo* studies in rats, the functional role of calcitonin in the field of skeletal and mineral metabolism as it relates to normal man is still conjectural at best.

This review will be concerned primarily with recent developments in the field of calcitonin research, with emphasis on those controversies that necessarily attend any scientific endeavor when species specificities and selective hormonal quantitation become an issue.

9.2. Calcitonin

Publications by Gray and Ontjes[14] and by Queener and Bell[15] afford an excellent concise historical background and updated review of the effects and mechanism of action of calcitonin, the factors that influence its synthesis and secretion, and the reported clinical uses of the hormone. It must be emphasized that since the discovery of this new hypocalcemic peptide, all would agree that calcitonins of ultimobranchial origin in lower animal species (e.g., reptiles, fish, birds) are more effective in lowering serum calcium than those produced by the thyroid parafollicular cells, or C cells, of mammals. Unlike the responses observed with peptidic fractions of parathyroid hormone, the entire 32-amino acid sequence of calcitonin is required for biological activity.[16] When the amino acid sequences of five calcitonins (porcine, ovine, salmon, bovine, and human) are compared, there are nine amino acids with common positions, seven of which are found in the *N*-terminal portion of the molecule. In the past, the increased biological activity of salmon calcitonin has been attributed to a greater affinity for the target tissue receptors and an increased resistance to biological degradation.[17,18] However, certain constraints within the calcitonin molecule may also contribute to the greater biological potency of salmon calcitonin. In 1974, Maier et al.[19] reported that the biological activity of human calcitonin could be improved by replacing the amino acids in positions 29 and 31 (valine and alanine) with those occurring in the corresponding positions of salmon calcitonin. In 1975, these same investigators reported on the hypocalcemic response of the rat to synthetic analogues of human calcitonin.[20]. Their results demonstrated that the replacement of methionine in position 8 and phenylalanine in position 22 of human calcitonin by valine and tryosine, respectively, either singly or together, yielded analogues with a potency 4–5 times, and a duration of action approximately 2 times, that of the original human calcitonin peptide.[20] In this study, a human calcitonin analogue with a β-mercaptopropionic acid in position 1 and valine in position 8 was also demonstrated to be 6 times more potent than human calcitonin, and longer-acting than the analogues with a valine substituted for methonine in position 8 of the peptide sequence. These studies are reminiscent of those in which substitution in the porcine calcitonin molecule of lysine and tyrosine at positions 14 and 19 for arginine and phenylalanine, respectively, led to a 2.5-fold increase in biological activity, and of others in which replacement of aspartic acid in position 15 of the bovine calcitonin molecule with asparagine resulted in a 3-fold increase in the hypocalcemic response.[21]

Investigations on the nature of rat calcitonin were also reported in 1975. In 1972, Milhaud and co-workers[22] reported that antibodies against human calcitonin developed in the rat cross-reacted well with rat calcitonin, but not with porcine or salmon calcitonin, and that antibodies against human calcitonin raised in the guinea pig cross reacted only slightly with rat calcitonin. The apparent immunological similarity of human and rat calcitonin was later confirmed, using immunofluorescent localization of rat thyroid C cells and different fragments of human calcitonin in binding–inhibition studies.[23] The derived data were consistent with the interpretation that the 17–32 amino acid sequences of rat and human calcitonin are identical. Purification and further characterization of rat calcitonin were later accomplished by Burford et al.,[24] using acid–acetone rat thyroid gland preparations. Utilizing guinea pig antisera and a radioimmunoassay sensitive enough to detect 2–3 ng calcitonin, these workers found rat thyroid venous plasma to contain 5–10 ng/ml. They also confirmed previous observations that either rat or human calcitonin can be used in the rat calcitonin radioimmunoassay, and that the rat and human antigenic determinants reside in the C-terminal region of the molecule (i.e., 10–32 or 22–32). Preliminary amino acid analyses of the homogenous rat calcitonin preparations were also consistent with the hypothesis that considerable structural similarities existed in human and rat calcitonin.[24] Using porcine calcitonin as the immunogen for rabbits, Kent and Retallack[25] also reported on a sensitive radioimmunoassay for rat calcitonin. Normal circulating levels of adult *female rats* were established as 0.8+0.25-ng equivalents of porcine calcitonin/ml; pentagastrin and calcium chloride, either parenterally (both chlorides) or orally (calcium chloride only), proved to be potent secretagogues for calcitonin in the rat. In contrast to the results of Milhaud *et al.*[22] and Burford *et al.*[24] cited earlier, cross-reactivity between porcine and rat calcitonin, but not human calcitonin, was noted in the assay. Kent and Retallack subsequently concluded that their antiserum was probably more specific for the *N*-terminal portion of the rat calcitonin molecule.[25] In early 1976, Cooper *et al.*[26] reported their results with a rat calcitonin radioimmunoassay. Chicken antisera to rat calcitonin were developed and the *in vivo* calcitonin response to a variety of pertubations studied in young *male rats*. This new rat calcitonin assay was reported to be sensitive to 0.1–2.0 ng of circulating calcitonin. Although challenges with either intravenous or oral calcium, thyroid cautery, and isoproterenol provoked the anticipated increments in blood calcitonin levels, pentagastrin (25 μg i.v.) or gastrin (50 μg i.v.) failed to elicit responses. However, in contrast to the findings of Kent and Retallack, who used an *N*-terminal radioimmunoassay,[25] Cooper *et al.*[26] were unable to detect calcitonin in the basal state in any animal. Thus, the specificity and sensitivity of presently available rat calcitonin assays appear to depend on the species source of the calcitonin immunogen and the nature of the antibody-producing species. These studies should be considered in the light of reports that human calcitonin fragments (from residue 11 to the *C*-terminal prolinamide) retain full immunological reactivity, although they are biologically inert.[27] Continued studies with *N*-terminal and *C*-terminal immunoassays using varied synthetic calcitonin derivatives and fragments should shed light on the relationship between immunological and biological activity in the rat and the ultimate fate of the calcitonin peptide *in vivo*.

The nature of circulating calcitonin in man and the specificity and sensitivity of reported radioimmunoassay systems had also been a matter of controversy since the discovery of this hypocalcemic peptide. In 1974, Singer and Habener[28] analyzed the nature of circulating calcitonin of patients with medullary carcinoma, using rabbit antiserum and a synthetic human calcitonin immunogen; four distinct peaks of immunoreactive calcitonin were isolated. Three of the plasma peaks isolated by gel filtration were of higher molecular weight than monomer human calcitonin or calcitonin M. Similar results were obtained by Moukhtar *et al.*[29] Subsequently, in 1975, Snider *et al.*[30] reported on their experience with circulating calcitonin in patients with medullary carcinoma. In their studies, at least five major immunoreactive calcitonin fractions were isolated, one of which cochromatographed with synthetic human calcitonin M, with an apparent molecular weight of 3400. The remaining immunoreactive material chromatographed at molecular weights of 14,000, 5200, and 2400, with immunoreactive material also demonstrated in the void volume. In experiments using synthetic fragments of calcitonin M, it was determined that the rabbit antisera used in these studies recognized antigenic sites between amino acids 11 and 32 of the calcitonin molecule. In contrast to the heterogenous circulating calcitonin profiles observed for patients with medullary carcinoma, most of the immunoreactivity of plasma obtained from patients with hypercalcemia or renal failure chromatographed between the void volume and the calcitonin M peak. The authors concluded that antisera to human calcitonin that recognized antigenic sites at the midportion of the molecule were more sensitive, and that "the divergent results reported by various investigators who have studied calcitonin by radioimmunoassay may be explained both by the heterogenerity of endogenous human calcitonin and by the varying affinities of different antibodies for the separate binding sites on the hormonal molecule."[30] Also published in 1975 were additional studies on the immunochemical heterogenerity of plasma calcitonin in normal subjects and patients with medullary carcinoma.[31,32] Using two different antisera, one produced in a goat by intradermal injections of synthetic human calcitonin M, the other prepared in a chicken by intradermal injection of a conjugate of the same calcitonin and human serum albumin, Sizemore *et al.*[31] demonstrated varied specifities of the N- and C-terminal radioimmunoassay systems. Five molecular species with molecular weights either greater than or equal to the intact human calcitonin molecule were recognized by radioimmunoassay using antiserum with predominant N-terminal binding affinity (which usually resulted in higher immunoreactive calcitonin activities using nonchromatographed samples), whereas the antiserum with predominent C-terminal binding affinity recognized only two molecular species, one with a molecular weight comparable to calcitonin M, the other in a position consistent with a calcitonin dimer.[31] When comparing the circulating calcitonin species in patients with medullary carcinoma and one with a calcitonin-producing islet cell carcinoma with two antisera, each of which was produced in rabbits immunized with human calcitonin, Deftos and co-workers[32] demonstrated immunological differences between circulating calcitonin of thyroid and nonthyroid origin in man. Although the sensitivity for the measurement of human calcitonin standards was comparable for both antisera, one gave higher values for calcitonin of patients with medullary carcinoma, the other demonstrating higher values in the patient with pancreatic carcinoma.[32]

Using a radioimmunoassay system that incorporated an antibody developed in a goat immunized with human synthetic calcitonin M, Morita *et al.*[33] reported on a "sensitive and reliable method" for quantitating human calcitonin. In these studies, basal calcitonin levels were normally less than 0.3 ng/ml, and values as high as 1, 10, and 1000 ng/ml were recorded for patients with malignant tumors, chronic renal failure, and medullary carcinoma, respectively.[33] Although it is tempting to associate the hypocalcemia of chronic or acute renal failure[33,34] with elevations in circulating calcitonin, hormonal heterogenity, varying degrees of antibody sensitivities, and a lack of correlation between immunoreactivity and bioactivity[27] should by necessity condition our enthusiasm in this regard. In the past, the "normal range" of plasma calcitonin in man has been controversial at best, with 1700–5000 pcg/ml cited by investigators using bioassay methods, and 5–1000 pcg/ml proposed by others utilizing radioimmunoassay systems.[14] These wide discrepancies are unacceptable, and should be resolved when the problem of nonspecific effects of human plasma in the radioimmunoassay on the binding between the labeled hormone and the antibody is settled, and when additional experience is gained with more sensitive and specific assay systems in which the hormone is extracted from plasma by either immunoabsorption or immunoprecipitation before radioimmunoassay quantitation.

Reports detailing the biological synthesis, release, degradation, and tissue response to calcitonin have also appeared. Studies of calcitonin biosynthesis using *in vitro* preparations of chicken ultimobranchial glands suggested the existence of a biologically active calcitonin precursor (procalcitonin) with a molecular weight of 13,000 daltons,[35] a finding consistent with the earlier report of Ross *et al.*,[36] which described a procalcitonin in trout C cells cultured *in vitro*. Although calcium has been traditionally considered as the primary secretagogue for calcitonin, various agents were proved to be capable in this regard in 1975. Earlier work by Cooper *et al.*,[37,38] Care *et al.*,[39] and Bell[40] defining the role of gastrin and pentagastrin as calcitonin secretagogues were repeatedly confirmed in a variety of *in vivo, in situ,* and *in vitro* experimental designs.[41–43] In addition to these observations, Wells *et al.*[41] reported the stimulation of calcitonin secretion in humans by ethanol, an effect independent of gastrin or plasma calcium concentration, and Ross *et al.*[42] confirmed that PGE_2 stimulated calcitonin release *in vitro,* an observation previously reported by Bell.[40] Using human thyroid tissue, Selawry *et al.*[43] showed that glucagon and dibutyryl cAMP were potent stimuli, confirming observations made in previous years by Avioli *et al.*[44–46] in man and dog, and by Bell[40,47] and Bell and Queener[48] in porcine thyroid tissue. Neither Ross *et al.*[42] nor Selawry *et al.*[43] were able to confirm earlier reports of magnesium-stimulated calcitonin release,[40,49] although Cooper[50] showed, in perfusions of porcine thyroid gland, that magnesium and strontium were able to stimulate calcitonin release. In direct contrast to these observations, Anast et al.[51] reported that induced hypermagnesemia (to plasma levels of 6 mg/dl) resulted in a rapid and striking *fall* in serum calcitonin levels of patients with medullary thyroid carcinoma. Internal feedback regulation of calcitonin secretion was also proposed by Orme and Pento,[52] who reported "calcitonin-induced self inhibition" in experiments with porcine thyroid slices.

Following the discovery of calcitonin, studies of the physiological role played by this hypocalcemic peptide in the rat proceeded with unbridled vigor. It soon became established that in this mammal (classically considered the ideal experimental model for humans by those with interests in skeletal and calcium research), calcitonin functioned primarily to suppress bone resorption. As a consequence of the skeletal action of calcitonin, it was proposed that the hormone also functioned to modulate or abort the tendency to postprandial hypercalcemia.[53-56] Further evidence for the physiological importance of calcitonin in the regulation of plasma calcium in rats was presented by Kalu et al.,[57] in a series of experiments using thyroidectomized, thyroparathyroidectomized, and nephrectomized animals. These investigators demonstrated that an immediate but transient hypercalcemia obtained when basal calcitonin secretion was abolished in old unfed rats, and that the relative importance of calcitonin and parathyroid hormone in the acute regulation of plasma calcium is age-related. Given these findings, they emphasized the essential role of calcitonin during the age-related skeletal maturational cycle of this species. Further delineation of the relationship of feeding, circulating calcium, and calcitonin secretion in the rat was presented in 1975 by Talmage et al.[53] In a series of well-designed experiments, these workers demonstrated that the calcitonin response to feeding was independent of changes in circulating calcium. Although plasma gastrin levels also rose in response to feeding, a cause–effect relationship between the rising gastrin and calcitonin levels observed during the feeding cycle could not be established in these studies. As noted earlier in this review, using an assay reportedly sensitive to 0.1–2.0 ng of circulating calcitonin in the rat, these same investigators were later unable to demonstrate changes in calcitonin during or following pentagastrin or gastrin infusions.[26]

It had been suggested in the early 1970's that calcitonin also protects the maternal rat skeleton from excessive resorption during pregnancy and lactation. The data of Taylor and colleagues are consistent with this hypothesis. These investigators also reported that calcitonin, unlike parathyroid hormone, was not essential for milk secretion in the rat.[58] The report of Taylor and colleagues should, however, be considered together with an earlier study of Samaan et al.[59] This group, reporting on the results of studies designed to quantitate calcitonin and parathyroid hormone levels in peripheral maternal and cord serum of 75 women at time of delivery, concluded that in the human fetus, calcitonin functions primarily to modulate bone growth and calcification. In their studies, serum calcitonin was higher in the umbilical artery than in the umbilical vein, indicating that it originated in the fetus and not the placenta.[59] The role of calcitonin in conditioning skeletal metabolism and circulating calcium and inorganic phosphate during and immediately following the gestational period was examined in other species in 1975. In 1967, it was suggested that the bovine parturient–hypocalcemic–hypophosphatemic–paretic syndrome resulted from excessive maternal calcitonin secretion.[60] Subsequent observations of Barlet[61] were in accord with this hypothesis, since he reported that thyroxine-supplemented, thyroidectomized goats fed low-calcium diets did not develop hypocalcemia or hypophosphatemia during parturition. In 1975, Garel and co-workers, reporting that the increases in maternal circulating calcitonin of mares and cows were unrelated to changes in plasma calcium,[62,63] advanced the hypothesis that prostaglandins might function as the major calcitonin secretagogue in pregnancy.[63] This conclusion was appropriate, since prostaglandins are potent secretagogues for calcitonin in porcine thyroid slice[40] and trout ultimobranchial gland[64] in vitro preparations. Moreover, postaglandin levels are elevated during parturition.[65] These tentative conclusions must now be reconciled with the report of Mayer and co-workers.[66] In a report of studies involving both cows with hypocalcemia and paturient paresis and nonparetic hypocalcemic animals, these investigators conclucded that the hypocalcemia of parturition was not the result of increased calcitonin secretion. In fact, the data suggested that the parturient hypocalcemic syndrome is associated with a *diminished* prepartal secretion of calcitonin.[66] In addition to studies detailing calcitonin levels in pregnant humans and farm animals, a publication describing changes in plasma calcitonin in spawning salmon also appeared in 1975. Watts *et al.*[67] reported that calcitonin levels increased progressively in the female salmon up to the time of spawning, after which they fell precipitously. Noting similar patterns in the male salmon, the authors concluded that "calcitonin may play an important role in the reproductive cycle of fish."[67] This reviewer is once again confronted with a confusing array of data regarding the role of calcitonin in pregnant females, parturient cows, and spawning salmon, and can only await clarification from more definitive agreement between investigative groups regarding the specificities of calcitonin immunoassays and the relationship between immunoassay and biological activities.

Further insight into the relationship between specific organ inactivation of the various calcitonins and the nature of the biological response was also gained in 1975. In 1972, Singer *et al.*,[68] using species-specific immunoassays, reported that porcine calcitonin was inactivated by the canine kidney, muscle, and bone, whereas salmon calcitonin and human calcitonin were inactivated primarily by the kidney. In that same year, Marx et al.,[17] discovered receptors in fetal rat calvaria and rat kidney cortex for salmon and mammalian (human and porcine) calcitonin(s), and reported that salmon calcitonin demonstrated the highest binding affinity for the receptors of either tissue. The following year, this same group of investigators reported the isolation of two independent orders of calcitonin receptor sites in the kidney and bone of rats: high-affinity/low capacity receptors that were not primarily sites of hormonal degradation, and low-affinity/high-capacity receptors that could be involved in the degradation process.[69] Hsu and Haymovits[70] later demonstrated that in rat kidney, porcine and salmon calcitonin competed with human calcitonin for a common degradation site. They were unable to demonstrate degradation of human calcitonin by bone cells obtained from the calvaria of 1-week-old rats.[70] In these experiments, as well as in those of Singer et al.[68] and Marx et al.,[69] loss of immunoreactivity was used as the determinant of degradation of the intact 1–32 calcitonin molecule. In 1975, Marx and Aurbach[71] showed that the high-affinity salmon calcitonin–binding sites of renal plasma membranes mediate the activation of the membrane-associated adenylate cyclase by calcitonin. In contrast to the results obtained using murine renal plasma membrane preparations, those obtained from the kidneys of man, dog, and cow were devoid of high-affinity binding sites for salmon calcitonin, and had little or no calcitonin-sensitive adenylate cyclase.[71] Of additional interest in this same report were the observations that destruction of plasma membrane receptor activity impaired the calcitonin-sensitive adenylate cyclase response, but *not* the fluoride-sensitive one. Other studies by Queener et al.[72] were more definitive in this regard. Using purified porcine renal cortical membranes, these investigators isolated a soluble adenylate cyclase that responded to porcine calcitonin and NaF, but not to parathyroid hormone or glucagon. They also equated the binding affinity of calcitonin with its ability to activate a specific solubilized adenylate cyclase.[72] These many studies detailing the renal binding of calcitonin with adenylate cyclase activity are consistent with the observations that calcitonin increases urinary cAMP excretion in thyroparathyroidectomized rats and in man, an effect that apparently precedes the phosphaturic response.[73] They also support the contention of some that the phosphaturic responses to parathyroid hormone and calcitonin reflect two distinct anatomical sites and adenylate cyclase systems.[73–76] The cAMP response of skeletal tissue to calcitonin and parathyroid hormone is also additive,[77,78] and the presence of separate target cells for each hormone was established by Wong and Cohn.[76] Thus, as demonstrated for the kidney, two distinct hormonal-specific adenylate cyclase systems probably also modulate the skeletal response to parathyroid hormone and calcitonin in mammals.

The effects of calcitonin on the kidney, gastrointestinal tract, and carbohydrate and fat metabolism were reviewed in detail in 1975 by Queener and Bell.[15] Gray and co-workers, having previously shown that infusions of salmon calcitonin resulted in jejunal secretion of water, sodium, potassium, and chloride in man,[80] were unable to document a similar intestinal response in rabbits.[81] The data of Barnett et al.[82] supported the concept that the diuretic and saluretic response to calcitonin in man was mediated by prostaglandins, and Blahos et al.[83] demonstrated a uricosuric action of calcitonin in man for the first time. The observations of Becker and co-workers that salmon calcitonin produced marked inhibition of gastric acid secretion and inhibited the gastrin response to feeding[84] were extended by Fahrenkrug et al.[85] These investigators reported that salmon calcitonin depressed basal, as well as food-stimulated, serum gastrin levels in man without associated changes in serum calcium.[85] They also showed that the effect of calcitonin on serum gastrin levels was restricted primarily to gastrin III and gastrin IV immunoreactive components, a result consistent with they hypothesis that calcitonin acts directly on the "gastrin cells" of the duodenum and gastric antrum.[85] A provocative report by Lupulescu[86] provided the first experimental in vivo evidence for calcitonin-stimulated DNA synthesis. Evidence of increased calcitonin secretion during the initial stages of hepatic regeneration in the rat was also presented.[87] The significance of these latter observations, as well as those demonstrating that calcitonin increases hepatic calcium uptake independent of cAMP,[88] has yet to be determined. Finally, while analyzing arteriovenous gradients of calcium, inorganic phosphate, hydroxyproline, oxygen, carbon dioxide and hydrogen ions across the femur, Singh et al.[89] studied the hypocalcemic response to porcine calcitonin in the dog. Observing no calcitonin-dependent increment in bone calcium uptake, these investigators concluded that calcitonin-induced hypocalcemia results entirely from decreased bone resorption. Reductions in femoral oxygen consumption and carbon dioxide production observed during limb perfusion with calcitonin were consistent with their assumption that in the dog, the skeletal effect of calcitonin is mediated directly or indirectly by factors that depress mitochondrial respiration.[89] These observations are obviously preliminary, but bear further consideration, since, as noted by Nagata et al.,[90] the hypocalcemic response to calcitonin may be dissociated from stimulated alterations in skeletal cAMP concentrations.

Scattered reports detailing the response of patients with Paget's disease of bone to calcitonin therapy have also appeared recently. Beneficial responses in this disorder have not been observed with weekly injections of salmon calcitonin,[91] and with human calcitonin preparations either alone[92,93] or combined with diphosphonates.[94] Symptomatic improvement was observed for up to 1 year following discontinuation of salmon calcitonin therapy.[95] Despite these results, as well as reports of stimulated release or suppression of immunoassayable calcitonin in patients with medullary carcinoma by nonphysiological doses of enteric hormones, calcium or magnesium, the case for calcitonin as an essential modulator of mineral and skeletal homeostasis in normal man has not yet been established.

References

1. Reiss, E., and Cantebury, J. M., 1974, Emerging concepts of the nature of circulating parathyroid hormones: Implications for clinical research, *Recent Prog. Horm. Res.* **30:**391–429.
2. Mayer, G. P., Habener, J. F., and Potts, J. T., Jr., 1976, Parathyroid hormone secretion *in vivo:* Demonstration of a calcium-independent nonsuppressible component of secretion, *J. Clin. Invest.* **57:**678–683.
3. Habener, J. F., Kemper, B., Potts, J. T., Jr., and Rich, A., 1975, Pre-proparathyroid hormone identified by cell-free translation of messenger RNA from hyperplastic human parathyroid tissue, *J. Clin. Invest.* **56:**1328–1333.
4. Hruska, K. A., Kopelman, R., Rutherford, W. E., Klahr, S., and Slatopolsky, E., 1975, Metabolism of immunoreactive parathyroid hormone in the dog: Role of the kidney and the effects of chronic renal disease, *J. Clin. Invest.* **56:**39–48.
5. Canterbury, J. M., Bricker, L. A., Levey, G. S., Kozlovskis, P. L., Ruiz, E., Zull, J. E., and Reiss, E., 1975, Metabolism of bovine parathyroid hormone; immunological and biological characteristics of fragments generated by liver perfusion, *J. Clin. Invest.* **55:**1245–1253.
6. Goltzman, D., Peytremann, A., Callahan, E. N., Segre, G. V., and Potts, J. T., Jr., 1976, Metabolism and biological activity of parathyroid hormone in renal cortical membranes, *J. Clin. Invest.* **57:**8–19.
7. Dziak, R., and Stern, P. H., 1975, Calcium transport in isolated bone cells III. Effects of parathyroid hormone and cyclic 3'5' AMP, *Endocrinology* **97:** 1281–1287.
8. MacGregor, R. R., Hamilton, J. W., and Cohn, D. V., 1975, The by-pass of tissue hormone stores during the secretion of newly synthesized parathyroid hormone, *Endocrinology* **97:**178–188.
9. Kemper, B., Habener, J. F., Rich, A., and Potts, J. T., Jr., 1975, Microtubules and the intracellular conversion of proparathyroid hormone to parathyroid hormone, *Endocrinology* **96:**903–912.
10. Hamburger, R. J., Lawson, N. L., and Schwartz, J. H., 1976, Response to parathyroid hormone in defined segments of proximal tubule, *Amer. J. Physiol.* **230:**286.
11. Forte, L. R., Nickols, G. A., and Anast, C. S., 1976, Renal adenylate cyclase and the interrelationship between parathyroid hormone and vitamin D in the regulation of urinary phosphate and adenosine cyclic 3'5'-monophosphate excretion, *J. Clin. Invest.* **57:**559–568.

12. Avioli, L. V., 1976, What's new—vitamins and minerals, *in: The Year in Metabolism, 1975–1976* (N. Freinkel, ed.), Chapter 9, Plenum Press, New York.

13. Hirsch, P. F., Gauthier, G. F., and Munson, P. L., 1963, Thyroid hypocalcemic principle and recurrent laryngeal nerve injury as factors affecting the response to parathyroidectomy in rats, *Endocrinology* **73:**244–252.

14. Gray, T. K., and Ontjes, D. A., 1975, Clinical aspects of thyrocalcitonin, *Clin. Orthop. Relat. Res.* **111:**238–256.

15. Queener, S. F., and Bell, N. H., 1975, Calcitonin: A general survey, *Metabolism* **24:**555.

16. Sieber, P., Brugger, M., Kamber, B., Riniker, B., Rittel, W., Maier, R., and Staehelin, M., 1969, Synthesis and biological activity of peptide sequences related to porcine α-thyrocalcitonin, *in: Calcitonin, Proceedings of the Second International Symposium* (S. Taylor, ed.), p. 28–40, Springer-Verlag, New York.

17. Marx, S. J., Woodard, C., Aurbach, G. D., *et al.*, 1972, Calcitonin receptors of kidney and bone, *Science* **178:**999–1001.

18. Marx, S. J., Woodard, C., and Aurbach, G. D., 1973, Calcitonin receptors for calcitonin: Binding and degradation of hormone, *J. Biol. Chem.* **248:**4797–4802.

19. Maier, R., Riniker, B., and Rittel, W., 1974, Analogues of human calcitonin. 1. Influence of modifications in amino-acid positions 29 and 31 on hypocalcaemic activity in the rat, *FEBS Lett.* **48:**68–71.

20. Maier, R., Kamber, B., Riniker, B., and Rittel, W., 1975, Analogues of human calcitonin II. Influence of modifications in amino acid positions 1, 8 and 22 on hypocalcemic activity in the rat, *Horm. Metab. Res.* **7:**511–514.

21. Guttmann, S. T., Ples, J., Huguenin, R., *et al.*, 1968, Syntheses des thyreocalcitonins, *Helv. Chim. Acta* **51:**1155–1161.

22. Milhaud, G., Tharaud, D., Jullienne, A., and Moukhtar, M. S., 1972, Radioimmunoassay of rat calcitonin, *in: Endocrinology, Proceedings of the 3rd International Symposium* (S. Taylor, ed.), p. 380–385, William Heinemann Medical Books, London.

23. Moukhtar, M. S., Tharaud, D., Jullienne, A., Raulais, D., Calmettes, C., and Milhaud, G., 1974, Immunological similarity of human and rat calcitonin confirmed by immunofluorescent methods, *Experientia* **30:**552–555.

24. Burford, H. J., Ontjes, D. A., Cooper, C. W., Parlow, A. F., and Hirsch, P. F., 1975, Purification, characterization and radioimmunoassay of thyrocalcitonin from rat thyroid glands, *Endocrinology* **96:**340–348.

25. Kent, G. N., and Retallack, R. W., 1975, Radioimmunoassay of the basal circulating level of calcitonin in the rat, *Biochem. Biophys. Res. Commun.* **66:**1251–1256.

26. Cooper, C. W., Obie, J. F., and Hsu, W. H., 1976, Improvement and initial *in vivo* application of the radioimmunoassay of rat thyrocalcitonin, *Proc. Soc. Exp. Biol. Med.* **151:**183–188.

27. Byfield, P. G. H., Clark, M. B., Turner, K., Foster, G. V., and MacIntyre, I., 1972, Immunochemical studies on human calcitonin M leading to information on the shape of the molecule, *Biochem. J.* **127:**199–206.

28. Singer, F. R., and Habener, J. F., 1974, Multiple immunoreactive forms of calcitonin in human plasma, *Biochem. Biophys. Res. Commun.* **61:**710.

29. Moukhtar, M. S., Jullienne, A., Taboulet, J., Calmettes, C., Raulais, D., and Milhaud, G., 1975, Hétérogéneité de la calcitonine immunoréactive dans le plasma de sujets avec cancer medullaire, *Pathol. Biol.* **23:**809–814.

30. Snider, R. H., Silva, O. L., Becker, K. L., and Moore, C. F., 1975, Heterogeneity of calcitonin, *Lancet* **1**:49–50.

31. Sizemore, G. W., and Heath, H., III, 1975, Immunochemical heterogeneity of calcitonin in plasma of patients with medullary thyroid carcinoma, *J. Clin. Invest.* **55**:1111–1118.

32. Deftos, J., Roos, B. A., Bronzert, D., and Parthemore, J. G., 1975, Immunochemical heterogeneity of calcitonin in plasma, *J. Clin. Endocrinol. Metab.* **40**:409–412.

33. Morita, R., Fukunaga, M., Yamamoto, I., Mori, T., and Torizuka, K., 1975, Radioimmunoassay for human calcitonin employing synthetic calcitonin M: Its clinical application, *Endocrinol. Jpn.* **22**:419–426.

34. Ardaillou, R., Beaufils, M., Nivez, M. P., Isaac, R., Mayaud, C., and Spaer, J. D., 1975, Increased plasma calcitonin in early acute renal failure, *Clin. Sci. Mol. Med.* **49**:301–304.

35. Moya, F., Nieto, A., and R.-Candela, J. L., 1975, Calcitonin biosynthesis: Evidence for a precursor, *Eur. J. Biochem.* **55**:407–413.

36. Ross, B. A., Okano, K., and Deftos, L. J., 1974, Evidence for a pro-calcitonin, *Biochem. Biophys. Res. Commun.* **60**:1134–1140.

37. Cooper, C. W., Schwesinger, W. H., Ontjes, D. A., Mahgoub, A. M., and Munson, P. L., 1972, Stimulation of secretion of pig thyrocalcitonin by gastrin and related hormonal peptides, *Endocrinology* **91**:1079–1089.

38. Hennessy, J. F., Wells, S. A., Jr., Ontjes, D. A., and Cooper, C. W., 1974, A comparison of pentagastrin injection and calcium infusion as provocative agents for the detection of medullary carcinoma of the thyroid, *J. Clin. Endocrinol. Metab.* **39**:487–495.

39. Care, A. D., Bates, R. F. L., Swaminathan, R., and Ganguli, P. C., 1971, The role of gastrin as a calcitonin secretagogue, *J. Endocrinol.* **51**:735–744.

40. Bell, N. H., 1975, Further studies on the regulation of calcitonin release *in vitro*, *Horm. Metab. Res.* **7**:77–83.

41. Wells, S. A., Jr., Cooper, C. W., and Ontjes, D. A., 1975, Stimulation of thyrocalcitonin secretion by ethanol in patients with medullary thyroid carcinoma—An effect apparently not mediated by gastrin, *Metabolism* **24**:1215–1219.

42. Ross, B. A., Bundy, L. L., Miller, E. A., and Deftas, L. J., 1975, Calcitonin secretion by monolayer cultures of human C-cells derived from medullary thyroid carcinoma, *Endocrinology* **97**:39–45.

43. Selawry, H. P., Becker, K. L., Bivins, L. E., Snider, R. H., and Silva, O. L., 1975, *In vitro* studies of calcitonin release in man, *Horm. Metab. Res.* **7**:432–437.

44. Birge, S. J., and Avioli, L. V., 1969, Glucagon-induced hypocalcemia in man, *J. Clin. Endocrinol. Metab.* **29**:213–218.

45. Avioli, L. V., Shieber, W., and Kipnis, D. M., 1971, Role of glucagon and adrenergic receptors in thyrocalcitonin release in the dog, *Endocrinology* **88**:1337–1340.

46. Avioli, L. V., Birge, S. J., Scott, S., and Shieber, W., 1969, Role of the thyroid gland during glucagon-induced hypocalcemia in the dog, *Amer. J. Physiol.* **216**:939–945.

47. Bell, N. H., 1970, The effects of glucagon, dibutyryl cyclic 3'5' adenosine monophosphate and theophylline on calcitonin-secretion *in vitro*, *J. Clin. Invest.* **49**:1368–1373.

48. Bell, N. H., and Queener, S., 1974, Stimulation of calcitonin synthesis and

release *in vitro* by calcium and dibutyryl cyclic AMP, *Nature London* **248**:343.

49. Care, A. D., Bell, N. H., and Bates, R. F. L., 1971, The effect of hypermagnesaemia on calcitonin secretion *in vivo*, *J. Endocrinol.* **51**:381–386.

50. Cooper, C. W., 1975, Ability of several cations to promote secretion of thyrocalcitonin in the pig, *Proc. Soc. Exp. Biol. Med.* **148**:449–454.

51. Anast, C., David, L., Winnacker, J., Glass, R., Baskin, W., Brubaker, L., and Burns, T., 1975, Serum calcitonin–lowering effect of magnesium in patients with medullary carcinoma of the thyroid, *J. Clin. Invest.* **56**:1615–1621.

52. Orme, A. L., and Pento, J. T., 1976, Evidence of calcitonin-induced inhibition of calcitonin secretion in porcine thyroid slices, *Proc. Soc. Exp. Biol. Med.* **151**:110–112.

53. Talmage, R. V., Doppelt, S. H., and Cooper, C. W., 1975, Relationship of blood concentrations of calcium, phosphate, gastrin and calcitonin to the onset of feeding in the rat, *Proc. Soc. Exp. Biol. Med.* **149**:855–859.

54. Swaminathan, R., Bates, R. F. L., and Care, A. D., 1972, Fresh evidence for a physiological role of calcitonin in calcium homeostasis, *J. Endocrinol.* **54**:525–526.

55. Cooper, C. W., Hirsch, P. F., and Munson, P. L., 1970, Importance of endogenous thyrocalcitonin for protection against hypercalcemia in the rat, *Endocrinology* **86**:406–415.

56. Kalu, D. N., Hadji-Georgopoulos, A., Sarr, M. G., Solomon, B. A., and Foster, G. V., 1974, The role of parathyroid hormone in the maintenance of plasma calcium levels in rats, *Endocrinology* **95**:1156–1165.

57. Kalu, D. N., Hadji-Georgopoulos, A., and Foster, G. V., 1975, Evidence for physiological importance of calcitonin in the regulation of plasma calcium in rats, *J. Clin. Invest.* **55**:722–727.

58. Taylor, T. G., Lewis, P. E., and Balderstone, O., 1975, Role of calcitonin in protecting the skeleton during pregnancy and lactation, *J. Endocrinol.* **66**:297–298.

59. Samaan, N. A., Wigoda, C., and Castillo, S. G., 1974, Human serum calcitonin and parathyroid hormone levels in the maternal, umbilical cord blood and postpartum, *Proceedings of the Fourth International Symposium*, London, 1974, p. 364.

60. Capen, C. C., and Young, D. M., 1967, Thyrocalcitonin: Evidence for release in a spontaneous hypocalcemic disorder, *Science* **157**:205–206.

61. Barlet, J. P., 1974, Role physiologique de la calcitonine chez la chevre gestante ou allaitante, *Ann. Biol. Anim. Biochim. Biophys.* **14**:447–457.

62. Garel, J. M., and Barlet, J. P., 1975, Plasma immunoreactive calcitonin and parathyroid hormone levels in parturient cows, *J. Endocrinol.* **66**:299–300.

63. Garel, J. M., Rosset, W. M., and Barlet, J. P., 1975, Plasma immunoreactive calcitonin levels in pregnant mares and newborn foals, *Horm. Metab. Res.* **7**:429–432.

64. Roos, B. A., Bundy, L. L., Bailey, R., and Deftos, L. J., 1974, Calcitonin-secretion *in vitro*. I. Preparation of monolayer C-cell cultures, *Endocrinology* **95**:1142–1149.

65. Zerobin, K., Jochle, W., and Steingruber, Ch., 1973, Termination of pregnancy with prostaglandins E_2 (PGE_2) and $F_{2\alpha}$ ($PGF_{2\alpha}$) in cattle, *Prostaglandins* **4**:891–901.

66. Mayer, G. P., Blum, J. W., and Deftos, L. J., 1975, Diminished prepartal plasma calcitonin concentration in cows developing parturient hypocalcemia, *Endocrinology* **96**:1478–1485.

67. Watts, E. G., Copp, D. H., and Deftos, L. J., 1975, Changes in plasma calcitonin and calcium during the migration of a salmon, *Endocrinology* **96:**214–218.
68. Singer, F. R., Habener, J. F., Greene, E., Godin, P., and Potts, J. T., Jr., 1972, Inactivation of calcitonin by specific organs, *Nature New Biol. London* **237:**269–270.
69. Marx, S. J., Woodward, C., Aurbach, G. D., Glossmann, H., and Keutmann, H. T., 1973, Renal receptors for calcitonin binding and degradation of hormone, *J. Biol. Chem.* **248:**4797–4802.
70. Hsu, H. H. T., and Haymovits, A., 1974, On the nature of degradation of calcitonin by mammalian cells, *Proc. Soc. Exp. Biol. Med.* **146:**1044–1049.
71. Marx, S. J., and Aurbach, G. D., 1975, Renal receptors for calcitonin: Coordinate occurrence with calcitonin-activated adenylate cyclase, *Endocrinology* **97:**448–453.
72. Queener, S. F., Fleming, J. W., and Bell, N. H., 1975, Solubilization of calcitonin-responsive renal cortical adenylate cyclase, *J. Biol. Chem.* **250:**7586–7892.
73. Kurokawa, K., Nagata, N., Sasaki, M., Nakane, K., 1974, Effects of calcitonin on the concentration of cyclic adenosine 3'5'-monophosphate in rat kidney *in vivo* and *in vitro*, *Endocrinology* **94:**1514–1518.
74. Bell, N. H., 1974, Evidence for a separate adenylate cyclase system responsive to beta-adrenergic stimulation in the renal cortex of the rat, *Acta Endocrinol.* **77:**604–611.
75. Melson, G. L., Chase, L. R., and Aurbach, G. D., 1970, Parathyroid hormone-sensitive adenyl cyclase in isolated renal tubules, *Endocrinology* **86:**511–518.
76. Haas, H. G., Dambacher, M. A., Guncaga, J., and Lauffenburger, T., 1971, Renal effect of calcitonin and parathyroid extract in man, *J. Clin. Invest.* **50:**2689.
77. Heersche, J. N. M., Marcus, R., and Aurbach, G. D., 1974, Calcitonin and the formation of 3'5'-AMP in bone and kidney, *Endocrinology* **94:**241–247.
78. Smith, D. M., and Johnston, C. C., Jr., 1974, Hormonal responsiveness of adenylate cyclase activity from separated bone cells, *Endocrinology* **95:**130–139.
79. Wong, G. L., and Cohn, D. V., 1975, Target cell in bone for parathormone and calcitonin are different: Enrichment for each cell type by sequential digestion of mouse calvaria and selective adhesion to polymeric surfaces, *Proc. Nat. Acad. Sci. U.S.A.* **72:**3167–3171.
80. Gray, T. K., Bieberdorf, F. A., and Fordtran, J. S., 1973, Thyrocalcitonin and the jejunal absorption of calcium, water and electrolytes in normal subjects, *J. Clin. Invest.* **52:**3084–3088.
81. Gray, T. K., Juan, D., and Powell, D. W., 1975, Salmon calcitonin and water and electrolyte transport in rabbit ileum, *Proc. Soc. Exp. Biol. Med.* **150:**151–154.
82. Barnett, D. B., Edwards, I. R., and Smith, A. J., 1975, Antagonism by indomethacin of diuretic response to calcitonin in man, *Br. Med. J.* (September 20), p. 686.
83. Blahos, J., Osten, J., Mertl, L., Kotas, J., Gregor, O., and Reisenauer, R., 1975, The uricosuric effect of calcitonin, *Horm. Metab. Res.* **7:**445–446.
84. Becker, H. D., Reeder, D. D., Scurry, M. T., and Thompsom, J. C., 1974, Inhibition of gastrin release and gastrin secretion by calcitonin in patients with peptic ulcer, *Amer. J. Surg.* **127:**71–75.

85. Fahrenkrug, J., Hornum, I., and Rehfeld, J. F., 1975, Effect of calcitonin on serum gastrin concentration and component pattern in man, *J. Clin. Endocrinol. Metab.* **41:**149–152.

86. Lupulescu, A., 1975, Effect of calcitonin on DNA synthesis in experimental wounds, *Proc. Soc. Exp. Biol. Med.* **150:**703–706.

87. MacManus, J. P., Youdale, T., and Braceland, B. M., 1975, Evidence for the release of calcitonin and parathyroid hormone during liver regeneration in the rat, *Horm. Metab. Res.* **7:**83–87.

88. Yamaguchi, M., Takei, Y., and Yamamoto, T., 1975, Effect of thyrocalcitonin on calcium concentration in liver of intact and thyroparathyroidectomized rats, *Endocrinology* **96:**1004–1008.

89. Singh, M., Lin, C., and Post, M., 1975, Calcitonin inhibition of bone cell metabolism *in vivo:* An experimental study in dogs, *Endocrinology* **96:**1468–1474.

90. Nagata, N., Sasaki, M., Kimura, N., and Nakane, K., 1975, Effects of porcine calcitonin on the metabolism of calcium and cyclic AMP in rat skeletal tissue *in vivo, Endocrinology* **97:**527–535.

91. Avramides, A., Flores, A., Derose, J., and Wallach, S., 1975, Treatment of Paget's disease of bone with once a week injections of salmon calcitonin, *Brit. Med. J.* (September 13), p. 632.

92. Rojanasathit, S., Rosenberg, E., Haddad, J. G., Jr., 1974, Paget's bone disease: Response to human calcitonin in patients resistant to salmon calcitonin, *Lancet* **2:**1412–1415.

93. Doyle, F. J., Woodhouse, N. J. Y., Glenn, A. C. A., Joplin, G. F., and MacIntyre, I., 1974, Healing of the bones in juvenile Paget's disease treated by human calcitonin, *Br. J. Radiol.* **47:**9–15.

94. Hosking, D. J., Aken, J. V., Bijvoet, O. L. M., and Will, E. J., 1976, Paget's bone disease treated with diphosphonate and calcitonin, *Lancet* **1:**615–616.

95. Avramides, A., Flores, A., DeRose, J., and Wallach, S., 1976, Paget's disease of the bone: Observations after cessation of long-term synthetic salmon calcitonin treatment, *J. Clin. Endocrinol. Metab.* **42:**459–463.

Ectopic Hormone Syndromes

Louis M. Sherwood

10.1. Introduction

The increasing focus on the diagnosis and management of patients with malignant disorders, the growth in investigative programs through governmental and private support, and the growing occupancy of hospital beds by patients with cancer have all given impetus to the accumulation of information concerning the production of proteins by tumors. For years, tumors have been associated with various clinical endocrine and metabolic disorders thought to be due to production of peptide hormones by the tumor. Advances in endocrine biochemistry and physiology, the enormous sensitivity of radioimmunoassay techniques, selective catheterization, and the use of *in vitro* methods for analysis of plasma and tumor tissue have facilitated the identification and clarification of some of these

LOUIS M. SHERWOOD • Department of Medicine, Michael Reese Hospital and Medical Center; and the Pritzker School of Medicine, University of Chicago, Chicago, Illinois.

disorders. Although this chapter will focus on recent developments in the area of ectopic hormone syndromes and multiple endocrine neoplasia, a more comprehensive approach to the subject requires a brief review of the major aspects of the history and development of these concepts.

10.2. Etiology and Mechanisms of Ectopic Hormone Production

While great progress has been made in examining and recognizing clinical syndromes and identifying related biochemical markers, much less progress has been made in uncovering the basic mechanisms responsible for the tumor syndromes. These syndromes are of intense interest, not only to the clinician, pathologist, and geneticist, but also to the developmental biologist, biochemist, and immunologist. Within an understanding of the causal mechanisms lie many basic concepts in cell differentiation and dedifferentiation, antigenic function, synthesis of hormones, and production of clinical manifestations.

It is generally accepted that these tumors undergo a process of dedifferentiation to a more primitive state in which proteins will be synthesized that are not normally produced by the differentiated cell. Since all somatic cells contain the same complement of DNA, this dedifferentiation is theoretically possible. However, this explanation is somewhat simplistic, and more tangible evidence of an etiological basis has been sought. Among the approaches taken have been the following:

1. It has been emphasized by Amatruda[1] and others that there is a close correspondence between histological tumor type and clinical syndrome. The ectopic hormone syndromes do not occur as random processes; rather, there are clear patterns of development of specific biochemical or clinical syndromes in association with discrete tumor types. Were the process of dedifferentiation completely random, it is unlikely that this association would occur. Table I indicates the association of syndromes with tumor type.

2. Definitive information concerning the chemical nature of the peptide hormones that are produced by the tumor tissues is still lacking; such information would enable investigators to determine whether these peptides represent normal or abnormal forms of the hormone. Synthesis of a hormone molecule identical to that produced by the normal gland is generally thought necessary to support the theory of derepression. The major problem is that the quantities of hormone that have been available from such tumors are small, adequate to characterize by bioassay, receptor assay, or radioimmunoassay, but generally not sufficient to permit determination of amino acid sequence. In the case of parathyroid hormone,[2,3] corticotropin (ACTH),[4-6] gastrin,[7,8] renin,[9] and others, there is evidence

Table I. Relationship of Tumor Type to Hormone Production[a]

Hormone	Tumor type
ACTH and lipoprotein (MSHβ)	Oat cell carcinoma of lung
	Thymoma
	Islet cell tumor
	Bronchial carcinoid
	Also: ovary, pheochromocytoma, gastrointestinal, prostate, neurogenic, parotid, and medullary thyroid
Growth hormone	Adenocarcinoma of the lung
Human placental lactogen	Undifferentiated carcinoma of the lung
	Hepatoma
	Lymphoma
	Pheochromocytoma
Prolactin	Renal cell
	Undifferentiated carcinoma of the lung
Gonadotropin	Hepatoblastoma, pancreatic, other gastrointestinal
	Undifferentiated adenocarcinoma of the lung
	Choriocarcinoma of male and female, other testicular
	Adenocarcinoma of ovary
	Melanoma
HCG β-subunit	Adenocarcinoma of the pancreas
HCG α-subunit	Carcinoid
Thyrotropin	Choriocarcinoma, hydatidiform mole
	Epidermoid carcinoma of the lung
	Mesothelioma
Vasopressin	Oat cell carcinoma of the lung
	Pancreatic adenocarcinoma
Parathyroid hormone	Epidermoid carcinoma of the lung
	Renal cell
	Other epidermoid tumors
Prostaglandin E₂	Renal cell carcinoma
	Lung tumors
Osteoclast-activating factor	Multiple myeloma
	Burkitt's lymphoma
Somatomedin (NSILA-s)	Mesodermal and mesenchymal tumors
Calcitonin	Oat cell of the lung, breast, pancreas, and other carcinomas
Glucagon	Non-beta islet cell tumors, undifferentiated lung cancer
Gastrin	Non-beta islet cell tumor
Vasoactive intestinal peptide	Non-beta islet cell tumor
Erythropoietin	Renal cell carcinoma
	Cerebellar hemangioblastoma
	Also: pheochromocytoma and hepatoma
Renin	Juxtaglomerular tumor
	Wilm's tumor
	Renal cell
Serotonin and 5-OH-tryptophan	Non-beta islet cell tumor
	Oat cell carcinoma of the lung
	Pancreatic adenocarcinoma

[a]Modified after Amatruda.[1]

that the tumors may produce forms of the hormones that differ from the native hormones in immunological characteristics, as well as in molecular weights. These differences do not necessarily imply that the tissues are synthesizing different forms of the hormone. Production of a precursor substance and its release (owing to lack in the tumor of an enzyme normally capable of converting precursor to hormone) or differences in the rate of metabolism or degradation of the hormone are possible factors. Since the problems related to heterogeneity of peptide hormones and to peptide hormone metabolism have now become increasingly recognized, the analysis of peptide hormones produced by tumors has become more complex. More definitive information is required, and immunological identity by radioimmunoassay does not necessarily prove biochemical or sequence identity, even though it implies sequence homologies.

3. Embryological studies performed *in vitro* provide evidence that embryonic induction can take place in tumors, lending additional support for the derepression hypothesis. Ellison and Wilson[10] showed that an undifferentiated rat renal cell carcinoma in organ coculture with mouse embryo spinal cord produced differentiated renal tubules. Thus, transformation from normal to neoplastic tissue could be a counterpart of normal differentiation. Ectopic hormone production could theoretically be explained as dedifferentiation of tumor cells and acquisition of previously competent function, followed by misprogramming and abnormal activation of genes. Tumors arising from different embryological layers would therefore undergo differentiation to varying degrees.[11] One group of tumors would acquire competence previously endowed in that germ layer; an example would be endodermal tumors that synthesize hormones characteristic of other endodermal tissues. A second group of mesodermal tumors would have to undergo more extensive dedifferentiation in order to assume secretory properties. A third group of ectodermal or mesodermal tumors would be extremely labile and acquire characteristics of endodermally derived glands by some nonrandom process.

4. Cell hybridization has also been suggested as a potential mechanism for the acquisition of new competence by tumors.[12] Experiments using cell hybridization techniques *in vitro* have emphasized the development of new characteristics by cells that have been hybridized; this possibility has been suggested for neoplastic tissue, although definitive evidence is lacking (e.g., fusion of a malignant cell with a normal neuroectodermal cell having secretory properties).

5. Weichert[13] proposed that the etiology of these tumors may be related to a common origin in neuroectodermal tissue. His arguments are based on the interesting and tantalizing observations of Pearse,[14] who defined the characteristics of a group of cells that he termed *APUD* (Amine-Precursor Uptake and Decarboxylation). The APUD cells have

secretory properties, contain neurosecretory granules, and are able to take up substances such as DOPA or 5-HT and convert them to amines; they also produce peptide hormones. Since these characteristics are found in neural cells, Pearse and Polak[15] suggested that neural crest cells migrate to the endodermal tissues during development and confer secretory properties on the developing endocrine organs. They based this observation on the fact that cells with APUD characteristics could be found in the endodermal secretory sites. In a unique set of experiments, they showed that quail neural crest cells grafted onto chicken embryos could migrate into the ultimobranchial body, giving rise to the calcitonin-producing C cell.[16] Using the APUD hypothesis, Weichert[13] suggested that endocrine cells with secretory characteristics in the alimentary tract were produced from neuroectodermal secretory cells, and that they migrated with endodermal cells of the pituitary, thyroid, parathyroid, pancreatic islet, ultimobranchial body, and thymus. Therefore, tumors that produce polypeptide hormones would have developed from APUD cells located in endodermal tissues, such as the lung. Weichert used this argument to support a common origin for the ectopic hormone syndromes, as well as multiple endocrine neoplasia.

Recently, however, doubt has been shed on the concept that all cells with APUD characteristics in the endodermal layer are derived from the neural crest. Le Douarin and Teillet[17] were unable to identify quail nuclei in endodermal gut derivatives other than the ultimobranchial body, contrary to what would have been predicted from the hypothesis of Pearse and Polak.[15] Pictet et al.[18] showed that embryos cultured in vitro in which the ectodermal layer had been removed prior to the development of the neural crest were still able to develop pancreatic beta cells that contained immunoreactive insulin. These studies suggest that enterchromaffin tissue does not necessarily develop from neural crest, but it is possible that ectodermal cells might have colonized the endoderm at an earlier stage of development.

Weichert's hypothesis is attractive as an explanation for the ectopic hormone syndromes and multiple endocrine tumors, since it is based on the association of specific tumors with biochemical characteristics, the frequent production of ectopic hormone syndromes in foregut derivatives, and the development of endocrine neoplasia in the same organs. Similarities in the histological characteristics of carcinoid tumors and some peptide-producing tumors, such as oat cell carcinoma, provide further support for this hypothesis. A note of caution has to be introduced into this concept, however, in view of the recent findings; APUD cells could develop from precursor cells in the endoderm not necessarily derived from the neural crest.

6. Using some aspects of the Weichert hypothesis in examining the

association of specific hormone syndromes with tumor histology, Levine and Metz[19] have approached the classification of tumors somewhat differently. They divided all tumors known to produce ectopic hormones into two groups; they also identified a third transitional group on the basis of tissue histology, developmental embryology, ultrastructure, and hormone secretion. Tumors in group 1 contain cells with APUD characteristics, and theoretically could be derived from the neural crest. They contain electron-dense, secretory granules similar to those in neurosecretory cells, and variously give rise to insulin, calcitonin, ACTH, melanocyte-stimulating hormone, vasopressin, gastrin, glucagon, secretin, catecholamines, and various biogenic amines, including serotonin and histamine. Among the tumors in this group are oat cell carcinoma, islet cell tumor, medullary thyroid carcinoma, malignant thymoma, tumors of the pancreas and biliary ducts, and foregut carcinoid.

In group 2, they included mesodermal tumors (such as hepatoma, hypernephroma, adrenal cortical tumors, gonadal tumors, vascular tumors and squamous cell carcinoma of the lung) that produce parathyroid hormone, erythropoietin, gonadotropin, human placental lactogen, prolactin, growth hormone, insulinlike activity, renin, and thyrotropin. The distinguishing feature of group 2 tumors is that they do not contain secretory granules, although they have other cellular inclusion bodies. Tumors of group 1 have the ability to synthesize all other hormones of group 1, but not of group 2.

In group 3, Levine and Metz classified transitional tumors, such as pheochromocytoma, paraganglioma, neuroblastoma, and ganglioneuroma, that produce hormones produced by tumors in both groups 1 and 2.

Their classification was based on information derived from a literature review; some of the information was inadequate, however, owing to limited or even speculative biochemical information or documentation.

10.3. Characteristics of the Ectopic Hormone Syndromes

It is important to review the following general characteristics of the ectopic hormone syndromes:

1. They are not isolated medical curiosities, but are being detected with increasing frequency in malignant disorders.
2. Recognition of hormone production or tumor markers is potentially of great importance in the early detection of cancer, as well as in the recognition of remission or recurrence of disease.

3. An understanding of the mechanisms by which these syndromes develop will lead to a better understanding of normal cell differentiation.
4. The metabolic or biochemical effects may be more devastating to the patient than the neoplasm itself.
5. Some patients have only biochemical abnormalities without clinical effects from the hormone or other proteins produced.
6. Endocrine or metabolic disorders that are common may coexist with the tumor and present a confusing picture (e.g., hyponatremia, hypercalcemia).
7. Selective venous catheterization with radioimmunoassay measurement of specific hormones may serve to localize the site of ectopic hormone production.
8. Documentation of the presence of an ectopic hormone syndrome may be accomplished by several methods:
    a. *Recognition of a clinical endocrine disorder or a biochemical abnormality* in a patient with a malignancy.
    b. *Disappearance or remission of the endocrine disorder or metabolic abnormality* following effective tumor therapy.
    c. *Recurrence of the metabolic abnormality in association with metastasis or recurrence* of the tumor.
    d. *Detection of hormone in blood at inappropriate concentrations.*
    e. *Extraction of the hormone from tumor tissue or metastasis, and detection* by bioassay or immunoassay.
    f. *Demonstration of production of hormone within the tumor by detecting increased concentration of hormone* on the venous side of the tumor.
    g. *Production of hormone by tumor tissue in vitro.*

In many reports of ectopic hormone syndromes in the literature, various criteria have been used. In some cases, biochemical or metabolic documentation is limited or even totally lacking. With the more recent development of methods of greater sensitivity, particularly radioimmunoassay, increased recognition and reporting of these abnormalities has been forthcoming.

10.4. Recent Developments in Specific Hormone Syndromes

The history of identified ectopic hormone syndromes dates back several decades, although the entities were recognized pathologically well before that time. Rather than a comprehensive review in all areas, a synopsis of recent developments in specific ectopic hormone syndromes will be provided below.

10.4.1. Ectopic Production of Corticotropin (ACTH)

This well-defined entity was appreciated almost 50 years ago, and to date, more than 200 patients have been reported. The hallmarks of the syndrome are the association of marked bilateral adrenal hyperplasia with tumor production of ACTH, greatly elevated plasma cortisol concentrations and urinary 17-ketosteroid and 17-hydroxysteroid excretion, with little or no suppression by dexamethasone. The disorder has been association primarily with oat cell carcinoma of the lung (60%), thymoma (15%), and islet cell carcinoma (10%), as well as with a variety of other tumors, including bronchial carcinoid, pheochromocytoma, medullary thyroid carcinoma, and others.[20]

In recent studies, radioimmunoassay has been used to examine tumor tissue and plasma samples in patients suspected of having the syndrome. Gewirtz and Yalow[6] suggested that ACTH production by tumors may be much more widespread than previously appreciated when they found significant quantities of hormone in extracts from 14 of 15 lung cancers from patients without clinical Cushing's syndrome. Of additional interest was the finding that the tumors contained principally or exclusively a big form of ACTH that was less retarded on gel filtration. The quantities of ACTH in these tumors (5–55 ng/g) were less than those found in patients with the clinical syndrome (1.75–2.5 μg/g). There was no particular relationship to histological type of tumor, ACTH being found in all varieties. This study stands in striking contrast to the association of the clinical syndrome with oat cell carcinoma of the lung.[20] Gewirtz and Yalow[6] also noted increases in plasma ACTH in some patients with chronic obstructive pulmonary disease, and suggested that markedly elevated levels in such patients might be an early marker for carcinoma of the lung. Big ACTH is considerably larger than the 39-amino-acid peptide, and has minimal biological activity, but it can be converted to active ACTH with trypsin.[5] These authors identified big ACTH as the predominant form in the tumor and plasma of patients with and without Cushing's syndrome. Orth et al.[21] did not find evidence of big ACTH in tumor extracts, but their procedures may have excluded big ACTH from the preparation. More recently, Ayvazian et al.[22] detected elevated concentrations of ACTH in the plasma of 21 of 24 patients with untreated carcinoma of the lung, and the hormone could be detected in tumor extracts or bronchial washings from the other 3. Only 10 of 38 treated patients had increases in ACTH, while those patients who had prolonged survival had low plasma ACTH. In a group of patients with obstructive lung disease who had mildly increased ACTH, 3 patients with the highest concentrations subsequently developed lung tumors.

The amino acid sequence of ectopic ACTH has not been determined

Upton and Amatruda[4] purified ACTH from at least 3 separate tumors, and the ectopic hormone chromatographed identically with pituitary ACTH, but had a different amino acid composition. Phenylalanine and isoleucine were present on analysis, despite their absence in human pituitary hormone, but the homogeneity of the preparation may not have been complete. Upton and Amatruda also identified peptides with corticotropin-releasing factor (CRF) activity in tumor extracts, a finding consonant with the clinical observation that patients with ectopic ACTH syndrome may respond to the adrenal-inhibitor metyrapone. The tumor stimulates both adrenal glands and pituitary through the CRF mechanism. Imura *et al.*[23] studied 6 tumors from patients with the ectopic ACTH syndrome, and found CRF-like activity in all of them, but the methodological details were not described. Hirata and colleagues[24] performed additional *in vitro* studies on ectopic ACTH tumor tissue, and noted variable physiological responses. One or more of the tumors released ACTH in response to norephinephrine, cAMP, or rat median eminence extract. One tumor generated increased cAMP in response to stimulators, with adenyl cyclase increasing the release of hormone. Synthetic studies showed that labeled hormone in these tumors was predominantly big ACTH, and the variable responses of the tumors to regulation suggested that some of the concepts of tissue autonomy in this syndrome may eventually need to be revised.

It is of interest that patients with the ectopic ACTH syndrome usually do not show the classical clinical features of Cushing's syndrome, and more commonly present the problems of diabetes, hypokalemia, muscle weakness, weight loss, edema, and hyperpigmentation. The management of such patients depends on the clinical state, the extent of the neoplasm, and the severity of the adrenal disease. In rare cases, surgical resection of the tumor is possible, with correction of the metabolic abnormalities; likewise, bilateral adrenalectomy has been used on occasion. More common is the use of inhibitors of adrenal synthesis, usually a combination of metyrapone and aminoglutethimide.[25]

10.4.2. Ectopic Production of Melanocyte-Stimulating Hormone (MSH)

Patients with tumors that produce ACTH are frequently hyperpigmented, and production of melanocyte-stimulating hormone (MSH) by their tumors has been demonstrated.[26] However, isolated production of MSH by tumors has not been reported. Most of the MSHβ activity being measured in tissue extracts may be of higher molecular weight than normal.[27] The pituitary gland synthesizes both β- and γ-lipotropin, higher-molecular-weight peptides that contain MSHβ in their sequences. Whether MSHβ being measured in the blood of man is actually lipotropin or whether it is a degradation product of larger molecules during extraction is not yet clear.[28] Most workers now feel that all MSHβ activity is actually in lipoprotein.

10.4.3. Ectopic Production of Growth Hormone

Growth hormone (GH) production by tumors is uncommon, and has been associated with pulmonary osteoarthropathy, particularly when the tumor is an adenocarcinoma. Steiner *et al.*[29] were the first to demonstrate, in the serum of patients with tumor of the lung, increased concentrations of GH that declined after the tumor was resected. Beck and Burger[30] reported increased GH concentrations in 7 of 18 bronchogenic and 5 of 8 gastric adenocarcinomas. Greenberg *et al.*[31] demonstrated clearly the synthesis and release of GH *in vitro* from a poorly differentiated large cell tumor of the lung in culture, in which synthesis was maintained for a period of 4 months. No additional studies of GH production by ectopic tumors have been reported recently.

10.4.4. Ectopic Production of Human Placental Lactogen (HPL) or Human Chorionic Somatomammotropin (HCS)

Strong homologies exist between certain placental hormones and pituitary hormones with respect to amino acid sequence, three-dimensional structure, and immunological and biological activity. Human placental lactogen (HPL), a hormone produced by normal human trophoblast, is identical to pituitary growth hormone in 86% of its amino acid sequence.[32] Ectopic production of placental-type hormones has been noted in a variety of tumors. Grumbach *et al.*[33] first demonstrated the presence of HPL in the serum of a male with undifferentiated carcinoma of the lung and gynecomastia; the tumor also contained gonadotropin. More definitive information was provided by Weintraub and Rosen and their co-workers,[34,35] who studied the frequency with which HPL could be detected in the serum of patients with trophoblastic or nontrophoblastic tumors. Among 128 patients in the latter category, HPL was detected in unconcentrated sera from 7 patients, including patients with carcinoma of the lung, hepatoma, lymphoma or leukemia, and malignant pheochromocytoma. Greater sensitivity was achieved by concentrating HPL by means of affinity chromatography. With this technique, HPL was detected in the serum of 4 of 9 patients with carcinoma of the lung. HPL was found in the unconcentrated sera from all of 8 patients with untreated trophoblastic tumors. Concentrations of HPL in this group were generally much higher than in patients with nontrophoblastic tumors, but were nonetheless well below those found during the third trimester peak of normal pregnancy. The immunological characteristics of tumor HPL and those of normal pregnancy were indistinguishable. Since HPL is absent from the serum of normal men and nonpregnant women, it may serve as an effective tumor marker in these groups.

Among patients with trophoblastic tumors, all displayed high concentrations of chorionic gonadotropin. The latter hormone was also detected in 5 patients with carcinoma of the lung. All had gynecomastia and increased serum estrogen concentrations, and 4 had detectable levels of HPL in serum concentrates. The concordance in the appearance in serum of these two ectopic hormones, and of other tumor markers, such as placental alkaline phosphatase, is of interest. It would appear that these three markers may be detectable in varying combination in the sera of patients with tumors,[36] and that they correlate closely with clinical course.[37] A "big" form of HPL has been detected in placental tissue and blood of pregnant women.[38] Such "big" HPL needs study in patients with the ectopic hormone syndrome, much as has been done in the studies of big ACTH.

10.4.5. Ectopic Production of Prolactin

A number of physiological and biochemical developments in recent years have proved the existence of a separate human prolactin, and there are biochemical similarities among GHHPL and pituitary prolactin. An increase in prolactin in the serum of a man with undifferentiated carcinoma of the lung and in a woman with renal cell carcinoma and galactorrhea was noted by Turkington.[39] The levels decreased after therapy with radiation and nephrectomy, respectively. Generation of prolactin *in vitro* was noted from the renal cell carcinoma in tissue culture. Rees *et al.*[40] also demonstrated an increase in radioimmunoassayable prolactin in a patient with a bronchogenic tumor. As the use of prolactin radioimmunoassay is extended, new patients with ectopic production of this hormone will almost certainly be identified.

10.4.6. Ectopic Production of Gonadotropins

Extensive interest has developed in recent years in the measurement of gonadotropins and their α- and β-subunits in the sera of patients with tumors. The two gonadotropins produced by the pituitary, follicle-stimulating hormone (FSH) and luteinizing hormone (LH), share biochemical properties with each other and with the chorionic gonadotropin produced by human trophoblastic tissue (HCG). They have in common an identical or nearly identical α-subunit, and discrete β-subunits, which confer specific biological and immunological properties.[35]

The association of clinical gynecomastia with tumors of the lung has been known for many years, and has now been defined in terms of gonadotropin production. In addition, a syndrome of precocious puberty in young males secondary to production of LH or a similar substance by tumors (particularly hepatoblastoma) has been reported.[41] These patients were all prepubertal and had other associated abnormalities, such as spina bifida and hemihypertrophy.

When gynecomastia occurs with carcinoma of the lung, it is sometimes associated with hypertrophic osteoarthropathy, and increased estrogen production has been noted in such patients.[42] Gynecomastia may be present even before the appearance of the tumor.[43] Definite evidence of tumor production of gonadotropin was found by Faiman et al.[44] who showed an arteriovenous difference across an adenocarcinoma of the lung. In addition to those patients who develop precocious puberty and gynecomastia, others may have elevated levels of gonadotropin in the serum without any clinical manifestations.[45] In addition to patients with carcinoma of the lung or hepatoblastoma, patients with tumors of the gonads, pineal, mediastinum, adrenal, breast, or bladder, or with melanoma, have been reported to produce gonadotropins.

Of interest is the source of the excess estrogen in patients with gonadotropin-producing tumors. Kirschner et al.[46] studied the source and rate of production of estrogens in 6 males in whom tumor mass could be correlated with the levels of gonadotropin. Estradiol production rates were increased, and although it might have seemed likely that this increase would occur through gonadotropic stimulation of estrogen production by the testis, such stimulation was not found to be the major cause. Studies of the conversion of administered dehydroepiandrosterone (DHEA) sulfate to estradiol, as well as in vitro studies of steroid metabolism by tumor tissue, demonstrated that gonadotropin-producing tumors can convert DHEA sulfate to estradiol, a property that is characteristic of trophoblastic tissue. This finding provided additional evidence that the ectopic tumors were closely related to the placenta in their biochemical functions.

Considerable emphasis has been placed of late on the measurement of specific subunits of the gonadotropins in order to differentiate FSH, LH, and HCG. This differentiation was not possible with the use of bioassays, which overlapped considerably, and many of the data in the older literature are therefore confusing. However, sensitive serum assays using the subunit antisera have now been developed. This development has led to the identification of some patients who produce only the subunit, rather than the intact hormone, as a tumor marker. Weintraub and Rosen[47] reported a patient with pancreatic adenocarcinoma who had an elevated level of HCGβ in serum (300 ng/ml); there was no evidence of complete hormone or α-subunit in tumor extracts or in serum, and the bioassay was negative. *In vitro* studies by Rabson *et al.*[48] with a bronchogenic tumor showed evidence that some clonal strains of the tumor produced varying amounts of the β-subunit. In the absence of pregnancy, demonstration of HCGβ is strongly suggestive of the presence of tumor. Using a radioimmunoassay capable of detecting both HCG and HCGβ, Braunstein *et al.*[49] studied the sera of 443 patients without tumors. Results were negative, except in 3 women who may have been pregnant. In the same series, HCG-like material was found in the sera of more than 7% of a large number of patients with malignant disorders.

Even though the α-subunit is not hormone-specific, its demonstration in serum may also be indicative of the presence of tumor.[50,51] The apparent secretion of a single subunit argues for the separate transcription of the α and β chains, but little is known about the mechanisms of normal subunit production and assembly of the whole hormone molecule. Nevertheless, as several authors have emphasized,[35,52] isolated subunits may serve as useful tumor markers.

In normal human testis, Braunstein *et al.*[53] identified material closely related to HCG, suggesting that the mechanisms for synthesizing HCG are still present in the adult human testis. This finding perhaps provides adequate explanation for the production of the gonadotropin by testicular tumors, but does not explain why adenocarcinoma of the pancreas, ovary, and stomach and hepatoblastomas can produce it with a frequency that ranges as high as 17–40%.[35,49,52–55]

10.4.7. Ectopic Production of Thyrotropin

Ectopic production of a thyrotropin has been well documented in patients with trophoblastic tumors.[56,57] These patients usually have only mild hyperthyroidism and biochemical parameters of the disease, but occasionally, more severe hyperthyroidism has been reported.[58] The material produced by these tumors is probably related to human chorionic thyrotropin (HCT). The two substances, though similar, are not identical.[59,60] The duration of action of HCT is similar to that of pituitary thyrotropin, with a peak action at 2–3 hr. There is slight immunological cross-reaction between the two, although HCT cross-reacts much better with bovine than with human thyrotropin. Molar thyrotropin, on the other hand, has a longer duration of action, cross-reacts poorly to human and bovine pituitary thyrotropin, and is a larger molecule than HCT.[58] Recent evidence suggests that molar thyrotropin may, in fact, be chorionic gonadotropin.[61]

In addition to trophoblastic tumors in the pregnant woman and testicular tumors in man, the syndrome has also been reported in patients with epidermoid carcinoma of the lung and mesothelioma.[62] Additional studies to identify ectopic thyrotropin need to be done, particularly with respect to the β-subunit of the hormone.

10.4.8. Ectopic Production of Antidiuretic Hormone (ADH)

The association of tumors with inappropriate antidiuretic hormone (ADH) secretion has been well recognized since it was emphasized by Schwartz and colleagues.[63] The wide variety of disorders, both malignant and nonmalignant that can produce the inappropriate ADH syndrome will not be reviewed here. The manifestations of the syndrome are present only when excess water is administered to the patient who already has a high level of circulating ADH. Much earlier studies have documented the presence of vasopressin activity in tumor extracts and in the serum of patients undergoing antidiuresis. The most definitive evidence for tumor production of hormone was provided by George *et al.*,[64] who demonstrated that the hormone could be synthesized *in vitro* by bronchogenic carcinoma; similar results have been reported for a uterine tumor by Martin *et al.*[65] The concentrations of ADH in tumors have been too small to permit biochemical characterization, but, from a variety of studies, it appears that the tumor hormone has chemical properties similar to those of ADH, and is inactivated by the same agents. In patients who present with hyponatremia and a concentrated urine, it is important to differentiate tumor production of vasopressin from other causes of inappropriate ADH, these causes include metastases to the hypothalamus, effects of a mediastinal tumor on volume receptors in the chest, renal tubular defects, CNS infection, cerebrovascular disease, other systemic illnesses, and the administration of drugs such as chlorpromamide and morphine. In addition, pain, stress, and increased smoking in patients with malignancy can lead to increased ADH secretion. No new findings in the biochemistry of the syndrome have been made in the last year, but it has been suggested that therapy with lithium carbonate[66] and demeclocycline[67] may be of some benefit as an adjunct to water restriction. Hamilton *et al.*[68] showed that neurophysin may also be present in some of these tumors.

10.4.9. Hypoglycemic Syndromes and Tumors

The association of hyperinsulinemia due to an islet cell tumor with clinical hypoglycemia is clear and well established. Patients with this disease have a low blood sugar in the fasting state, produce increased quantities of insulin relative to the plasma glucose, and are frequently symptomatic. The cause of hypoglycemia in a second group of patients, who have tumors of other tissues, is much less clear. The problems related to this issue were well outlined a decade ago by Unger in a thoughtful editorial.[69] A heterogeneous basis for the hypoglycemia in this group adds to the confusion. A variety of tumor types may be associated with hypoglycemia, and to date more than 180 such patients have been reported.[70] Among the tumors associated with hypoglycemia are: (1) *very large mesodermal or mesenchymal tumors in the abdomen and thorax,* such as fibrosarcoma, mesothelioma, neurofibroma, and leiomyosarcoma; (2) *hepatoma or hepatocellular carcinoma:* (3) *adrenal cortical carcinoma;* (4) *lymphoma;* (5) *gastrointestinal carcinoma;* and (6) *miscellaneous tumors of the lung, ovary, nervous system and kidney.*

No clear-cut evidence for insulin production by these tumors has been obtained, although there are occasional reports suggesting the presence of insulin or insulinlike activity on immunofluorescent staining of the tissue.[71] Therefore, the evidence that these tumors actually produce insulin is minimal. A recent report by Lyall *et al.*[72] presented evidence of increased insulin secretion in a patient with a hemangiopericytoma. Following removal of the tumor, blood glucose returned to normal. The tumor contained no immunoreactive insulin or neurosecretory-type granules, however. The authors suggested that the tumor might be stimulating insulin release and possibly suppressing glucagon secretion.

Although the hypoglycemogenic tumors generally do not produce insulin, they clearly are associated with an increase in insulinlike activity in the serum.[70] Such activity is not suppressible with insulin antibodies, and can be measured in *in vitro* systems, such as the rat diaphragm or epididymal fat pad. This so-called nonsuppressible insulinlike activity (NSILA) is distinct immunologically from insulin, and probably represents a group of different peptides. There is now considerable evidence to suggest that NSILA is a form of somatomedin (formerly known as "sulfation factor"), a protein molecule, or protein molecules, produced in response to GH, which carries out some of the effects of GH on intermediary metabolism.[73] NSILA-s or a form of NSILA that is soluble in acid ethanol[74,75] has been shown to be elevated in the sera of some patients with extrapancreatic tumors and hypoglycemia (fibrosarcoma, pheochromocytoma, adrenal carcinoma, hepatoma). The hypoglycemic activity in the sera of these patients is equivalent in biological terms to that of the increased levels of insulin in patients with islet cell tumors. NSILA-s is a peptide of 7400 mol. wt. that, like other somatomedins, has both insulin like and GH activity. It does not react with insulin antibodies, and liver plasma membranes have separate receptors for NSILA-s and insulin. Much of the NSILA-s is reversibly bound to larger protein molecules.

Marks *et al.*[70] studied several tumors associated with hypoglycemia, including Hodgkin's lymphoma, melanotic melanosarcoma, and fibrosarcoma, and found no evidence of insulin, although there was increased insulinlike activity in the serum. Recent evidence for NSILA-s production by these tumors is tantalizing, and suggests that a hormonal etiology for the syndromes may finally be uncovered.

Nevertheless, it is likely that no single mechanism accounts for the hypoglycemia in these patients. Possible causes include production of NSILA-s or other insulinlike factors, production by tumors of a factor that stimulates insulin release, excessive glucose consumption by the tumor, production of metabolites that interfere with gluconeogenesis (e.g., tryptophan), acquired glycogen-storage disease (hepatocellular carcinoma), malnutrition, chemotherapy, and suppression of counterregulatory mechanisms. The differentiation between islet cell tumors and non-pancreatic tumors associated with hypoglycemia is straightforward. The management of patients with islet cell tumors has recently been reviewed in detail.[76] The management of patients with extrapancreatic causes of hypoglycemia is more difficult since, in these disorders, agents such as dioxide and streptozotocin are less helpful.

10.4.10. Ectopic Production of Parathyroid Hormone (PTH) and Other Calcium-Mobilizing Substances

Hypercalcemia is commonly observed in patients with malignant disease and often becomes a clinically important metabolic abnormality, owing to its effects on the gastrointestinal and nervous systems and on cardiovascular and renal function. Differential diagnosis is usually straightforward, although the separation of primary hyperparathyroidism from a latent malignancy with or without bone metastases can, on occasion, be extremely difficult. Since hyperparathyroidism is now thought to have a prevalence of almost 1 per 1000, it may coexist with other potential causes of hypercalcemia.

The concept of ectopic parathyroid hormone (PTH) production in association with malignant disorders dates back over 30 years, but there are still fewer than 25 patients in whom the presence of immunoassayable PTH has actually been documented in tumor tissue. In other studies using radioimmunoassay,[2,3] it has been thought to be more frequent than previously appreciated.

Current research in the area of malignant disease and hypercalcemia is concerned with the prevalence of PTH production and other bone-mobilizing factors that have been identified as alternative causes of the hypercalcemia syndrome. Much of the earlier literature involves descriptions of patients with hypercalcemia and malignancy without obvious bone metastasis who either had remission of hypercalcemia after surgical or medical treatment of the tumor or developed hypercalcemia with tumor recurrence. In these patients, it was postulated, but not usually proved, that the tumors were making PTH.[77] Munson et al.[78] and Sherwood et al.[79] detected the presence of a PTH-like substance in a number of tumors from patients with the syndrome. Sherwood and co-workers used a radioimmunoassay, and found from 0.75 to 8.3 ng/g dry weight of tumor; its molecular weight by sucrose density-gradient analysis was also identical to that of bovine hormone. In a subsequent report, Knill-Jones et al.[80] demonstrated production of PTH from a liver tumor on the basis of a positive arteriovenous difference in hormone concentration across the tumor. Occasional reports of immunoreactive PTH in tumors have appeared subsequently. Riggs et al.[81] examined the nature of the hormone in the serum of patients with the ectopic PTH syndrome. These studies indicated that the hormone in patients with ectopic hyperparathyroidism was less immunoreactive than glandular PTH. More detailed studies of 6 patients by the same group[2,3] showed that the lower immunological activity of the ectopic hormone was accounted for by smaller quantities of circulating carboxyl-terminal fragments. The carboxyl-terminal fragment is the major form of circulating PTH; it is not active biologically.[82] Benson et al.[2,3] suggested the possibility of synthesis of an altered polypeptide, secretion of an intermediate form or precursor of the hormone, abnormal metabolism of the hormone in serum or tissues, or possibly release of factors that might interfere with the radioimmunoassay. They also provided some evidence that there might be larger forms of the hormone in the blood of patients with the syndrome. These studies did not involve examination of tumor tissue extracts, and intensive additional study is necessary. Recent findings suggest, furthermore, that the metabolism of PTH may be affected by the degree of hypercalcemia.[83] Selective catheterization has been applied extensively in locating the site of parathyroid adenomas in primary hyperparathyroidism,[84] and Blair et al.[85] used the same technique to prove that a renal cell tumor was the source of PTH. Synthesis of PTH in vitro by a squamous cell tumor was demonstrated by Hartman et al.[86] in studies that suggested the tumor produced a hormone similar to, but not necessarily identical with, the natural hormone.

Considerable emphasis has been placed in the last two years on substances other than PTH that might cause hypercalcemia in patients with malignant disorders. An epidemiological survey of tumors and hypercalcemia is urgently needed in order to determine how often PTH or one of the other substances is the responsible agent. Strong evidence suggesting that there might be factors other than PTH producing hypercalcemia was also provided by Powell et al.,[87] who reported 11 patients without metastatic bone disease who had hypercalcemia and hypophosphatemia, and showed improvement of hypercalcemia with therapy. The tumor extracts contained bone-resorbing activity, but all assays in the blood and tissue for PTH were negative. One likely hypercalcemic factor is a prostaglandin, particularly PGE_2. Initial observations giving rise to this suggestion were made by Tashjian and colleagues,[88] who found evidence that hypercalcemia in a mouse sarcoma model was produced by a prostaglandin, PGE_2. Evidence to support this view was provided by the following findings: development of hypercalcemia in the absence of tumor metastases, presence of bone-resorbing activity and PGE_2 in tumor extracts, release of PGE_2 and bone-resorbing activity into tissue culture medium, decrease in the production of prostaglandin and hypercalcemia with indomethacin, arteriovenous differences in PGE_2 content, and production of hypercalcemia by infusion of prostaglandin. In addition to these findings in the mouse model, the rabbit VX_2 carcinoma was also shown to produce a prostaglandin that was responsible for hypercalcemia.[88,89] Several studies showed prostaglandins to be a demonstrable cause of clinical hypercalcemia, particularly in patients with renal carcinoma.[90-92] In an extensive study by Seyberth et al.,[93] 29 patients with solid tumors, 14 of whom were hypercalcemic, were examined for the presence of prostaglandin and PGE_M, a specific metabolite of the prostaglandin E series. Elevations of PGE_M were noted in the urine of 12 of 14 hypercalcemic patients, while there was only a modest elevation in 7 of the 15 patients without hypercalcemia. No control subjects had abnormalities in the metabolite, and no PTH was detectable in the sera of the hypercalcemic patients. The 14 with hypercalcemia included 10 with carcinoma of the lung, 2 with pancreatic adenocarcinoma, and 2 with adenocarcinoma of unknown source. The response to therapy in these patients was variable, although the patients reported by Brereton et al.[90] and Ito et al.[92] responded to indomethacin.

A possible explanation for the hypercalcemia in multiple myeloma has been provided by the identification of osteoclast-activating factor (OAF), a new bone-resorbing factor identified in human lymphocytes.[94] This protein (or proteins) was found in the supernatant fluid of human lymphocytes grown in tissue culture in the presence of phytomitogen; it stimulated osteoclastic resorption from labeled fetal rat bones in an organ culture system. A similar substance has been found in cultured cells from patients with multiple myeloma, Burkitts's lymphoma, and one with malignant lymphoma, but not from patients with other tumors.[95] The activity of OAF can be separated from that of prostaglandin, PTH, or vitamin D–like compounds, and is inhibited by cortisol. Past suggestions that hypercalcemia might also be due to an osteolytic vitamin D–like sterol produced by tumors have not been substantiated.

10.4.11. Ectopic Production of Other Hormones

10.4.11.1. Calcitonin

Elevations of calcitonin in 2 patients with oat cell carcinoma have recently been reported by Silva et al.[96] In one patient, an elevated concentration was found in the thymic vein draining the tumor, while the other tumor itself contained a high concentration of calcitonin. Both patients had a normal serum calcium concentration; usually, this is also the case in patients with medullary carcinoma of the thyroid. The same authors[97] extended their series to 26 patients with bronchogenic carcinoma, of whom 62% (16 patients) had elevated levels of calcitonin, in the range of 100–16,000 ng/ml. The concentrations were quite high in patients with oat cell carcinoma and adenocarcinoma of the lung. Two causes of elevated calcitonin concentrations were noted, production of calcitonin by the tumor and increased calcitonin secretion from the thyroid. Because these patients were in general quite ill, selective catheterization studies were not possible in many, and postmortem analysis of the tumor tissue was not always accomplished. The reason for thyroid secretion of increased calcitonin in these patients with pulmonary tumors is unknown, but the finding has also been made by others.[98,99] Two other patients with ectopic production of calcitonin from oat cell carcinoma were reported by Cattan et al.[100]; they also had ectopic production of vasopressin. In addition, Coombes et al.[101] demonstrated that tumors of the nonectoderm from the pancreas, maxillary antrum, prostate, uterus, bladder, and breast can also be associated with elevated serum calcitonin concentrations.

10.4.11.2. Erythropoietin

Sherwood and Goldwasser[102] recently demonstrated the synthesis and release of erythropoietin from three renal cell carcinomas maintained in tissue culture. Polycythemia has classically been described in association with both malignant and benign lesions of the kidney, cerebellar hemangioblastoma, uterine fibroma, adrenal cortical tumors, ovarian neoplasms, hepatomas, and pheochromocytomas. Further progress in the field will be made by the development of a radioimmunoassay to improve on bioassay for use in tumor screening.

10.4.11.3. Renin-Secreting Tumors

Hollifield et al.[103] recently reported a renal cell tumor associated with excessive production of renin and with hypertension. This was the first report of a renal cell carcinoma producing this syndrome. Earlier reports included tumors of the juxtaglomerular apparatus (or hemangiopericytomas), Wilms' tumor, and at least one patient with oat cell carcinoma of the lung. The degree of hypertension has varied in these patients, although some have had severe hypertension, hypokalemia, increased peripheral vein renin activity, and secondary aldosteronism. Selective catheterization of the renal veins with differential renin measurements is the principal method of establishing the diagnosis.

10.4.11.4. Other Prostaglandins

Sussman et al.[36] demonstrated the production of prostaglandin A in a patient with an anaplastic renal tumor who developed severe hypertension and hemiparesis 1 year after removal of the tumor. Presumably, the loss of a vasodilating PGA permitted underlying severe hypertension to emerge. With increased availability of assays for prostaglandin A, E, and F, additional patients with tumor syndromes related to prostaglandins are likely to be reported.

10.4.11.5. Osteomalacia, Hypophosphatemia, and Hyperphosphaturia

A number of patients with hypophosphatemia, marked hyperphosphaturia, and osteomalacia in association with mesenchymomas, pleomorphic sarcomas, neurofibromas, and sclerosing or cavernous hemangiomas have been reported.[104] These patients have marked phosphaturia and metabolic bone disease. The precise nature of the factor causing the phosphaturia is as yet unclear.

10.4.11.6. Glucagon and Skin Disease; Vasoactive Intestinal Peptide (VIP)

The association of glucagon-producing tumors with a necrolyzing bullous skin eruption has recently been described.[105] Other islet-cell tumors produce gastrin and possibly VIP, which has been linked theoretically with the production of pancreatic cholera and diarrhea of other tumors.[106]

10.5. Production of Nonhormonal Proteins and Other Syndromes by Malignant Disorders

10.5.1. Ectopic Production of Other Proteins

It is likely that tumors produce a wide variety of abnormal proteins. In those instances in which the tumor produces a protein that is associated with a distinct clinical syndrome or biochemical abnormality, it is usually readily detectable. In the case of tumor antigens, ectopic enzymes, or other abnormal proteins produced by tumors, the abnormality will go undetected unless a specific search for the antigen or protein is made. Where intensive search for tumor hormones has been made with more sensitive radioimmunoassays, affinity chromatography, selective catheterization, and other specialized techniques, increased frequency of abnormalities has always been detectable. The same is likely to be true for other tumor proteins.

Considerable interest has been generated in tumor antigens, such as alpha fetoprotein and the carcinoembryonic antigen. Although a discussion of these proteins is beyond the scope of this chapter, the reader is referred to a comprehensive 1975 review on the subject of carcinofetal proteins.[107] Of considerable interest has been the identification of a placental form of alkaline phosphatase in ectopic tumors, particularly those of the lung and other tissues that produce other trophoblastic hormones.[36] Placental alkaline phosphatase is heat-stable and can be separated electrophoretically. No evidence of this enzyme was detectable in 50 control sera from patients with nonneoplastic diseases.[36] Recent studies suggest that the amino-terminal amino acid sequence and peptide maps of placental and tumor alkaline phosphatase are similar.[35] Concordance of enzyme elevation with the presence of gonadotropin and HPL markers has been useful in following the progress of trophoblastic or ectopic tumors producing these hormones.[35] Four patients with hepatocellular carcinoma producing a new variant of alkaline phosphatase have recently been described.[108]

10.5.2. Tumor Syndromes Not Known to Be Associated with Definite Humoral Substances

Malignant diseases are protean in their manifestations, specific findings usually depending on the tissue of origin and the presence or absence of local or distant metastases. In addition to those manifestations due to the physical presence of tumor, a variety of extraneoplastic manifestations could be due to the production of ectopic proteins or other factors. Among these are fever, anorexia, weight loss and other disturbances of metabolism, and disorders of the immunological and connective tissue systems, nervous system, vasculature, skin, and kidney.

In most instances, these fascinating manifestations have not definitely been associated with the production of a specific protein by the tumor. Suggestive evidence has been provided, however, that certain tumors may produce pyrogens, anorexigenic substances, tumor antigens leading to immune complex disease, and thromboplastic substances causing accelerated coagulation. Extensive characterization or purification of such tumor proteins has not yet been accomplished. Continued investigation in this area will likely lead to more specific association of tumor products with these syndromes. The subject has been reviewed extensively in a conference on paraneoplastic syndromes,[109] to which the reader is referred.

ACKNOWLEDGMENT

The author wishes to thank Ms. Nicolina Litteria for her excellent assistance in the preparation of this manuscript.

References

1. Amatruda, T. T., Jr., 1974, Non-endocrine secreting tumors, *in: Duncan's Diseases of Metabolism* (P. K. Bondy and L. E. Rosenberg, eds.), pp. 1629–1650, W. B. Saunders Co., Philadelphia.
2. Benson, R. C., Riggs, B. L., Pickard, B. M., and Arnaud, C. D., 1974, Radioimmunoassay of parathyroid hormone in hypercalcemic patients with malignant disease, *Amer. J. Med.* **56:**821–826.
3. Benson, R. C., Riggs, B. L., Pickard, B. M., and Arnaud, C. D., 1974, Immunoreactive forms of circulating parathyroid hormone in primary and ectopic hyperparathyroidism, *J. Clin. Invest* **54:**175–181.
4. Upton, G. V., and Amatruda, T. T., Jr., 1971, Evidence for the presence of tumor peptides with corticotropin-releasing-factor-like activity in the ectopic ACTH syndrome, *N. Engl. J. Med.* **285:**419–424.
5. Gewirtz, G., Schneider, B., Krieger, D. T., and Yalow, R. S., 1974, Big ACTH: Conversion to biologically active ACTH by trypsin, *J. Clin. Endocrinol. Metab.* **38:**227–230.
6. Gewirtz, G., and Yalow, R. S., 1974, Ectopic ACTH production in carcinoma of the lung, *J. Clin. Invest.* **53:**1022–1032.
7. Gregory, R. A., and Tracy, H. J., 1972, Isolation of two "big gastrins" from Zollinger-Ellison tumor tissues, *Lancet* **2:**797–799.
8. Yalow, R. S., and Berson, S. A., 1973, Characteristics of "big ACTH" in human plasma and pituitary extracts, *J. Clin. Endocrinol. Metab.* **36:**415–423.
9. Day, R. P., Leutscher, J. A., and Gonzalez, C. M., 1975, Occurrence of big renin in human plasma, amniotic fluid and kidney extracts, *J. Clin. Endocrinol. Metab.* **40:**1078–1084.
10. Ellison, E. H., and Wilson, S. D., 1967, Ulcerogenic tumor of the pancreas, *Prog. Clin. Cancer* **3:**225–244.
11. Sherbet, G. V., 1974, Epigenetic mechanisms and paraneoplastic phenomena, *Ann. N. Y. Acad. Sci.* **230:**516–532.
12. Warner, T. F., 1974, Cell hybridization in the genesis of ectopic hormone secreting tumors, *Lancet* **1:**1259–1260.
13. Weichert, R. F., III, 1970, The neural ectodermal origin of the peptide secreting endocrine glands, *Amer. J. Med.* **49:**232–241.
14. Pearse, A. G. E., 1969, The cytochemistry and ultrastructure of polypeptide hormone–producing cells of the APUD genes and the embryologic, physiologic and pathologic implications of the concept, *J. Histochem. Cytochem.* **17:**303–313.
15. Pearse, A. G. E., and Polak, J. M., 1971, Neural crest origin of the endocrine polypeptide (APUD) cells of the gastrointestinal tract and pancreas, *Gut* **12:**783–788.
16. Polak, J. M., Pearse, A. G. E., LeLièvre, C., Fontaine, J., and Le Douarin, N.

M., 1974, Immunocytochemical confirmation of the neural crest origin of avian calcitonin-producing cells, *Histochemistry* **40**:209–214.

17. Le Douarin, N. M., and Teillet, M. A., 1973, The migration of neural crest cells to the wall of the digest tract in amino embryo, *J. Embryol. Exp. Morphol.* **30**:31–48.

18. Pictet, R. L., Rall, L. B., Phelp, P., and Rutter, W., 1976, The neural crest and the origin of the insulin-producing and other gastrointestinal hormone–producing cells, *Science* **191**:191–192.

19. Levine, R. J., and Metz, S. A., 1974, A classification of ectopic hormone producing tumors, *Ann. N. Y. Acad. Sci.* **230**:533–546.

20. Amatruda, T. T., Jr., and Upton, G. V., 1974, Hyperadrenocorticism and ACTH-releasing factor, *Ann. N. Y. Acad. Sci.* **230**:168–180.

21. Orth, D. N., Nicholson, W. E., Mitchell, W. M., Island, D. P., and Liddle, G. W., 1973, Biologic and immunologic characterization and physical separation of ACTH and ACTH fragments in ectopic ACTH syndrome, *J. Clin. Invest.* **52**:1756–1769.

22. Ayvazian, L. F., Schneider, B., Gewirtz, G., and Yalow, R. S., 1975, Ectopic production of big ACTH in carcinoma of the lung, *Amer. Rev. Respir. Dis.* **111**:279–287.

23. Imura, H., Matsukura, S., Yamamota, H., Hirata, Y., Nakai, Y., Endo, J., Tanaka, A., and Nakamura, M., 1975, Studies on ectopic ACTH-producing tumors: II. Clinical and biochemical features of 30 cases, *Cancer* **35**:1430–1437.

24. Hirata, Y., Yamamoto, H., Matsukura, S., and Imura, H., 1975, *In vitro* release and biosynthesis of tumor ACTH in ectopic ACTH-producing tumors, *J. Clin. Endocrinol. Metab.* **41**:106–114.

25. Carey, R. M., Orth, D. N., and Hartmann, W. H., 1973, Malignant melanoma with ectopic production of adrenocorticotropic hormone: Palliative treatment with inhibitors of adrenal steroid biosynthesis, *J. Clin. Endocrinol. Metab.* **36**:482–487.

26. Abe, K., Nicholson, W. E., Liddle, G. W., Island, D. P., and Orth, D. N., 1967, Radioimmunoassay of beta-MSH of human plasma and tissues, *J. Clin. Invest.* **46**:1609–1616.

27. Bloomfield, G. A., Scott, A. P., Lowry, P. J., Gilkes, J. J. H., and Rees, L. H., 1974, A reappraisal of human beta-MSH, *Nature* **252**:492–493.

28. Gilkes, J. J. H., Bloomfield, G. A., Scott, A. P., Lowry, P. J., Ratcliffe, J. G., Landon, J., and Rees, L. H., 1975, Development and validation of a radioimmunoassay for peptides related to beta-melanocyte-stimulating hormone in human plasma: Lipotropins, *J. Clin. Endocrinol. Metab.* **40**:450–457.

29. Steiner, A. L., Goodman, A. D., and Powers, S. R., 1968, Study of a kindred with pheochromocytoma medullary thyroid carcinoma, hyperparathyroidism and Cushing's disease: Multiple endocrine neoplasia, type II, *Medicine* **47**:371–409.

30. Beck, C., and Burger, H. G., 1972, Evidence for the presence of immunoreactive growth hormone in cancers of the lung and stomach, *Cancer* **30**:75–79.

31. Greenberg, P. B., Martin, T. J., Beck, C., and Burger, H. G., 1972, Synthesis and release of human growth hormone from lung carcinoma in cell culture, *Lancet* **1**:350–352.

32. Sherwood, L. M., Handwerger, S., McLaurin, W. D., and Lanner, M., 1971, Amino acid sequence of human placental lactogen, *Nature* **233**:59–61.

33. Grumbach, M. M., Kaplan, S. L., Sciarra, J. J., and Burr, I. M., 1968, Chorionic growth hormone-prolactin: Secretion, distribution, biologic activity in man; and postulated function as the "growth hormone" of the second half of pregnancy, *Ann. N.Y. Acad. Sci.* **148:**501–531.
34. Weintraub, B. D., and Rosen, S. W., 1971, Ectopic production of human chorionic somatomammotropin by non-trophoblastic cancers, *J. Clin. Endocrinol. Metab.* **32:**94–101.
35. Rosen, S. W., Weintraub, B. D., Vaitukaitis, J. L., Sussman, H. H., Hershman, J. M., and Muggia, F. M., 1975, Placental proteins and their subunits as tumor markers, *Ann. Intern. Med.* **82:**71–83.
36. Sussman, H. H., Weintraub, B. D., and Rosen, S. W., 1974, Relationship of ectopic placental alkaline phosphatase to ectopic chorionic gonadotropin and placental lactogen, *Cancer* **33:**820–823.
37. Muggia, F. M., Rosen, F. W., Weintraub, B. D., and Hansen, H. H., 1975, Ectopic placental proteins in non-trophoblastic tumors, *Cancer* **36:**1327–1337.
38. Schneider, A. B., Kowalski, K., and Sherwood, L. M., 1975, Identification of "big" human placental lactogen in placenta and serum, *Endocrinology* **97:**1364–1372.
39. Turkington, R. W., 1971, Ectopic production of prolactin, *N. Engl. J. Med.* **285:**1455–1458.
40. Rees, L. H., Bloomfield, G. A., and Reese, G. M., 1974, Multiple hormones in a bronchial tumor, *J. Clin. Endocrinol. Metab.* **38:**1090–1097.
41. McArthur, J. W., Toll, G. D., Russfield, A. B., Reiss, A. M., Quinby, W. C., and Baker, W. H., 1973, Sexual precocity attributable to ectopic gonadotropin secretion by hepatoblastoma, *Amer. J. Med.* **54:**390–403.
42. Ginsburg, J., and Brown, J. B., 1961, Increased estrogen excretion in hypertrophic pulmonary osteoarthropathy, *Lancet* **2:**1274–1276.
43. Rosen, W. S., Becker, C. E., Schlaff, S., Easton, J., and Gluck, M. C., 1968, Ectopic gonadotropin production before clinical recognition of bronchogenic carcinoma, *N. Engl. J. Med.* **279:**640–641.
44. Faiman, C., Colwell, J. A., Ryan, R. J., Hershman, J. M., and Shields, T. W., 1967, Gonadotropin secretion from a bronchogenic carcinoma. Demonstration by radioimmunoassay, *N. Engl. J. Med.* **277:**1395–1399.
45. Vaitukaitis, J. L., 1973, Immunologic and physical characterization of human chorionic gonadotropin (HCG) secreted by tumors, *J. Clin. Endocrinol. Metab.* **37:**505–514.
46. Kirschner, M. A., Cohen, F. B., and Jespersen, D., 1974, Estrogen production and its origin in men with gonadotropin-producing neoplasms, *J. Clin. Endocrinol. Metab.* **39:**112–118.
47. Weintraub, B. D., and Rosen, S. W., 1973, Ectopic production of the isolated beta subunit of human chorionic gonadotropin, *J. Clin. Invest.* **52:**3135–3142.
48. Rabson, A. S., Rosen, S. W., Tashjian, A. H., Jr., and Weintraub, B. D., 1973, Production of human chorionic gonadotropin *in vitro* by cell line derived from a carcinoma of the lung, *J. Nat. Cancer Instit.* **50:**669–674.
49. Braunstein, G., Vaitukaitis, J. L., Carbone, P. P., and Ross, G. T., 1973, Ectopic production of human chorionic gonadotropin by neoplasms, *Ann. Intern. Med.* **78:**39–45.
50. Franchimont, P., Gaspard, U., Rueter, A., and Heynen, T., 1972, Polymorphism, protein and polypeptide hormones, *Clin. Endocrinol.* **1:**315–319.
51. Rosen, S. W., and Weintraub, B. D., 1974, Ectopic production of the isolated

alpha subunit of the glycoprotein hormone: A quantitative marker in certain cases of cancer, *N. Engl. J. Med.* **290:**1441–1447.

52. Vaitukaitis, J. L., 1976, Peptide hormones as tumor markers, *Cancer* **37:**567–572.

53. Braunstein, G. D., Rasor, J., and Wade, M. E., 1975, Presence in normal human testes of a chorionic-gonadotropin-like substance distinct from human luteinizing hormone, *N. Engl. J. Med.* **293:**1339–1343.

54. Golde, D. W., Schambelan, M., Weintraub, B. D., and Rosen, S. W., 1974, Gonadotropin secreting renal carcinoma, *Cancer* **33:**1048–1053.

55. Vaitukaitis, J. L., 1974, Human chorionic gonadotropin as a tumor marker, *Ann. Clin. Lab. Sci.* **4:**276–280.

56. Odell, W. D., Bates, R. W., Rivlin, R. S., Lipsett, M. B., and Hertz, R., 1963, Increased thyroid function without clinical hyperthyroidism in patients with cardiocarcinoma, *J. Clin. Endocrinol. Metab.* **23:**658–664.

57. Hershman, J. M., and Higgins, H. P., 1971, Hydatidiform mole—a cause of clinical hyperthyroidism. Two cases with evidence that the molar tissue secreted a thyroid stimulator, *N. Engl. J. Med.* **284:**573–577.

58. Hershman, J. M., Higgins, H. P., and Starnes, W. R., 1970, Differences between thyroid stimulator in hydatidiform mole and human chorionic thyrotropin, *Metabolism* **19:**735–744.

59. Hennen, G., Pierce, J. G., and Freychet, P., 1969, Human chorionic thyrotropin: Further characterization and study of its secretion during pregnancy, *J. Clin. Endocrinol. Metab.* **29:**581–594.

60. Hershman, J. M., and Starnes, W. R., 1969, Extraction and characterization of thyrotrophic material in the human placenta, *J. Clin. Invest.* **48:**923–929.

61. Kenimer, J. G., Hershman, J. M., and Higgins, H. P., 1974, The thyrotropin in hydatidiform moles is human chorionic gonadotropin, *J. Clin. Endocrinol. Metab.* **40:**482–491.

62. Devroede, G. J., and Tirol, A. F., 1968, Giant pleural mesothelioma associated with hypoglycemia and hyperthyroidism, *Am. J. Surg.* **116:**130–134.

63. Schwartz, W. B., Bennett, W., Curelop, E. S., and Bartter, S. C., 1957, A syndrome of renal sodium loss and hyponatremia probably resulting from inappropriate secretion of antidiuretic hormone, *Amer. J. Med.* **23:**529–542.

64. George, J. M., Capen, C. C., and Phillips, A. S., 1972, Biosynthesis of vasopressin *in vitro* and ultrastructure of a bronchogenic carcinoma, *J. Clin. Invest.* **51:**141–148.

65. Martin, T. J., Greenberg, P. B., Beck, C., and Johnston, C. I., 1973, Synthesis of peptide hormones by human tumors in cell cultures, *Endocrinology, Proceedings of the Fourth International Congress* (R. O. Scow, ed.), *Excerpta Med. Int. Congr. Ser.,* 1198–1204.

66. White, M. G., and Fetner, C. D., 1975, Treatment of the syndrome of inappropriate secretion of antidiuretic hormone with lithium carbonate, *N. Engl. J. Med.* **292:**390–392.

67. Cherill, D. A., Stote, R. M., Birge, J. R., and Singer, I., 1975, Demeclocycline treatment in the syndrome of inappropriate antidiuretic hormone secretion, *Ann. Intern. Med.* **83:**654–656.

68. Hamilton, B. P. M., Upton, G. V., and Amatruda, T. T., Jr., 1972, Evidence for the presence of neurophysin in tumors producing the syndrome with inappropriate antidiuresis, *J. Clin. Endocrinol. Metab.* **35:**764–767.

69. Unger, R. H., 1966, The riddle of tumor hypoglycemia, *Amer. J. Med.* **40:**325–330.

70. Marks, L. J., Steinke, J., Podolsky, S., and Egdahl, R. H., 1974, Hypogly-

cemia associated with neoplasia, *Ann. N. Y. Acad. Sci.* **230:**147–160.

71. Saeed, S. M., Fine, G., and Horn, R. C., Jr., 1969, Hypoglycemia associated with extrapancreatic tumors. Immunofluorescent study, *Cancer* **24:**158–166.

72. Lyall, S. S., Marieb, N. J., Wise, J. K., Cornog, J. L., Neville, E. C., and Felig, P., 1975, Hyperinsulinemic hypoglycemia associated with a neurofibrosarcoma, *Arch. Intern. Med.* **135:**865–867.

73. Van Wyk, J. J., Underwood, L. E., Hintz, R. L., Clemmons, D. R., Voina, S. J., and Weaver, R. P., 1974, The somatomedins: A family of insulinlike hormones under growth hormone control, *Recent Prog. Horm. Res.* **30:**259–318.

74. Megyesi, K., Kahn, C. R., Roth, J., and Gorden, P., 1974, Hypoglycemia in association with extrapancreatic tumors: Demonstration of elevated plasma NSILA-s by a new radioreceptor assay, *J. Clin. Endocrinol. Metab.* **38:**931–934.

75. Megyesi, K., Kahn, C. R., Roth, J., and Gorden, P., 1975, Circulating NSILA-s in man: Preliminary studies of stimuli *in vivo* and of binding to plasma components, *J. Clin. Endocrinol. Metab.* **41:**475–484.

76. Schein, P. S., Delellis, R. A., Kahn, C. R., Gorden, P., and Kraft, A. R., 1973, Islet cell tumors: Current concepts in management, *Ann. Intern. Med.* **79:**239–257.

77. Lafferty, F. W., 1966, Pseudohyperparathyroidism, *Medicine* **45:**247–260.

78. Munson, T. L., Tashjian, A. H., Jr., and Levine, L., 1965, Evidence of parathyroid hormone in non-parathyroid tumors associated with hypercalcemia, *Cancer Res.* **25:**1062–1067.

79. Sherwood, L. M., O'Riordan, J. L. H., Aurbach, G. D., and Potts, J. T., Jr., 1967, Production of parathyroid hormone by non-parathyroid tumors, *J. Clin. Endocrinol. Metab.* **27:**140–146.

80. Knill-Jones, R. P., Buckle, R. M., Parson, V., Calne, R. Y., and Williams, R., 1970, Hypercalcemia and increased parathyroid-hormone activity in a primary hepatoma: Studies before and after hepatic transplantation, *N. Engl. J. Med.* **282:**704–708.

81. Riggs, B. L., Arnaud, C. D., Reynolds, J. C., and Smith, L. H., 1971, Immunologic differentiation of primary hyperparathyroidism from hyperparathyroidism due to non-parathyroid cancer, *J. Clin. Invest.* **50:**2079–2083.

82. Segre, G. V., Habener, J. F., Powell, D., Tregear, G. W., and Potts, J. T., Jr., 1972, Parathyroid hormone in human plasma: Immunochemical characterization and biological implications, *J. Clin. Invest.* **51:**3163–3172.

83. Canterbury, J. M., Bricker, L. A., Levey, G. S., Kozlovskis, P. L., Ruiz, E., Zull, J. E., and Reiss, E., 1975, Metabolism of bovine parathyroid hormone: Immunological and biological characteristics of fragments generated by liver perfusion, *J. Clin. Invest.* **55:**1245–1253.

84. Eisenberg, H., Pallotta, J., and Sherwood, L. M., 1974, Selective arteriography, venography and venous hormone assay in diagnosis and localization of parathyroid lesions, *Amer. J. Med.* **56:**810–820.

85. Blair, A. J., Jr., Hawker, C. D., and Utiger, R. D., 1973, Ectopic hyperparathyroidism in a patient with metastatic hypernephroma, *Metabolism* **22:**147–154.

86. Hartman, C. R., MacGregor, R. R., Chu, L. L. H., McGregor, D. H., Cohn, D. D., and Hamilton, J. N., 1975, Evidence for the biosynthesis of PTH-like peptides by a human squamous cell carcinoma, Abstract of the Endocrine Society, 57th Meeting, New York, No. 2.

87. Powell, D., Singer, F. R., Murray, T. M., Minkin, C., and Potts. J. T., Jr., 1973, Non-parathyroid humoral hypercalcemia in patients with neoplastic diseases, *N. Engl. J. Med.* **289**:176–181.
88. Tashjian, A. H., Jr., Voelkel, E. F., Goldhaber, P., and Levine, L., 1974, Prostaglandins and calcium metabolism in cancer, *Fed. Proc. Fed. Amer. Soc. Exp. Biol.* **33**:81–86.
89. Voekel, E. F., Tashjian, A. H., Jr., Franklin, R., Wasserman, E., and Levine, L., 1975, Hypercalcemia and tumor-prostaglandin: The VX$_2$ carcinoma model in the rabbit, *Metabolism* **24**:973–986.
90. Brereton, H. D., Halushka, P. V., Alexander, R. W., Mason, D. M., Keiser, H. R., and DeVita, V. T., Jr., 1974, Indomethacin-responsive hypercalcemia in a patient with renal cell adenocarcinoma, *N. Engl. J. Med.* **291**:83–85.
91. Robertson, R. P., Baylink, D. J., Marini, J. J., and Adkison, H. W., 1975, Elevated prostaglandins and suppressed parathyroid hormone associated with hypercalcemia and renal cell carcinoma, *J. Clin. Endocrinol. Metab.* **41**:164–167.
92. Ito, H., Sanada, T., Katavama, T., and Shimazaki, J., 1975, Indomethacin-responsive hypercalcemia, *N. Engl. J. Med.* **293**:558–559.
93. Seyberth, H. W., Segre, G. V., Morgan, J. L., Sweetman, B. J., Potts, J. T., Jr., and Oates, J. A., 1975, Prostaglandins as mediators of hypercalcemia associated with certain types of cancer, *N. Engl. J. Med.* **293**:1278–1283.
94. Luben, R. A., Mundy, G. R., Trummel, C. L., and Raisz, L. G., 1974, Partial purification of osteoclast-activating factor from phytohemagglutinin-stimulated human leukocytes, *J. Clin. Invest.* **53**:1473–1480.
95. Mundy, G. R., Luben, R. A., Raisz, L. G., Oppenheim, J. J., and Buell, D. N., 1974, Bone-resorbing activity in supernatants from lymphoid cell lines, *N. Engl. J. Med.* **290**:867–871.
96. Silva, O. L., Becker, K. L., Primack, A., Doppman, J., and Snider, R. H., 1974, Ectopic secretion of calcitonin by oat-cell carcinoma, *N. Engl. J. Med.* **290**:1122–1124.
97. Silva, O. L., Becker, K. L., Primack, A., Doppman, J. L., and Snider, R. H., 1976, Increased serum calcitonin levels in bronchogenic cancer, *Chest* **69**:495–499.
98. Milhaud, G., Calmette, C., Taboulet, J., Julienne, A., and Moukhtar, M. S., 1974, Letter: Hypersecretion of calcitonin in neoplastic conditions, *Lancet* **1**:462–463.
99. Voelkel, E. F., Tashjian, A. H., Jr., Davidoff, F. F., Cohen, R. B., Perlia, C. P., and Wurtman, R. J., 1973, Concentrations of calcitonin and catecholamines in pheochromocytomas, a mucosal neuroma and medullary thyroid carcinoma, *J. Clin. Endocrinol. Metab.* **37**:297–307.
100. Cattan, D., Vesin, P., Rougier, P. H., Kalifat, R., Belaiche, J., Parrot, M., Milhaud, G., and Beardwell, C. G., 1974, Letter: Hyperthyrocalcitoninaemia, Schwartz-Bartter syndrome, and oat-cell carcinoma, *Lancet* **1**:938.
101. Coombes, R. C., Hillyard, C., Greenberg, P. B., and MacIntyre, I., 1974, Plasma-immunoreactive-calcitonin in patients with non-thyroid tumours, *Lancet* **1**:1080–1083.
102. Sherwood, J. B., and Goldwasser, E., 1976, Erythropoietic production by human renal tumor cells in culture, *Endocrinology* **99**:504–510.
103. Hollifield, J. W., Page, D. L., Smith, C., Michelakis, A. M., Staab, E., and Rhamy, R., 1975, Renin-secreting clear cell carcinoma of the kidney, *Arch. Intern. Med.* **135**:859–864.
104. Stanbury, S. W., 1972, Osteomalacia, *Clin. Endocrinol. Metab.* **1**:239–266.

105. Mallinson, C. N., Bloom, S. K., Warin, A. P., Salmon, P. R., and Cox, B., 1974, A glucagonoma syndrome, *Lancet* **2:**7871–7875.
106. Said, S. I., and Faloona, G. R., 1975, Elevated plasma and tissue levels of vasoactive intestinal peptide in the watery diarrhea syndrome due to pancreatic bronchogenic and other tumors, *New Eng. J. Med.* **293:**155–160.
107. Hirai, H., and Alpert, E. (eds.), 1975, Carcinofetal proteins: Biology and chemistry, *Ann. N.Y. Acad. Sci.* **259:**1–452.
108. Higashino, K., Ohtani, R., Kudo, S., Hashinotsume, M., Hada, T., Kang, K.-Y., Ohkochi, T., Takahashi, Y., and Yamamura, Y., 1975, Hepatocellular carcinoma and a variant alkaline phosphatase, *Ann. Intern. Med.* **83:**74–78.
109. Hall, T. C., 1974, Paraneoplastic syndromes, *Ann. N.Y. Acad. Sci.* **230:**1–577.

11

Current Concepts in Steroid Hormone Action

Bert W. O'Malley and Richard E. Buller

11.1. Introduction

Steroid hormones play a central role in a multitude of homeostatic mechanisms in man and animals. The sex steroids (androgens, estrogens, and progestins) are intimately involved in cytodifferentiation, as well as in initiation and regulation of the reproductive processes. Glucocorticoids play a role in fetal lung and liver maturation, the ability of organisms to withstand stress, glucose intermediary metabolism, and many other processes. Mineralocorticoids, such as aldosterone, are essential for regulation of salt and water balance, and thus have been implicated in various forms of hypertension. Vitamin D, which is also a steroid, is of major importance in calcium and phosphate metabolism.

Because of their importance, the relatively large class of small

BERT W. O'MALLEY and RICHARD E. BULLER • Department of Cell Biology, Baylor College of Medicine, Houston, Texas 77030.

(mol. wt. approximately 300) polycyclic organic compounds called *steroid hormones* has been subject to intense research scrutiny over the past 50 years. Initial studies were directed at the chemical characterization and structure determination of these compounds secreted by the body's endocrine glands. Subsequently, many physiological studies were carried out in order to identify tissue responses to steroids and the biochemical nature of these responses. Since the early 1960's, when high-labeled radioactive steroids were first available, it has been possible to investigate the subcellular distribution of hormones within hormone-responsive or target tissues. Protein molecules termed *receptors,* which play the central intermediary role in the action of all steroid hormones, have been isolated. These actions include increased RNA and protein synthesis. While some attention has been directed to methods of posttranscriptional control of steroid-induced protein synthesis, it seems likely that steroid hormones exert their primary effects at the level of transcription. The reason is that steroid administration results first in increased RNA synthesis at genes that are otherwise not expressed or are transcribed at a low rate.

It is the purpose of this review to present the data that have been accumulated to support the hypothesis that intracellular steroid hormone action is mediated through specific receptor proteins. With these data as background, it will be possible to delve into those recent advances in the molecular endocrinology of steroid hormone action that allow us to postulate a generalized step-by-step detailed scheme of steroid hormone action. Finally, we will use the body of evidence assimilated in numerous research laboratories to explain some of the interesting endocrine phenomena that have been observed with regard to the role of steroid hormones in various disease states.

11.2. Autoradiography

Injection of [^{3}H]estradiol into rats by Jensen and co-workers resulted in the observation that the steroid was retained preferentially by some tissues.[1,2] Similar experiments with other hormones revealed that estrogens were retained by the uterus and vagina[1-3]; progesterone was retained by the oviduct[4,5]; testosterone was retained by the ventral prostate and seminal vesicles[6-8]; aldosterone was retained by the kidney and urinary bladder[9,10]; and vitamin D was retained by the intestine and parathyroid glands.[11,12]

To determine the subcellular distributions of steroid hormones, two lines of research have been pursued. Following *in vivo* injections of labeled hormone, target tissues were isolated and various subcellar fractions prepared. The evidence suggested nuclear and cytoplasmic localization of radioactivity.[13-16] No specific binding to nucleoli was found.[17]

Because of the inherent difficulty in preparing pure subcellular fractions and the possibility of isolation artifacts pointed out by Williams and Gorski,[18] evidence from a second line of investigation has been extremely important in the unequivocal determination of the nucleus as the subcellular site of preferential hormone retention. The technical aspects of this second method, autoradiography, were discussed by Stumpf.[19] Using autoradiography, several workers observed the selective concentration of [^{3}H]17β-estradiol by various anterior pituitary cell nuceli,[20,21] certain hypothalamic nuclei, [21,22] and nuclei of uterine endometrial, stromal, and myometrial cells.[14,23,24] Similar results have been obtained from autoradiographic studies of the intra-cellular localization of [^{3}H]aldosterone in the nuclei of kidney and bladder epithelia,[25] and the nuclear accumulation of [^{3}H]progesterone by the uterus[26] and certain neurons of the hypothalamus.[27] Nuclear localization of steroid was shown to be specific in that the concomitant administration of the same steroid, unlabeled and in excess, blocked the nuclear accumulation of the tritium label. Coadministration of unrelated steroids did not block nuclear accumulation of labeled steroid by target tissues.[27] These experiments provided direct visual evidence that steroids are preferentially accumulated by nuclei of target cells.

11.3. Receptor-Mediated Steroid Translocation to Nuclei

The discovery of receptor proteins shed considerable light on the mechanism by which target cell nuclei selectively accumulate steroids. Classic pharmacology defines a receptor as a biological transducer that converts input information, in this case circulating hormones, into a biological response (e.g., increased RNA and protein synthesis). Biochemically, a receptor is a protein molecule that selectively binds a ligand in a saturable fashion and with high affinity (K_D approximately $10^{-8}-10^{-10}$ M). Jensen first postulated the existence of such a binding molecule for estrogen in the rat uterus.[28,29] His observations were substantiated and extended by other researchers.[13-16] Similar steroid-specific binding proteins were described for progesterone,[30,31] dihydrotestosterone,[32,33] glucocorticoids,[34,35] aldosterone,[36,37] and most recently for vitamin D.[38-40] In the absence of hormone, these receptor proteins were located in the cytoplasm.

When whole tissues were incubated with labeled steroid under appropriate *in vitro* conditions, subsequent examination of nuclear and cytoplasmic fractions showed that much of the label had been accumulated by the nuclear fraction, and that the cytoplasmic fraction had been depleted of its original capacity to specifically bind hormone.[41,42] Alternatively, target tissues were homogenized and binding studies carried out on purified cytoplasmic and nuclear fractions. In unstimulated target cells, selective high-affinity binding of steroid occurred only in the cytoplasmic fraction. The addition of labeled hormone–receptor complexes to nuclei under appropriate *in vitro* conditions resulted in a selective nuclear accumulation of hormone–receptor complexes, coupled with a concomitant decrease in cytoplasmic hormone–receptor complexes. These observations were highly suggestive of receptor-mediated nuclear accumulation of steroid.

Various model systems have been used to provide additional evidence that receptor proteins are required to effect specific binding of hormones to nuclei. Cytoplasmic receptors were shown to be present in lymphoblasts sensitive to the cytolytic actions of glucocorticoids.[43,44] Conversely, cells resistant to the cytolytic actions of glucocorticoids contained few cytoplasmic receptor sites.[43,45] Glucocorticoid-sensitive fibroblasts contained receptors,[46,47] whereas insensitive fibroblasts contained markedly diminished numbers of cytoplasmic glucocorticoid-binding molecules.[47] Diminished cytoplasmic levels of androgen receptor protein in the kidney of the androgen-insensitive adult Tfm mouse and rat were reported by Bullock *et al.*[48] and Gehring *et al.*[49] Hepatic responses to 5α-dihydrotestosterone failed to occur in animals deficient in liver receptor for this steroid.[50] Thus, several lines of evidence from many different model systems indicate that steroid hormones bind to nuclear acceptor sites through reactions dependent on specific receptors.

11.4. Quantitation of Nuclear Receptors by Nuclear Exchange

The nuclear exchange assay for estradiol, developed by Clark and co-workers, has been a particularly useful methodological advance.[51–56] Injection of estradiol (E_2) *in vivo* drives cytoplasmic estrogen receptors into target tissue nuclei in a dose-dependent fashion. The extent to which nuclear translocation of cytoplasmic receptor had occurred was assayed *in vitro* by "exchange" of tritium-labeled estradiol with the cold estradiol complexed with receptor in the nuclei. With the use of this assay, tissues that did not contain cytoplasmic estrogen receptor were shown to be devoid of specifically bound nuclear E_2 in an exchangeable form.[51]

The sensitivity of the nuclear exchange assay was such that variations in nuclear estrogen–receptor complex were detected in response to physiological variations in circulating estrogens. A 6-fold increase in nuclear-bound receptor occurred cyclically between metestrus and proestrus in the cycling female rat.[52] The variation in nuclear receptor closely paralleled the secretion of estrogen during the estrous cycle.[52]

Because the exchange assay depended on the *in vivo* binding of unlabeled steroid–receptor complexes to nuclei, it was possible to examine the actions of various antiestrogens. While evidence from other laboratories has documented the fact that some steroid antagonists function by binding to the cytoplasmic receptor and preventing nuclear uptake of the complex,[57,58] this cannot be the only mechanism of steroid hormone antagonism. Clark *et al.* used the nuclear exchange assay to examine the antiestrogenic actions of CI-628, nafoxidine, and clomiphene.[55,56] These three compounds apparently bound to uterine cytoplasmic estrogen receptor, and were then translocated to the nuclear compartment in a normal fashion.[55,56] Initial uterotropic responses were observed, and these responses were maintained over prolonged periods of time. However, a subsequent restimulation or challenge with estradiol was completely ineffective. This result was explained by the observation that in addition to the prolonged nuclear retention of estrogen receptor mediated by these antiestrogens, cytoplasmic receptor resynthesis may have been blocked.[56]

11.5. Cell-Free Binding Studies

Measurement of nuclear or acceptor site capacity and binding constants has been achieved in several laboratories, Binding of hormone–receptor complex to chromatin or nuclei appeared to involve high-affinity binding to several thousand sites per cell (see Buller and O'Malley[59] for a review). We recently studied the kinetics of the chick oviduct progesterone receptor interaction with nuclei[60] and chromatin.[61] The results were remarkably similar, and suggested that the nuclear membrane did not play an essential role in the equilibrium binding distribution of receptors. Moreover, we obtained essentially the same results using receptor purified to homogeneity by affinity chromatography.[61,62] Figure 1 represents a saturation curve and Scatchard plot analysis of nuclear binding of a purified homogeneous preparation of progesterone receptors to highly purified chick oviduct nuclei. The K_D for this system was 1.1×10^{-9} M, and there were 10,000 binding sites per nucleus. Oviduct contained more binding sites than other tissues, but the binding affinity varied little from tissue to tissue.[60,61] One surprising finding involved the elucidation of apparent nuclear binding site heterogeneity. In addition to a large num-

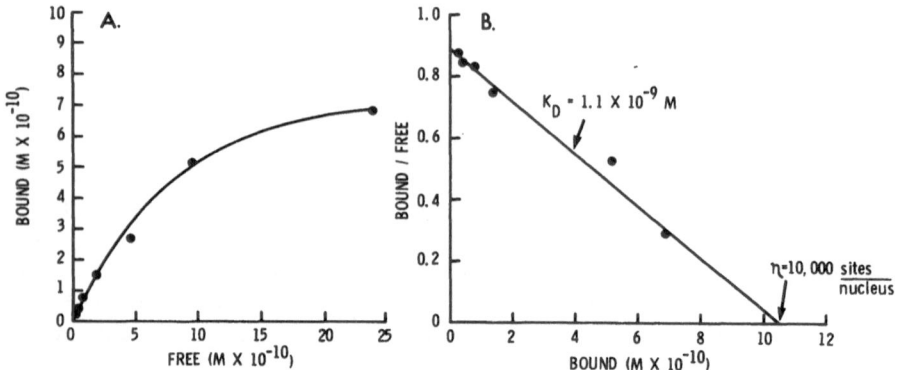

Fig. 1. Binding of purified progesterone receptors to purified chick oviduct nuclei. Nuclei were purified by sedimentation through heavy sucrose and incubated with progesterone receptor that had been purified to homogeneity by affinity chromatography. After washing, the nuclear bound counts of the pellets were determined by ethanol extraction. Details of the analysis can be found in Buller *et al.*[60] (A) Saturation curve for receptor bindings; (B) Scatchard analysis of the data in A used to determine K_D, the dissociation constant, and η the number of sites per nucleus. (Reproduced with permission of Kuhn *et al.*[62])

ber (approximately 9000) of high-affinity binding sites (K_D approximately 10^{-8} M), Scatchard analysis suggested the presence of at least one other class of binding sites of even higher affinity.[60] Because this very-high-affinity binding component was present in such low titers, it was difficult to quantitate binding parameters for it. The K_D approximated 10^{-11} M, and the sites per nucleus were on the order of a few hundred.

11.6. Nature of the Nuclear Acceptor Site

The extent to which DNA participated in the binding of hormone–receptor complexes to chromatin varied somewhat depending on the hormone studied, and has not yet been adequately explained. The regions of the genome to which aldosterone, glucocorticoid, and estrogen receptors[63-67] bound were apparently much more susceptible to digestion by DNase than the corresponding regions to which progesterone receptors bound in the chick oviduct.[68] In the latter case, both the number of acceptor sites and the binding constant remained constant, even with prior digestion of up to 60% of the nuclear DNA content (Buller, unpublished observations). By studying the kinetics of receptor interaction with nuclei, it was possible to show that during the initial period of receptor interaction with nuclei, the reaction was linear with respect to receptor

(Fig. 2A) and with respect to nuclear DNA (Fig. 2B). This finding was consistent with a reaction that followed overall second-order kinetics, but, more important, showed that the receptors were binding to some specific nuclear constituent. Since Triton X-100 treatment of nuclei that had been incubated with receptors did not diminish nuclear receptor content despite removal of the outer nuclear membrane, it seemed likely that the receptors were binding intranuclearly. Moreover, neither pretreating oviduct chromatin with mung bean nuclease, which is specific for single-strand DNA, nor incubation with specific antibody for single-strand DNA blocked subsequent chromatin binding of progesterone receptors.[61] Thus, chick oviduct progesterone receptors do not bind to single-strand DNA, or to double-strand regions of DNA that are accessible to digestion by DNase I. These findings did not support Crick's general model for gene control, which required that regulatory macromolecules interact with single-strand regions of the genome.[69]

It did not seem likely that DNA was the sole determinant of receptor binding to the genome. While it is true that not all tissues contain receptors, mixing experiments performed in cell-free systems showed that receptors isolated from target tissues bound preferentially to target tissue

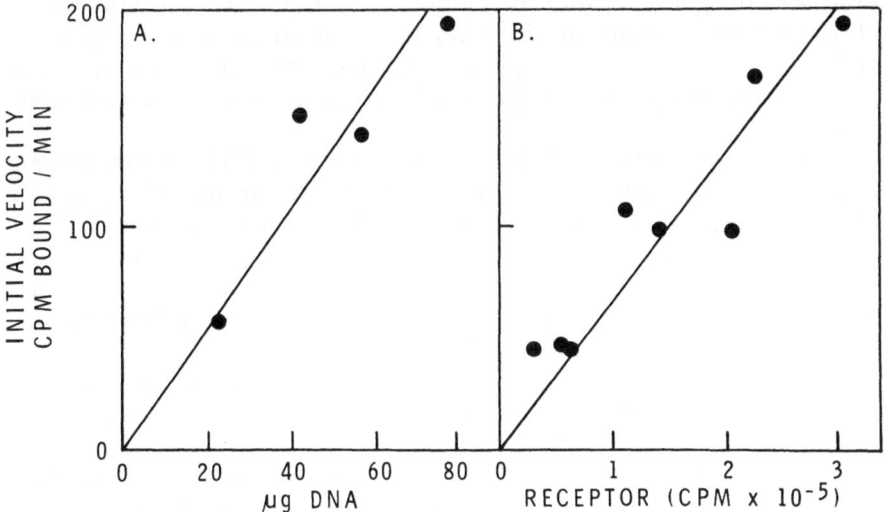

Fig. 2. Kinetics of receptor interaction with nuclei. Incubations were carried out for various short time intervals and bound counts of [³H]progesterone–receptor complex determined. The slopes (initial velocity) from plots of the bound counts vs. time were plotted: (A) as a function of nuclear DNA with receptor concentration held constant, and (B) as a function of receptor concentration with nuclear DNA held constant. (Buller, unpublished observations.)

nuclei and chromatin.[60,61,68-70,72] Since all tissues within a given animal contain the same DNA, such a finding would require either that specific regions of the DNA in nontarget tissues be masked by nuclear proteins or that nuclear proteins participate in a cooperative fashion with DNA in defining specific nuclear acceptor sites. Evidence in support of the first possibility comes from reports of saturable binding of hormone–receptor complexes to purified DNA.[64,66] Baxter *et al.*[66] found that chromatin with receptors bound to it was more resistant to digestion by DNase, suggesting that receptors were covering up exposed DNA. Receptor interaction with DNA has even been shown to be hormone-dependent.[73] However, except for the preliminary suggestion that unique and middle repetitive sequence DNA may be involved in receptor binding,[74] no firm proof exists that specific acceptor sites are defined by a specific sequence of nucleotides. Indeed, glucocorticoid receptors apparently bind equally well to single- and double-strand homologous DNA, as well as to *Escherichia coli* DNA.[17] Estrogen receptor binding to DNA has been similarly character- ized.[64,75-77] Yamamoto and Alberts showed that estrogen receptors bind equally well to heterologous DNA and synthetic polynucleotides, but not to double-strand RNA.[75] The binding affinity these authors reported was much lower than that reported by other workers. Thus, it would seem likely that chromosomal proteins play an active role in receptor interac- tions with the genome. Indeed, a more recent report discusses the role of chromosomal proteins in the binding of glucocorticoid receptors to DNA.[78] Strong evidence in support of this hypothesis has been offered by two laboratories working independently on different hormone-responsive systems.

Puca *et al.*[79] reported the identification of a high-affinity nuclear acceptor site for the estrogen receptor of calf uterus. The apparent acceptor was present within a subfraction of the nuclear proteins at levels 5–10 times in excess of cytoplasmic receptors. Studies of receptor interac- tions with acceptor were carried out by means of affinity chromatography. These studies revealed that the interactions were influenced by salt and dependent on hormone.

Our laboratories have previously implicated nonhistone (acidic) pro- tein involvement in the nuclear acceptor site for the progesterone recep- tor of chick oviduct.[80-82] Several lines of reasoning suggest that nonhi- stone proteins are a logical choice to confer acceptor-site specificity. First, they are a very heterogeneous class of proteins resolved by size, charge, and immunological procedures. This heterogeneity contrasts with the relative homogeneity of the histones. Second, unlike histones, nonhistone chromosomal proteins turn over rapidly. Third, tissue specificity of non- histones has been shown.[83] Fourth, specific changes in the nonhistone protein population of cells have been demonstrated in response to hormone administration.[84,85] Fifth, Spelsberg *et al.* have performed chromatin reconstitution studies demonstrating that chromatin-associated receptor binding capacity can be transferred to nontarget tissue chromatin by transfer of a particular fraction of the nonhistone chromosomal proteins.[81,82] Finally, these reconstitution studies have recently been extended using an *in vitro* transcription assay (see Section 11.10) to show that control of the expression of a specific gene is modified by acidic proteins.[86] Thus, it seems probable that the actual chromatin-associated acceptor sites consist of a DNA backbone that is structurally modified by chromatin-associated nonhistone proteins.

11.7. Hormone Dependency of Nuclear Binding Receptors

Analogous to the receptor requirement of hormone accumulation by nuclei, there is a hormone requirement for nuclear retention of receptors. High-salt extracts prepared from highly purified estrogen-primed chick oviduct nuclei contained little progesterone binding activity.[41] The same observation was made with regard to the absence of receptors in nuclei prepared from immature rat uterus[23] and adrenalectomized rat liver.[87] Similarly, *in vitro* incubation of receptors with chromatin or purified nuclei in the absence of hormone resulted in little high-affinity binding of receptor to the genome.[66,88,89] Figure 3 shows the sucrose-gradient sedimentation profile of extracts prepared from oviduct nuclei that had been incubated with progesterone receptor with and without progesterone. All extracts were labeled with excess [^{3}H]progesterone prior to centrifugation. Macromolecular bound [^{3}H]progesterone was present only in the extract prepared from nuclei that had been incubated with receptor–hormone complexes. Such studies strongly suggest an absolute hormone requirement for nuclear and chromatin binding of receptors. It is possible that *in vitro*, receptors are distributed freely throughout both the cytoplasm and nucleoplasm, but are retained by nuclei only in the presence of hormone. Such a distribution would suggest a hormone-induced modification of receptor conformation that effects an alteration in the equilibrium distribution of receptors in favor of the nuclear compartment.

11.8. Receptor Activation for Nuclear Binding

Virtually all steroid hormone–receptor complexes, including the vitamin D receptor–hormone complex,[90] undergo temperature-sensitive

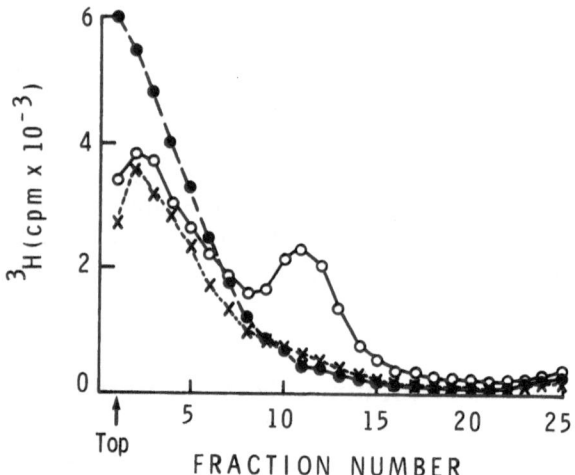

Fig. 3. Hormone dependence of receptor binding to nuclei. High salt extracts were prepared from purified nuclei incubated with [³H]progesterone-labeled receptor (O---O), progesterone-free receptor (X---X), or buffer alone (●---●). The extracts were labeled with excess [³H]progesterone and briefly treated with dextran-coated charcoal prior to centrifugation on sucrose gradients at 48,000 rpm (SW 50.1) for 16 hr. (Reproduced with permission of Buller et al.[68])

nuclear binding. Experiments under cell-free, low-salt conditions indicate very little receptor binding to nuclei or chromatin at 0°C.[65,68,91,92] In contrast, incubation of receptors with nuclei at 22–37°C results in significant binding to nuclei or chromatin. This finding is consistent with the observation that *in vitro* incubation of hormone with tissue slices requires elevated temperatures (37°C) for the nuclear localization of hormone to occur.[3,23,42] Multiple possible explanations for these observations may be offered. First, temperature may induce changes in cytoplasmic receptors that facilitate nuclear binding. Second, the nuclear uptake process itself may be influenced by temperature. Third, temperature may influence the availability of nuclear acceptor sites. Fourth, the interaction of receptor with acceptor may be facilitated by elevated temperatures. Fifth, activation may be an *in vitro* artifact without *in vivo* relevance. Finally, some combination of the effects enumerated above may occur *in vivo*.

The effects of salt and temperature on receptors apparently result in the exposure of increased regions of positive charge. These alterations in the physical properties of receptors were readily detected by chromatographic procedures,[89,93–95] and less readily detectable by gross procedures, such as surcrose-gradient centrifugation,[68,93] although exceptions exist.[96,97]

It was interesting to find that in chick oviduct nuclei, there are

considerably more nuclear acceptor sites exposed at elevated temperatures.[60] Complicated kinetic arguments allowed us to conclude that the
rate of the nuclear binding process showed minimal temperature dependency over the range 0–25°C. This finding was consistent with a simple
diffusion-limited uptake of oviduct progesterone receptors, and contrasts
with the active transport process suggested by other authors.[98]

In summary, the important observation that the *in vitro* interaction
of receptors with the genome is facilitated by elevated temperatures has
led to publication of a large number of papers concerning "activation
processes" that may be temperature-, salt-, and/or enzymatically
mediated.[99,100] It is essential to realize that activation is simply any process
that facilitates the rate or extent of nuclear binding *in vitro*. Although no
significant relevance to *in vivo* response has been proven, a recent report
shows that *in vitro* nuclear synthetic responses are stimulated best by
"activated receptors."[101]

11.9. Correlation of Nuclear Binding with Biological Response

Studies that have attempted to correlate nuclear binding of receptors
with biological responses have been inferential. Two recent lines of work
have been strongly suggestive that such a correlation is indeed appropriate. Spirolactones are known antagonists of aldosterone. Normally, aldosterone promotes renal tubular readsorption of Na^+. However, in the
presence of spirolactones, the antinatriuretic effects of aldosterone are
greatly diminished. Marver *et al.*[58] recently demonstrated that the spirolactone SC-26304 can competitively bind to kidney cytoplasmic aldosterone receptors, thus creating a spirolactone–receptor complex that is
incapable of binding to nuclear acceptor sites. Thus, in the absence of the
receptor–acceptor interaction, the antinatriuretic effects of aldosterone
were blocked. These findings confirmed those reported earlier by Kaiser
et al.[57] with regard to the inhibition of nuclear binding of glucocorticoid
receptors and the absence of glucocorticoid responses in the presence of
cortexalone.

A second line of evidence that argues strongly for a correlation
between nuclear binding of receptors and biological response resulted
from the studies of Anderson *et al.*[53] using nuclear exchange methods.
The details of this method were outlined in Section 11.4. These authors
correlated estrogen-induced uterotropic and growth responses with
nuclear receptor content. They found that cytoplasmic receptor was
present in excess of that required to produce maximal uterotropic
responses. In general, growth responses were proportional to the quantity

of estrogen–receptor complex that remained bound to the nucleus for 6 hr, and not to the amount of complex that was driven into the nucleus immediately after administration of large doses of estradiol *in vivo*. Analogous work with antiestrogens[55,56] showed that prolonged nuclear retention of antiestrogen–receptor complex resulted in prolonged uterotropic responses. Also, exchangeable nuclear estradiol has been shown to correlate with induction of a specific protein, IP.[102] Thus, nuclear retention, rather than initial nuclear uptake of receptors, probably determines more complex responses such as cellular growth and replication.

11.10. Cell Genetic Variants in Hormone Response

Recent work has demonstrated that even nuclear retention of hormone–receptor complexes does not guarantee responses. Cell hybridization studies produced cells that contain glucocorticoid receptors indistinguishable from parental receptors.[103] Nuclear binding in the hybrid clones was also observed; however, tyrosine aminotransferase (TAT) induction did not occur. Such a finding is susceptible to several possible explanations. Because glucocorticoids have other functions in addition to induction of TAT, production of hybrid clones may simply have resulted in the deletion of the TAT gene, leaving behind many other genes the expression of which remained influenced by glucocorticoids. Alternatively, the nuclear acceptor site that was occupied by receptor and thus induced TAT may have been altered so that TAT became uninducible. Isolation of TAT mRNA and hybridization studies could differentiate between these hypotheses.

A most interesting finding was reported by Lippman *et al.*[104] They cloned human and mouse leukemic cell lines that contained glucocorticoid receptors in amounts comparable to those of normal tissues. No unusual findings were made with regard to affinity and specificity of these receptors. Saturable high-affinity nuclear binding of receptors was also demonstrated. Nevertheless, the cells were totally unresponsive to steroid administration. No changes in growth, macromolecular synthesis, amino acid uptake, or glucose utilization were detected. These results expanded on an earlier observation by Gehring *et al.*[105] of a mouse lymphoma cell line that contained glucocorticoid receptors, but was unresponsive to the steroid. Using special techniques to isolate lymphoma cell variates resistant to killing by glucocorticoids,[101] Sibley and Tomkins succeeded in characterizing cell lines the steroid resistance of which can be attributed to each of the following three classes of defects: (1) absence of a cytoplasmic receptor, (2) deficient nuclear transfer of otherwise normal cytoplasmic receptors, and (3) failure of reactions subsequent to nuclear localization of receptor–hormone complex.[106] Yamamoto and co-workers went one step further and showed altered DNA-binding properties of glucocorticoid receptors that could not be driven to the nucleus by administering glucocorticoid to whole cells in culture.[107] Thus, the presence of receptors is a necessary, but not sufficient, condition for hormone responsiveness.

11.11. Quantitation of Transcriptional Events in Vitro

There have been numerous attempts to study the *in vitro* effects of steroid hormones on RNA synthesis. Such studies have usually consisted of *in vivo* administration of hormone and isolation of nuclei or chromatin, followed by measurement of endogenous RNA polymerase I (nucleolar) and RNA polymerase II (nucleoplasmic) activities. Accordingly, it has been found that dihydrotestosterone,[108–110] E_2,[111–115] glucocorticoids,[116,117] progesterone,[118] and vitamin D[119] increase either or both polymerase I and polymerase II activity assayed *in vitro*.

Davies and Griffiths incubated androgen receptors with prostatic nuclei and chromatin *in vitro*.[120,121] They demonstrated a putative receptor-mediated, hormone-dependent, tissue-specific enhancement of prostatic nucleolar polymerase activity. More recently, these investigators also described receptor-mediated increases in nucleoplasmic RNA polymerase activity. Unfortunately, all such studies have been limited by the inability to separate the various steps involved in RNA synthesis and the lack of purified homogeneous receptor preparations. Therefore, most investigators have been unable to determine the precise step at which steroid hormone–receptor complexes act to elicit differential gene response.

The events that may be involved in determining alterations in differential gene expression include: (1) RNA polymerase binding to the genome, (2) RNA polymerase search for initiation sites, (3) formation of stable RNA polymerase–DNA initiation complexes, (4) initiation of RNA chain synthesis, (5) RNA chain propagation rate, (6) RNA chain size, (7) termination of RNA chain synthesis, and (8) repetition or reinitiation of the previous sequence of events. It was conceivable that any of these events might be altered by steroid hormones, resulting in the previously well-described increases in RNA synthesis and RNA polymerase activity. A recent series of papers from our laboratories has utilized previously published procedures adopted from studies in bacterial and bacteriophage systems[122,123] to investigate the effect of estrogen and progesterone on RNA synthesis in the chick oviduct.[124–132] This methodology permitted assessment of each of the parameters mentioned above.

This basic procedure is represented diagramatically in Fig. 4. Increasing amounts of RNA polymerase were incubated with a fixed amount of DNA or chromatin at 37°C. The RNA polymerase molecules interact rapidly and reversibly with the template in several different ways, e.g., (1) nonspecifically, (2) to form a closed preinitiation complex, or (3) to form a stable or "open" preinitiation complex. Formation of stable preinitiation complexes occurs by a well-characterized time- and temperature-dependent process that is thought to involve a local opening or destabilizing of the DNA duplex at specific sites in the DNA.[133] The next step involves the addition of the 4 nucleoside triphosphates (NTPs) rifampicin, and heparin, the latter being added to inhibit RNase activity. The drug rifampicin acts as a competitive inhibitor of RNA synthesis *prior to* the formation of the first phosphodiester bond, and has no effect on RNA chain elongation.[134,135] Only RNA polymerase molecules bound in an open preinitiation complex can utilize the NTP substrates to begin RNA synthesis in the presence of rifampicin. All other RNA polymerase mole-

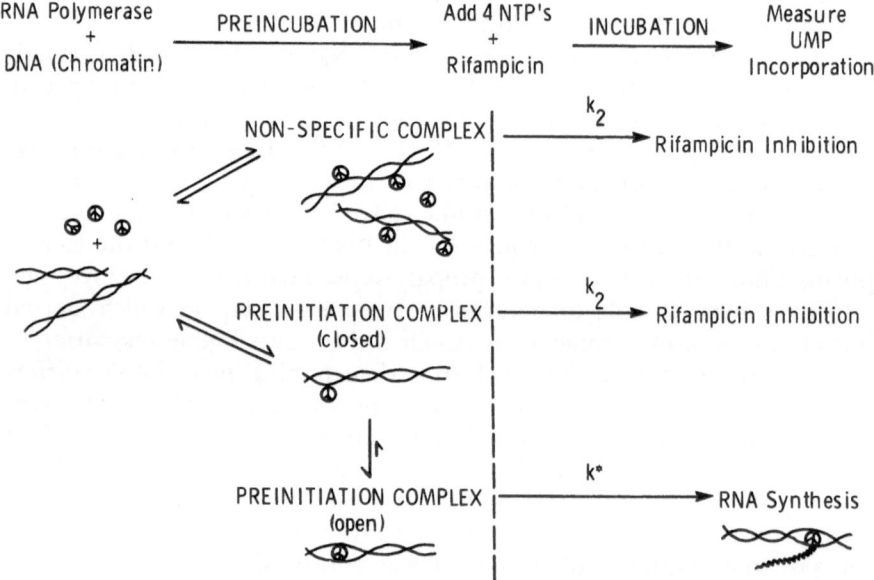

Fig. 4. Schematic representation of the rifampicin-challenge assay. RNA polymerase ($\otimes$) is combined with DNA or chromatin(xxxx) for a preincubation that results in formation of nonspecific complexes, closed preinitiation complexes, and open preinitiation complexes. When rifampicin and nucleoside triphosphates (NTPs with [³H]UTP label) are incubated with these complexes, rifampicin rapidly inhibits (k_2) RNA synthesis from all but the open preinitiation complexes (k^*). The products are collected by filtration, and the UMP label incorporated into RNA is determined. (Reproduced with permission of Towle, unpublished observations.)

cules are inhibited by the drug. When the product RNA has been isolated and its size determined in sucrose gradients, one can calculate an average size of the RNA chain synthesized. From this parameter and the amount of RNA synthesized, it is possible to calculate the number of initiation sites per unit amount of chromatin.[124] Moreover, using short synthetic periods, on the order of 1 min, it is also possible to calculate elongation rates. Use of this "rifampicin-challenge" transcription assay permits control and assessment of all the parameters involved in RNA synthesis. One must only determine which parameters are altered by steroid hormone administration.

11.12. Gene Expression in the Chick Oviduct Model System

The chick oviduct provides an excellent model system for the study of the hormonal control of cellular differentiation and gene expression. When newly hatched chicks receive daily injections of the synthetic estrogen diethylstilbesterol (DES) for 10–14 days, their oviducts grow from tiny 50-mg undifferentiated structures to large 2–3 g well-differentiated organs. Thousands of new proteins are synthesized during this time.[4,136,137] By far the most spectacular induction is that of the specific egg-white protein ovalbumin; over 60% of the cellular protein is represented by ovalbumin in the differentiated oviduct.[137] By way of contrast, this protein is undetectable initially. Hybridization experiments[136,138] have demonstrated increases in repetitive and unique sequence RNA during this time period. Thousands of new polyA-containing mRNAs are synthesized in response to estrogen stimulation.[139] Thus, we would predict that the expression of thousands of new oviduct genes is induced by steroid hormone administration to chicks.

During this hormone response, there are also well-documented increases in the biologically active messenger RNA that codes for ovalbumin.[140–142] Using viral reverse transcriptase and purified ovalbumin mRNA, Harris et al.[140] prepared highly radioactive complementary DNA copies of part of the gene responsible for ovalbumin mRNA synthesis ($[^3H]cNDA_{ov}$). This part served as an extremely sensitive hybridization probe for ovalbumin messenger RNA, and was therefore used to determine the ovalbumin messenger RNA content of oviduct cells during estrogen stimulation. Essentially no copies of the ovalbumin mRNA were found in the unstimulated oviduct, or in the oviduct of an animal that had been estrogen-stimulated but subsequently withdrawn from all hormone.[140] Moreover, readily measured increases in ovalbumin mRNA were detected as early as 30 min after secondary stimulation with estrogen. The absence of blocked or partially degraded ovalbumin mRNAs in unstimulated and stimulated–withdrawn animals suggested that estrogen induced *de novo* synthesis of ovalbumin message.

When daily injections of estrogen were halted for a subsequent 10–12 day period, the rate of ovalbumin synthesis dropped off to less than 1% of that observed during maximal hormone stimulation.[140] Readministration of estrogen (secondary stimulation) resulted in a very rapid accumulation of the mRNA for ovalbumin,[140,143,144] as well as the mRNAs for other egg-white proteins.[143] Similarly, when a differentiated chick oviduct was withdrawn from estrogen and subsequently presented with a progesterone challenge, it responded by increasing RNA synthesis, including mRNAs for egg-white proteins, as if challenged with estrogen.[144,145] Peripheral conversion of estrogen to progesterone has been ruled out (Schwartz, unpublished observations). Moreover, no such response occurred if testosterone was substituted for estrogen or progesterone.[145] Thus, either progesterone or estrogen can be utilized to study induction of gene expression in oviducts of prestimulated chicks that have subsequently been withdrawn from all hormone.

11.13. *In Vivo* Steroid-Induced Alterations in Chromatin Transcription Assayed *in Vitro*

The availability of a well-controlled transcription assay set the stage for the further investigation of steroid inductions of specific RNA synthesis in the chick oviduct. The first point of attack was the determination of the transcriptional event altered by steroids. Animals withdrawn from hormone were reinjected with estrogen and killed at various times after hormone administration. The rifampicin-challenge assay described in Section 11.10 was utilized to study the initiation of transcription by *E. coli* RNA polymerase on chromatin isolated from these animals.[125,129] The results of this experiment appear as Fig. 5. The number of initiation sites increased nearly 100% within 30 min of hormone administration. There was no significant alteration in elongation rate or the number average chain length of the RNA product.[125] In simultaneous studies, the level of nuclear bound hormone was assayed by a [^{3}H]estradiol exchange assay similar to that described earlier. This study revealed that optimum nuclear levels of bound receptor–hormone complex were attained by 20 min postinjection. An additional parameter measured in this study was the appearance of ovalbumin mRNA molecules in the cell's cytoplasmic compartment. The earliest detectable increase in ovalbumin mRNA occurred between 30 and 60 min following hormone administration.

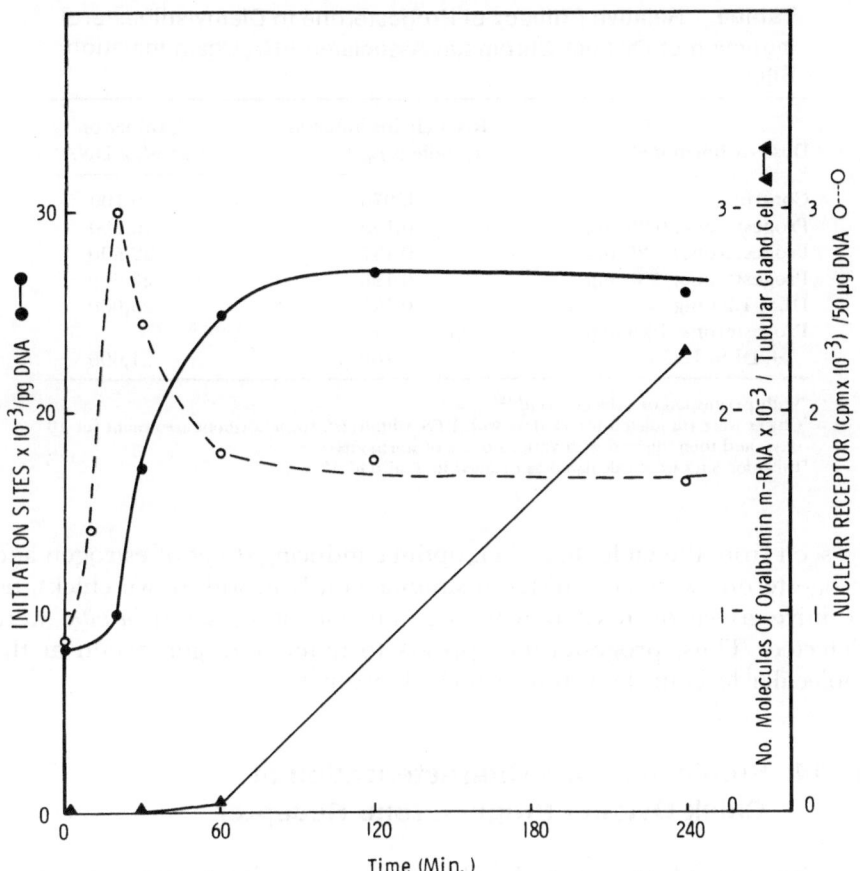

Fig. 5. Secondary response of chick oviduct to estrogen stimulation. Withdrawn chicks were injected with DES (2.5 mg) and killed at the indicated times. Nuclear estradiol was measured by the [³H]estradiol exchange assay. Initiation sites for RNA synthesis were quantitated using *E. coli* polymerase under rifampicin conditions. Ovalbumin mRNA titers were determined by RNA hybridization to [³H]cDNA. (Reproduced with permission of Tsai *et al.*[125])

Thereafter, linear increases in cellular ovalbumin mRNA were observed. These observations suggested a temporal sequence of events in hormone–responsive tissues that consisted of: (1) nuclear binding of hormone–receptor complex, (2) creation of new RNA polymerase initiation sites, and (3) synthesis of many new species of both unique and repetitive sequence RNA.

The administration of progesterone to hormone–deprived animals brought about similar increases in chromatin transcription.[126] Table I compares the efficacy of estrogen and progesterone in this process. It can

Table I. Relative Efficacy of Progesterone to Diethylstilbesterol Induction of Oviduct Chromatin-Associated RNA Chain Initiation Sites[a]

Dose of hormone[b]	RNA chains initiated (pmole/5 μg DNA)	Initiation sites/pg DNA[c]
Control	0.076	9,100
Progesterone, 0.25 mg	0.135	16,200
Progesterone, 1.25 mg	0.187	22,500
Progesterone, 2.0 mg	0.196	23,600
DES, 1.25 mg	0.191	23,000
Progesterone, 1.25 mg, + DES, 1.25 mg	0.180	21,600

[a]With permission of Schwartz et al.[126]
[b]Chicks were stimulated for 12 days with DES, withdrawn from hormone treatment for 10 days, and then injected with various doses of hormone(s).
[c]Initiation sites were calculated as detailed in Tsai et al.[124]

be seen from the table that when optimal inducing doses of estrogen and progesterone were administered simultaneously to withdrawn chicks, no additive effects on RNA polymerase initiation sites assayed *in vitro* were detected. Thus, progesterone appears to mimic estrogen action at the molecular level in the withdrawn chick oviduct.

11.14. Purification and Characterization of Chick Oviduct Progesterone Receptor

Because of the central role of receptors in dictating hormone responses, it was essential to have homogeneous receptor preparations available. These preparations could then be used in cell-free reconstitution studies for further investigations of the process by which steroid hormones alter differential gene expression. We, therefore, undertook purification and characterization of the chick oviduct progesterone receptor.

Progesterone-binding activity in chick oviduct cytosol can be traced to several apparently different receptor forms. Using sucrose gradients and low-salt conditions,[95] we detected hormone-binding species sedimenting at 6S and 8S. The 8S species was not present in progesterone-responsive immature oviducts, suggesting that the 6S form may be the functional form of the receptor. Only 4S forms were found when the same samples were centrifuged on high salt gradients. This observation suggested that the 6S and 8S species might be some sort of molecular aggregate of the 4S population. Using various chromatographic techniques, it has been possible to show that the 4S population consists of two progesterone binders, each with somewhat different molecular properties.[95,146-148] These binders have previously been classified as the A and B proteins on the basis of their different affinities for nuclear constituents.[147,148] The A protein binds to DNA, but not to chromatin; conversely, the B protein binds well to chromatin, and less readily to DNA. Both proteins have identical hormone-binding specificities and kinetics.[146]

The B protein has recently been purified to homogeneity from hen oviducts.[149] Earlier hydrodynamic studies of the crude 4S cytoplasmic receptors had shown that they behaved as highly asymmetrical molecules in solution.[41] The purified B protein retained this asymmetry. It was therefore of interest to examine the shape of this particle by an independent method. High-resolution transmission electron microscopy was performed by Dr. Michael Conn in our laboratories. These studies demonstrated particles with a prolate elipsoidal shape: approximately 114 Å long and 38 Å across the minor axis. Using these particle dimensions and estimating the partial specific volume at 0.73 m³/g, one can calculate a molecular weight of approximately 106,000 g/mole.[150] This value was in close agreement with molecular weight estimates obtained by sodium dodecyl sulfate gel electrophoresis and the Siegal and Monty equation.

The purity of the B protein preparations was estimated at greater than 95% on the basis of its electrophoretic properties in several polyacrylamide gel systems. Moreover, amino-terminal analysis by dansylation procedures showed only a single amino acid: lysine. Significantly, it was also possible to show that [³H]progesterone and the B protein comigrated on nondenaturing gels. The purified B component retained its biologically important affinity for nonhistone proteins of chromatin.

Spectral analysis of the purified B protein revealed additional important findings.[151] Circular dichroic spectra suggested an α-helical content of about 12%. When the protein was denatured with guanidine hydrochloride and subsequently renatured in the presence and absence of progesterone, there was no detectable difference in the helix content. UV absorption spectra were also obtained. Because of the absorbance of free progesterone at 250 nm and the changes in the region of the absorption curve when intact B protein–hormone complex was compared with denatured B protein, it was possible to calculate the amount of progesterone associated with the B protein. It has been shown now, for the first time, that 1 progesterone molecule associates with each B protein molecule. In contrast to studies using less purified receptor,[150] no binding sites for ATP or cAMP were detected.

The A protein has also been purified to near homogeneity.[152] It also possesses a significant degree of asymmetry and retains many of the properties found in less highly purified preparations. Specifically, it has little affinity for chromosomal proteins, but reacts strongly with pure DNA.

When the A and B proteins were isolated together using affinity chromatography,[62] the sedimentation pattern on low-salt sucrose gradients showed predominantly 6S species. If high-salt conditions were used, the 6S molecule could be dissociated into one A subunit and one B subunit. These subunits were not interconvertible. From less purified forms of the A and B subunits, it has been possible to recombine the two 4S species to yield significant amounts of 6S species.[95] Partial copurification (200- to 1000-fold pure) of the two progesterone-binding forms under sal- conditions that prohibited aggregation also permitted significant reformation of 6S species from 4S constituents when the salt was removed.[128] No 8S species were observed. At present, we have been unable to recombine A and B proteins that have been isolated separately and purified to homogeneity. Thus, there may be some small additional cofactor required for stabilization of 6S receptor A B dimers. Nevertheless, it is the 6S species consisting of one A and one B subunit that we consider to be the functional progesterone receptor.

11.15. *In Vitro* Studies of Receptor-Mediated Alterations in Chromatin Transcription

In the transcription studies described previously, it was found that *in vivo* administration of steroid to hormone-deprived chicks resulted in the production of increased numbers of RNA chain initiation sites on oviduct chromatin.[124,125,127] As yet, no direct proof could be offered that interaction of steroid receptor with the genome *in vivo* was directly responsible for the increase in initiation sites assayed *in vitro*. Steroids might, for example, have as their primary effect the production of activator RNA molecules such as those proposed by Britten and Davidson.[153] These species in turn might be responsible for increasing RNA synthesis. To explore this possibility and therefore understand more clearly the role of receptors in the transcription process, progesterone receptors that had been purified to homogeneity[62] were tested *in vitro* for effects on chromatin transcription.

A fixed concentration of withdrawn oviduct chromatin was preincubated with increasing quantities of purified progesterone receptor for 30 min at room temperature. The chromatin receptor complexes were next incubated for an additional 30 min with a saturating amount of RNA polymerase to allow for the formation of stable initiation complexes. Finally, rifampicin, nucleotides, and heparin were added for a 15-min period of RNA synthesis. A dose-dependent increase in detectable RNA synthesis was found with the addition of increasing amounts of receptor. Half-maximal increases occurred at a progesterone receptor concentration of 0.5×10^{-8} M (see Fig. 6). At higher receptor concentrations, some decrease in RNA synthesis was sometimes detected. Subfractions from other tissues that did not contain progesterone receptor were unable to increase transcription.[128]

We reported previously that crude receptor preparations could spuriously stimulate RNA synthesis by a template-independent mechanism.[154] To rule out such a possibility in the current studies, the experiments shown in Table II were performed. It can be seen that the increase in RNA synthesis was dependent on all the following components: (1) an intact receptor–hormone complex (boiled receptor was ineffective); (2) receptor (hormone alone was ineffective); (3) chromatin template (actinomycin D completely inhibited synthesis); (4) *E. coli* RNA polymerase (effect still present when α-amanitin, an inhibitor of avian polymerase, was

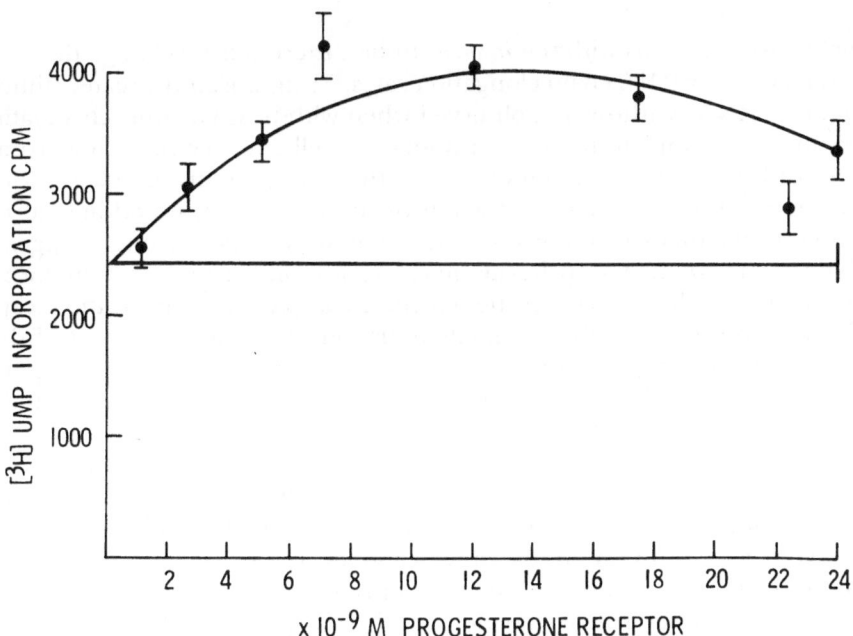

Fig. 6. Effects of purified progesterone receptor on chromatin rifampicin-resistant RNA synthesis. Oviduct chromatin was incubated with progesterone receptor that had been purified to homogeneity using affinity chromatography. RNA polymerase and various salts were added, and then RNA synthesis was started with the addition of nucleotides, rifampicin, and heparin. The amount of [³H]UMP incorporated into trichloracetic acid precipitable material (O––O) was measured by filtration. The straight line represents control values. (Reproduced with permission of Schwartz *et al.*[126])

Table II.   Determinants in Progesterone Receptor Induction of RNA Synthesis for Oviduct Chromatin *in Vitro*[a]

Components added to assay	[³H]UMP incorporated into RNA/5 μg chromatin DNA (cpm)[b]	Activity (%)
Background		
RNA polymerase only	230	8
Progesterone–receptor complex plus RNA polymerase	400	14
Chromatin alone	200	7
Control		
Chromatin + RNA polymerase	2730	100
Chromatin + boiled progesterone–receptor complex	2860	105
Chromatin + 10⁻⁸ M progesterone alone	2430	89
Experimental		
Chromatin + RNA polymerase + 10⁻⁸ M progesterone–receptor complex	4100	150
+ α-amanitin (10 μg)	3740	137
+ actinomycin D (10 μg)	320	12

[a]With permission of Schwartz *et al.*[126]
[b]RNA synthesis was assayed in the presence of nucleotides and rifampicin as detailed in Tsai *et al.*[124]

included). Again, as with the *in vivo* studies, there was no change in RNA product size or RNA chain elongation rates.[126] Significantly greater stimulation of RNA synthesis was observed when withdrawn oviduct chromatin was used as template than when nontarget cell chromatin, such as from liver or erythrocytes, was employed. If the cells were prestimulated with hormone *in vivo* prior to extraction of the chromatin, no additional *in vitro* stimulation by receptor was noted. This observation strongly suggests that the sites regulated by hormone *in vivo* are similar to those influenced *in vitro* by purified progesterone–receptor complex. Moreover, the receptor had no effect on DNA template initiation sites. Ultimate proof of the specificity of receptor–stimulated chromatin transcription will require product analysis by hybridization with a specific probe for ovalbumin mRNA (see Section 11.12).

Using less highly purified progesterone receptor isolated by entirely different procedures, it was also possible to demonstrate similar increases in chromatin transcription measured by the rifampicin-challenge assay.[126,128] Optimization of these changes required the addition of receptor–hormone complex 30–40 min prior to the onset of RNA synthesis. To test for the role of hormone in the receptor-stimulated transcriptional changes, receptor fractions were prepared in the absence of hormone. Half the preparation was then labeled with progesterone, and the other half was kept free of hormone. Table III shows the results assayed by the rifampicin-challenge transcription assay. More rifampicin-resistant RNA chains were synthesized in the presence of hormone ($P < 0.005$). The receptor concentration in this assay was 5×10^{-9} M and corresponded to that required for a half-maximal response. Therefore, it was not surprising to observe a 20% increase in rifampicin-resistant RNA synthesis, compared with the 40–60% stimulations noted at saturating concentrations of hormone–receptor complex. Thus, transcription proceeds to a greater extent in the presence of hormone, and the receptor-mediated RNA synthetic events are indeed hormone-dependent as predicted.

There were four important correlations between our previously published nuclear and chromatin binding studies[60,61,68] and the more recent transcription studies. First, the time required to optimize *in vitro* binding of receptors incubated with nuclei or chromatin at 23°C was 30–40 min. We have also found that optimal differences in chromatin transcription occurred after 30–40 min of receptor incubation with chromatin.[128] Second, the receptor concentration $(2–7 \times 10^{-9}$ M) that brought about a half-maximal increase in chromatin transcription measured by the rifampicin-challenge assay[126,128] was indistinguishable from the equilibrium dissociation constant $(2–10 \times 10^{-9}$ M) for the binding of chick oviduct progesterone receptors to nuclei or chromatin.[60,61] These correlations suggest that numerous *in vitro* studies in other hormone-response systems (see Buller and O'Malley[59] for a review) that have reported saturable binding of receptors to nuclei and chromatin have been reporting functional binding. It is difficult to reconcile these findings with those of other workers who have claimed that saturable binding of receptors is an *in vitro* artifact.[78,155,156] Third, the number of new chains initiated (relative to new chains initiated on oviduct chromatin) following receptor incubation with liver or erythrocyte chromatins was roughly proportional to the amount of receptor bound to these chromatins. Finally, our observation that only receptor that was complexed with hormone was able to promote initiation

Table III. Hormone Influence on Receptor Chromatin-Mediated Transcription[a]

Condition[b]	[^{3}H] UMP incorporated (cmp)[c]
No hormone	3655±205
Progesterone	444±200

[a]With permission of Buller *et al.*[128]
[b]Progesterone receptors were prepared in the absence of hormone. Excess progesterone was added to half the preparation, which was labeled overnight and desalted by Sephadex chromatography. The receptor–progesterone complex or hormone-free fraction was incubated at a concentration of 5×10^{-9} M with 10 μg DNA as oviduct chromatin.
[c]RNA synthesis was carried out as detailed in Tsai *et al.*[124] Values reported are mean ± S.E.M. for 32 samples.

of transcription on chromatin was consistent with our previous observations that receptor binding to nuclei was a hormone-dependent phenomenon.[68]

11.16. Induction of Specific Gene Sequences by Progesterone Receptors *in Vitro*

Nucleic acid hybridization techniques using $[^3H]cDNA_{ov}$ were used to detect the production of minute amounts of ovalbumin mRNA sequences synthesized *in vitro*. It was possible to show that ovalbumin mRNA was synthesized *in vitro* only from oviduct chromatin isolated from animals that had received steroid stimulation *in vivo*.[130] Thus, it appeared technically possible to examine the *in vitro* effects of purified progesterone receptor on the production of ovalbumin messenger RNA from chromatin isolated from hormonally withdrawn animals. Bulk amounts of RNA were synthesized both from control withdrawn chromatin and from withdrawn chromatin incubated in the presence of saturating amounts of purified progesterone receptor (10^{-8} M). The hybridization data showed that the RNA synthesized in the presence of pure receptor–hormone complex contained a 10- to 50-fold enrichment of ovalbumin mRNA sequences, as compared with control chromatins.* These data are consistent with the hypothesis that steroid hormone–receptor complexes act directly on chromatin to enhance the number of initiation sites for RNA synthesis. It should be noted that the gene coding for the ovalbumin message is present only as one copy per haploid genome, so that the receptor effects on chromatin open the initiation sites for many thousands of unique sequence genes.

11.17. Relationship of the Progesterone Receptor Subunit Structure to Its Effects on Differential Gene Expression

Earlier, we discussed the fact that the progesterone receptor perhaps consisted of two similar but nonidentical subunits A and B in the form of a species that sedimented on (low-salt) sucrose gradients at approximately 6S. The studies of the *in vitro* effects of progesterone receptor on RNA chain initiation were carried out utilizing receptor preparations that contained large amounts of the 6S receptor dimer species. The next logical step in the investigation of the role that steroid receptors play in altering

*Chang, C., Schwartz, R. J., and O'Malley, B. W. (manuscript in preparation).

chromatin transcription was evaluation of the subunit effects of the receptor individually. If, as we postulated, the A subunit is truly a regulatory protein, it might be expected to alter transcription, but to do so less efficiently than the intact dimer. Conversely, if the B subunit of the dimer is merely a specifier protein that carries the A protein to the neighborhood of responsive genes, it should be ineffective in stimulating chromatin transcription. Figure 7 shows the results of adding homogeneous A or B or partially purified 6S A·B dimer to chromatin prior to transcription assay. The intact 6S dimer was again capable of stimulating RNA chain initiation at low concentrations. The isolated B subunit was ineffective in stimulating transcription from oviduct chromatin at any concentration tested. At very high concentrations (10^{-7} M), inhibitory effects were often noted.[128] The isolated A subunit, on the other hand, was capable of stimulating transcription, but only at significantly higher concentrations (approximately 10- to 15-fold) than those required for the intact dimer. Thus far, it has not been possible to recombine homogeneous A and B

OVIDUCT CHROMATIN TRANSCRIPTION BY RECEPTOR DIMERS AND ISOLATED SUBUNITS

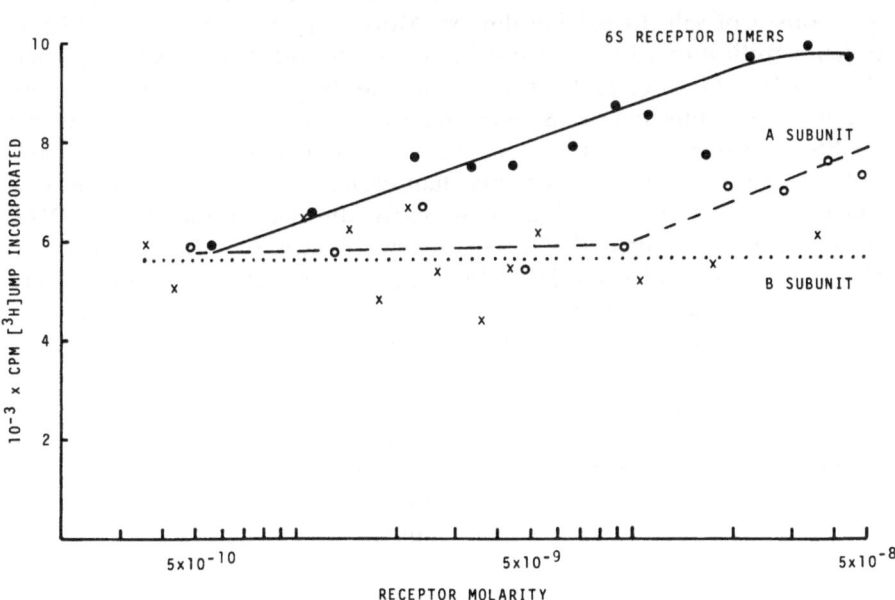

Fig. 7. Influence of progesterone receptor subunit structure on rifampicin-resistant chromatin RNA synthesis. Progesterone receptor A subunit (O---O),[152] B subunit (×--×),[149] or 6S A·B dimer (●---●),[128] was added to chromatin, and their effects on rifampicin-resistant RNA synthesis were measured as before. (Reproduced with permission of Buller et al.[128])

subunits to reform 6S dimers. Transcription experiments combining A and B without recombination showed no cooperative effect. Clearly, the 6S form is necessary for optimal activity. These data support, but do not yet prove, our hypothesis[81,95,157] that the active form of the chick oviduct progesterone receptor is a 6S dimer consisting of a specifier subunit (B) complexed with a regulatory subunit (A).

The question of the ubiquity of steroid receptor dimers consisting of an A-like DNA-binding regulatory subunit and a B-like chromatin-binding specifier subunit should be considered. This idea was originally formulated for the progesterone receptor by our laboratory.[81,95,146,157] However, glucocorticoid,[128] estrogen (Schrader, unpublished observations), and androgen[158] binding activity can be eluted from various ion-exchange resins as pairs of peaks reminiscent of the oviduct progesterone system. Such behavior should not be equated with the progesterone receptor studies until rigorously proven, but the 7S–10S to 3S–5S transition on sucrose gradients originally reported for estrogen receptor by Toft and Gorski[159] appears to be ubiquitous phenomenon. Similar salt-mediated transformations have been reported for every other steroid hormone receptor characterized to date. Such a transition and biphasic chromatographic elution profiles would be expected if all steroid receptors consist of salt-dissociable dimers. Moreover, there is apparent functional significance to such a transition. Nozu and Tamaoki[160] reported that nuclear binding of 9S rat prostatic androgen receptors was more extensive than binding of 5S receptors. Davies and Griffiths[121] found that an 8S rat prostatic androgen receptor stimulated endogenous nuclear polymerase much more efficiently than either a 3S (salt-treated) or 4.5S nuclear form. Hu et al.[161] have similarly showed stimulation of DNA transcription by a purified 3S prostatic cytosol receptor. Their purification procedure selected for the DNA-binding character of receptors that were initially in an 8S form. Thus, they may have purified only an "A-like" regulatory subunit of an 8S dimer. Finally, Kaiser et al.[57] and Marver et al.[58] have characterized, respectively, aldosterone antagonists and glucocorticoid antagonists. In both cases, the antagonist appeared to function by binding to the appropriate steroid hormone receptor protein and preventing nuclear translocation of the complex. Significantly, in the presence of antagonist, receptors no longer formed 7S–8.5S species, but were observed only as 3S–4S species on sucrose gradients.

11.18. A Model for Steroid Hormone Action

The data presented above are consistent with the model of steroid hormone action presented schematically in Fig. 8, and described below.

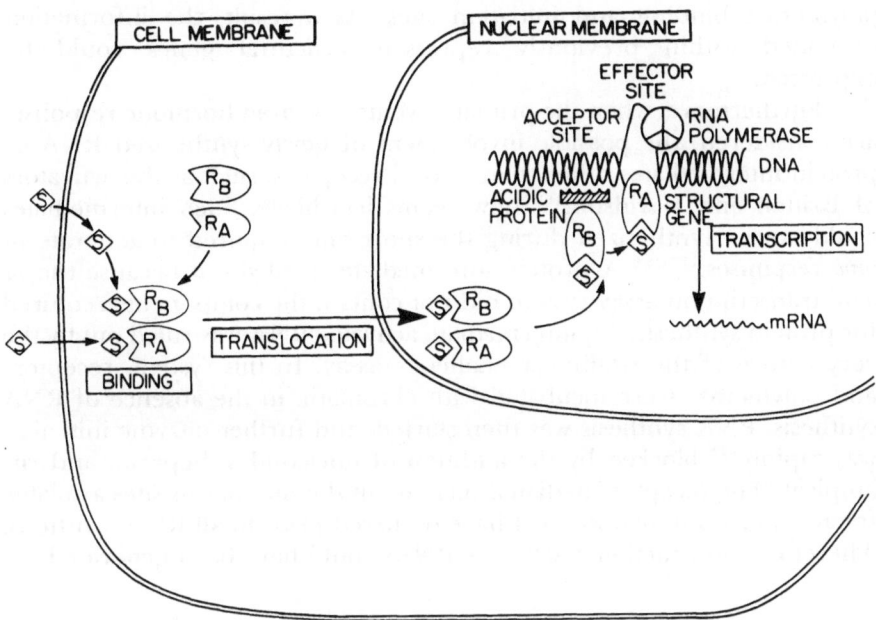

Fig. 8. Molecular mechanism of steroid hormone action: (S) Steroid; (R$_A$) A subunit of receptor dimer; (R$_B$) B subunit of receptor dimer. (Reproduced with permission of Buller et al.[128])

Steroids (S) enter target cells, probably by passive diffusion, and bind to cytoplasmic receptor dimers. An unusual feature of this model is the requirement of two bound hormone molecules per intact functional receptor dimer. Following translocation to the cell nucleus, the receptor dimer binds through its B or specifier subunit to chromatin acceptor sites consisting of DNA and chromatin-associated nonhistone proteins. This mechanism allows the concentration of active receptor molecules in areas of the genome that are under hormonal control. Because the DNA-binding site of the A or regulatory subunit is apparently occluded when it is combined with the B subunit in the intact dimer,[152] it may be necessary to postulate the release of the A subunit from the dimer after its localization on chromatin. The A subunit would then be free to search the adjacent genome for specific effector sites that presumably lie in the neighborhood of the acceptor sites. The search may be conducted by one-dimensional diffusion along the chromatin lattice, as previously postulated.[59,60] Binding of the A subunit to an effector site could then promote a destabilization of the DNA duplex, and thus create new potential RNA polymerase binding and initiation sites. As a result, the information contained within previously repressed structural genes could be expressed.

Furthermore, when the primary events in steroid hormone responses are considered, the possible involvement of newly synthesized RNA or protein intermediates other than steroid receptors, such as the activators of Britten and Davidson,[153] now seems less likely. Such intermediates could not be synthesized during the short time required to generate *in vivo* responses.[125,126] A protein intermediate is ruled out because the *in vitro* transcription assay system did not contain the components required for protein synthesis. An intermediate activator RNA was ruled out by the very nature of the rifampicin-challenge assay. In this system, receptors and polymerase were incubated with chromatin in the absence of RNA synthesis. RNA synthesis was then started, and further enzyme initiation was rapidly[131] blocked by the addition of nucleotides, heparin, and rifampicin. The receptor-mediated increase in the number of sites available for RNA chain initiation must have occurred prior to all RNA synthesis. Therefore, no functional activator RNAs could have been generated.

11.19. Medical Relevance

The elucidation of the central role that receptor proteins play in steroid hormone action has provided for exciting progress in endocrinology and extended this field of medicine to a molecular level. The syndrome of testicular feminization has long been explained simply as an "end-organ defect" similar to that postulated in pseudohypoparathyroidism and nephrogenic diabetes insipidus. Patients with this syndrome are genetic males who possess a female phenotype that includes well-developed breasts and typical female body build and external genitalia. However, they also possess intraabdominal or inguinal testes and have normal male circulating levels of androgens and estrogens. The extension of animal model studies from the Tfm mouse[60] and rat[61] to humans with the disease permits explanation of this enigma on the basis of defective cytoplasmic androgen receptor proteins.

The susceptibility of breast cancer to endocrine manipulation has been known since 1896.[162] In the premenopausal female, endocrine manipulation can consist of any or a combination of oophorectomy, adrenalectomy, hypophysectomy, antiestrogen drugs, and androgen therapy.[163] Unfortunately, these methods of treatment are at best palliative, often do not work at all, and can cause serious side effects. The recent advances in the field of molecular endocrinology discussed in this review provide a mechanistic rationale for the selection and therapeutic benefits to patients with hormone-sensitive tumors. The major contributions toward understanding this area were made originally by Jensen and co-workers[164] and more recently by McGuire and co-workers.[165,166] Their work and that of other investigators suggests that only those patients whose tumors contain estrogen receptors will be good candidates for endocrine manipulation. Table IV emphasizes this point. Approximately 47.4% of those responses reported had significant estrogen receptor titers. Of this group, 32 of 41, or 78%, responded to endocrine manipulation. On the other hand, only 3 of 63, or 4.7% without receptor showed a favorable response to endocrine therapy. Results such as these have led McGuire and others to point out that every breast cancer patient taken to surgery should have a tumor sample analyzed for receptor content.[166] Then, if mastectomy does not cure the patient, and the tumor contains receptor, there will be hope of inducing a remission by treatment with endocrine ablative therapy. In the absence of significant receptor titers, some other mode of therapy such as X-irradiation and cytotoxic agents should be employed.

In principle, receptor assays could also be used to classify patients with prostatic cancers and lymphosarcomas. Various animal model systems can also be used to design safer and more effective contraceptive agents that will bind to cytoplasmic receptor proteins, excluding endogenous steroids, and do so in a fashion that prevents nuclear transfer of the receptor–drug complex, thus inhibiting response. These are but a few of the possible advances within our reach as clinical endocrinology evolves into a molecular biological science.

Table IV. Correlation of Tumor Receptor Titer with Response to Endocrine Manipulation[a]

Investigator	Receptor-positive tumors[b]	Receptor-positive responders[c]	Receptor-negative responders
Korenman and Dukes[167]	7/15	—	—
Jensen et al.[164]	13/40	10/13	1/27
Maass et al.[168]	67/164	6/7	0/14
Engelsman et al.[169]	14/37	14/17	2/20
Leung et al.[170]	28/53	—	—
McGuire et al.[166]	36/64	—	—
Savlov et al.[171]	68/118	2/4	0/2

[a]Taken from Buller[172] with permission.
[b]Investigators vary somewhat in their definition of receptor-positive.
[c]A response is defined minimally as a 50% reduction in tumor size following some form of endocrine manipulation.

References

1. Jensen, E. V., and Jacobson, H. I., 1960, Fate of steroid estrogens in target tissues, *in: Biological Activities of Steroids in Relation to Cancer* (G. Pincus and E. P. Vollmer, eds.), pp. 161–178, Academic Press, New York.
2. Jensen, E. V., and Jacobson, H. I., 1962, Basic guides to the mechanism of estrogen action, *Recent Prog. Horm. Res.* **18**:387–414.
3. Gorski, J., Toft, D., Shyamala, G., Smith, D., and Notides, A., 1968, Hormone receptors: Studies on the interaction of estrogen with the uterus, *Recent Prog. Horm. Res.* **24**:45–80.
4. O'Malley, B. W., McGuire, W. L., Kohler, P. O., and Korenman, S. G., 1969, Studies on the mechanism of steroid hormone regulation of synthesis of specific proteins, *Recent Prog. Horm Res.* **25**:105–160.
5. Falk, R. J., and Bardin, C. W., 1970, Uptake of tritiated progesterone by the uterus of the ovariectomized guinea pig, *Endocrinology* **86**:1059–1063.
6. Bruchovsky, N., and Wilson, J. D., 1968, The conversion of testosterone to 5α-androstan-17β-ol-3-one by rat prostate *in vivo* and *in vitro*, *J. Biol. Chem.* **243**:2012–2021.
7. Anderson, K. M., and Liao, S., 1968, Selective retention of dihydrotestosterone by prostatic nuclei, *Nature London* **219**:277–279.
8. Fang, S., Anderson, K. M., and Liao, S., 1969, Receptor proteins for androgens: On the role of specific proteins in selective retention of 17β-hydroxy-5α-androstan-3-one by rat ventral prostate *in vivo* and *in vitro*, *J. Biol. Chem.* **244**:6584–6595.
9. Edelman, I. S., Bogoroch, R., and Porter, G. A., 1963, On the mechanism of action of aldosterone on sodium transport: The role of protein synthesis, *Proc. Nat. Acad. Sci. U.S.A.* **50**:1169–1177.
10. Fanestil, D. D., and Edelman, I. S., 1966, Characteristics of the renal nuclear receptors for aldosterone, *Proc. Nat. Acad. Sci. U.S.A.* **56**:872–879.
11. Stohs, S. J., and DeLuca, H. F., 1967, Subcellular location of vitamin D and its metabolites in intestinal mucosa after a 10-IU dose, *Biochemistry* **6**:3338–3349.
12. Henry, H. L., and Norman, A. W., 1975, Studies on the mechanism of action of calciferol VII. Localization of 1,25-dihydroxy-vitamin D_3 in chick parathyroid glands, *Biochem. Biophys. Res. Commun.* **62**:781–788.
13. Noteboom, W. D., and Gorski, J., 1965, Stereospecific binding of estrogens in the rat uterus, *Arch. Biochem. Biophys.* **111**:559–568.
14. King, R. J. B., Gordon, J., and Inman, D. R., 1965, The intracellular localization of oestrogen in rat tissues, *J. Endocrinol.* **32**:9–15.
15. Talwar, G. P., Segal, S. J., Evans, A., and Davidson, O. W., 1964, The binding of estradiol in the uterus: A mechanism for depression of RNA synthesis, *Proc. Nat. Acad. Sci. U.S.A.* **52**:1059–1066.
16. Cousins, R. J., DeLuca, H. F., Suda, T., Chen, T., and Tanaka, Y., 1970, Metabolism and subcellular location of 25-hydroxycholecalciferol in intestinal mucosa, *Biochemistry* **9**:1453–1459.
17. Beato, M., Kalimi, M., Konstam, M., and Feigelson, P., 1973, Interaction of glucocorticoids with rat liver nuclei. II. Studies on the nature of the cytosol transfer factor and the nuclear acceptor site, *Biochemistry* **12**:3372–3379.
18. Williams, D., and Gorski, J., 1972, A new assessment of subcellular distribution of bound estrogen in the uterus, *Biochem. Biophys. Res. Commun.* **45**:258–264.

19. Stumpf, W. E., 1970, Localization of hormones by autoradiography and other histochemical techniques, *J. Histochem. Cytochem.* **18**:21–29.
20. Anderson, C. H., and Greenwald, G. S., 1969, Autoradiographic analysis of estradiol uptake in the brain and pituitary of the female rat, *Endocrinology* **85**:1160–1165.
21. Stumpf, W. E., 1968, Cellular and subcellular ^{3}H-estradiol localization in the pituitary by autoradiography, *Z. Zellforsch, Mikrosk. Anat.* **92**:23–33.
22. Stumpf, W. E., 1968, Estradiol-containing neurons: Topography in the hypothalamus by dry-mount autoradiography, *Science* **162**:1001–1003.
23. Jensen, E. V., Suzuki, T., Kawashime, T., Stumpf, W. E., Jungblut, P. W., and DeSombre, E. R., 1968, A two-step mechanism for the interaction of estradiol with rat uterus, *Proc. Nat. Acad. Sci. U.S.A.* **59**:632–638.
24. Stumpf, W., 1968, Subcellular distribution of ^{3}H-estradiol in rat uterus by quantitative autoradiography—a comparison between ^{3}H-estradiol and ^{3}H-norethynodrel, *Endocrinology* **83**:777–782.
25. Bogoroch, R., 1969, Studies on the intracellular localization of tritiated steroids, *in: Autoradiography of Diffusible Substances* (L. J. Roth and W. E. Stumpf, eds.), pp. 99–111, Academic Press, New York.
26. Stumpf, W. E., and Sar, M., 1973, Cellular and subcellular localization of ^{3}H-progesterone and its metabolites in rat uterus studied by autoradiography, *J. Steroid Biochem.* **4**:477–481.
27. Sar, M., and Stumpf, W. E., 1973, Neurons of the hypothalamus concentrate [^{3}H]progesterone or its metabolics, *Science* **182**:1266–1268.
28. Jensen, E. V., 1965, Metabolic fate of sex hormones in target tissues with regard to tissue specificity. *Proceedings of the Second International Congress of Endocrinology*, London, 1964, pp. 420–433, Excerpta Med. Found., Amsterdam.
29. Jensen, E. V., 1966, Mechanism of estrogen action in relation to carcinogenesis, *Proc. Can. Cancer Res. Conf.* **6**:143–165.
30. Sherman, M. R., Corvol, P. L., and O'Malley, B. W., 1970, Progesterone-binding components of chick oviduct. I. Preliminary characterization of cytoplasmic components, *J. Biol. Chem.* **245**:6085–6096.
31. Milgrom, E., and Baulieu, E. E., 1968, C$_{19}$-stéroides conjugués substrats des 17β-hydroxystéroide oxydo-réductases. Un mécanisme pouvant contrôler l'oxydation de la testosterone, *Ct. Rd. Acad. Sci. Série D* **266**: 1529–1531.
32. Mainwaring, W. I. P., 1960, A soluble androgen receptor in the cytoplasm of rat prostate, *J. Endocrinol.* **45**:531–541.
33. Baulieu, E.-E., and Jung, I., 1970, A prostatic cytosol receptor, *Biochem. Biophys. Res. Commun.* **38**:599–606.
34. Baxter, J. D., and Tomkins, G. M., 1970, The relationship between glucocorticoid binding and tyrosine aminotransferase induction in hepatoma tissue culture cells, *Proc. Nat. Acad. Sci. U.S.A.* **65**:709–715.
35. Baxter, J. D., and Tomkins, G. M., 1971, Specific cytoplasmic glucocorticoid hormone receptors in hepatoma tissue culture cells, *Proc. Nat. Acad. Sci. U.S.A.* **68**:932–937.
36. Herman, T. S., Fimognari, G. M., and Edelman, I. S., 1968, Studies on renal aldosterone-binding proteins, *J. Biol. Chem.* **243**:3849–3856.
37. Swaneck, G. E., Chu, L. L. H., and Edelman, I. S., 1970, Stereospecific binding of aldosterone to renal chromatin, *J. Biol. Chem.* **245**:5382–5389.
38. Brumbaugh, P. F., and Haussler, M. R., 1974, 1α,25-Dihydroxycholecalci-

ferol receptors in intestine I. Association of 1α, 25-dihydroxycholecalciferol with intestinal mucosa chromatin, *J. Biol. Chem.* **249:**1251–1257.

39. Tsai, H. C., and Norman, A. W., 1973, Studies on calciferol metabolism: VIII. Evidence for a cytoplasmic receptor for 1,25-dihydroxy-vitamin D_3 in the intestinal mucosa, *J. Biol. Chem.* **248:**5967–5975.

40. Brumbaugh, P. F., Hughes, M. R., and Haussler, M. R., 1975, Cytoplasmic and nuclear binding components for 1α-25-dihydroxyvitamin D_3 in chick parathyroid glands, *Proc. Nat. Acad. Sci. U.S.A.* **72:**4871–4875.

41. O'Malley, B. W., Toft, D. O., and Sherman, M. R., 1971, Progesterone binding components of chick oviduct. II. Nuclear components, *J. Biol. Chem.* **246:**1117–1122.

42. O'Malley, B. W., Sherman, M. R., and Toft, D. O., 1970, Progesterone "receptors" in the cytoplasm and nucleus of chick oviduct target tissue, *Proc. Nat. Acad. Sci. U.S.A.* **67:**501–508.

43. Lippman, M., Halterman, R., Perry, S., Leventhal, B., and Thompson, E. B., 1973, Glucocorticoid binding proteins in human leukaemic lymphoblasts, *Nature New Biol.* **242:**157, 158.

44. Rosenau, W., Baxter, J. D., Rousseau, G. C., and Tomkins, G. M., 1972, Mechanism of resistance to steroids: Glucocorticoid receptor defect in lymphoma cells, *Nature London New Biol.* **237:**20–24.

45. Baxter, J. D., Harris, A. W., Tompkins, G. M., and Cohn, M., 1971, Glucocorticoid receptors in lymphoma cells in culture: Relationship to glucocorticoid killing activity, *Science* **171:**189–191.

46. Hackney, J. F., Gross, S. R., Aronow, L., and Pratt, W. R., 1970, Specific glucocorticoid-binding macromolecules from mouse fibroblasts growing *in vitro*. A possible steroid receptor for growth inhibition, *Mol. Pharmacol.* **6:**500–512.

47. Pratt, W. B., and Ishii, D. N., 1972, Specific binding of glucocorticoids *in vitro* in the soluble fraction of mouse fibroblasts, *Biochemistry* **11:**1401–1410.

48. Bullock, L. P., Bardin, C. W., and Ohno, S., 1971, The androgen insensitive mouse: Absence of intranuclear androgen retention in the kidney, *Biochem. Biophys. Res. Commun.* **44:**1537–1543.

49. Gehring, U., Tomkins, G. M., and Ohno, S., 1971, Effect of the androgen-insensitivity mutation on a cytoplasmic receptor for dihydrotestosterone, *Nature London New Biol.* **232:**106, 107.

50. Roy, A., Milin, B. S., and McMinn, D. M., 1974, Androgen receptor in rat liver: Hormonal and developmental regulation of the cytoplasmic receptor and its correlation with the androgen-dependent synthesis of α_{2u}-globulin, *Biochim. Biophys. Acta* **354:**213–232.

51. Anderson, J., Clark, J. H., and Peck, E. J., Jr., 1972, Oestrogen and nuclear binding sites: Determination of specific sites by [^{3}H]oestradiol exchange, *Biochem. J.* **126:**561–567.

52. Clark, J. H., Anderson, J., and Peck, E. J., Jr., 1972, Receptor–estrogen complex in the nuclear fraction of rat uterine cells during the estrous cycle, *Science* **176:**528–530.

53. Anderson, J. N., Peck, E. J., Jr., and Clark, J. H., 1973, Nuclear receptor-estrogen complex: Relationship between concentration and early uterotrophic responses, *Endocrinology* **92:**1488–1495.

54. Anderson, J. N., Peck, E. J., Jr., and Clark, J. H., 1973, Nuclear receptor-estrogen complex: Accumulation, retention and localization in the hypothalamus and pituitary, *Endocrinology* **93:**711–717.

55. Clark, J. H., Anderson, J. N., and Peck, E. J., Jr., 1973, Estrogen receptor anti-estrogen complex: Atypical binding by uterine nuclei and effects on uterine growth, *Steroids* **22**:707–718.
56. Clark, J. H., Peck, E. J., Jr., and Anderson, J. N., 1974, Oestrogen receptors and antagonism of steroid hormone action, *Nature London* **251**:446–448.
57. Kaiser, N., Milholland, R. J., Turnell, R. W., and Rosen, F., 1972, Cortexolone: Binding to glucocorticoid receptors in rat thymocytes and mechanism of its antiglucocorticoid action, *Biochem. Biophys. Res. Commun.* **49**:516–521.
58. Marver, D., Stewart, J., Funder, J. W., Feldman, D., and Edelman, I. S., 1974, Renal aldosterone receptors: Studies with [^{3}H]aldosterone and the anti-mineralocorticoid [^{3}H]spirolactone (SC-26304), *Proc. Nat. Acad. Sci. U.S.A.* **71**:1431–1435.
59. Buller, R. E., and O'Malley, B. W., 1976, The biology and mechanism of steroid hormone receptor interaction with the eukaryotic nucleus, *Biochem. Pharmacol.* **25**:1–12.
60. Buller, R. E., Schrader, W. T., and O'Malley, B. W., 1975, Progesterone-binding components of chick oviduct. IX. The kinetics of nuclear binding, *J. Biol. Chem.* **250**:809–818.
61. Jaffe, R. C., Socher, S. H., and O'Malley, B. W., 1975, An analysis of the binding of the chick oviduct progesterone-receptor to chromatin, *Biochim, Biophys. Acta* **399**:403–419.
62. Kuhn, R. W., Schrader, W. T., Smith, R. G., and O'Malley, B. W., 1975, Progesterone binding components of chick oviduct. X. Purification by affinity chromatography, *J. Biol. Chem.* **250**:4220–4228.
63. Higgins, S. J., Rousseau, G. G., Baxter, J. D., and Tomkins, G. M., 1973, Nature of nuclear acceptor sites for glucocorticoid and estrogen-receptor complexes, *J. Biol. Chem.* **248**:5873–5879.
64. King, R. J. B., and Gordon, J., 1972, Involvement of DNA in the acceptor mechanism for uterine oestradiol receptor, *Nature London New Biol.* **240**:185–187.
65. Marver, D., Goodman, D., and Edelman, I. S., 1972, Relationships between renal cytoplasmic and nuclear aldosterone-receptors, *Kidney Int.* **1**:210–223.
66. Baxter, J. D., Rousseau, G. G., Benson, M. C., Garcea, R. L., Ito, J., and Tomkins, G. M., 1972, Role of DNA and specific cytoplasmic receptors in glucocorticoid action, *Proc. Nat. Acad. Sci. U.S.A.* **69**:1892–1896.
67. Harris, G. S., 1971, Nature of oestrogen specific binding sites in the nuclei of mouse uteri, *Nature London New Biol.* **231**:246–248.
68. Buller, R. E., Toft, D. O., Schrader, W. T., and O'Malley, B. W., 1975, Progesterone-binding components of chick oviduct, VIII. Receptor activation and hormone-dependent binding to purified nuclei, *J. Biol. Chem.* **250**:801–808.
69. Crick, F., 1971, General model for the chromosomes of higher organisms, *Nature London* **234**:25–27.
70. Mainwaring, W. I. P., and Peterken, B. M., 1971, A reconstituted cell-free system for the specific transfer of steroid–receptor complexes into nuclear chromatin isolated from rat ventral prostate gland, *Biochem. J.* **125**:285–295.
71. Schrader, W. T., Socher, S. H., and Buller, R. E., 1975, Steroid hormone-receptor interactions with nuclear constituents, *in: Methods in Enzymology* (B. W. O'Malley and J. Hardman, eds.), Vol. 36, pp. 292–312, Academic Press, New York.
72. King, R. J. B., Beard, V., Gordon, J., Pooley, A. S., Smith, J. A., Steggles, A.

W., and Vértes, M., 1971, Studies on estradiol-binding in mammalian tissues, *in: Advances in the Biosciences, 1971* (G. Raspé, ed.), Vol. 7, pp. 21–44, Pergamon Press, Oxford.

73. Rousseau, G. G., Baxter, J. D., and Tomkins, G. M., 1972, Glucocorticoid receptors: Relations between steroid binding and biological effects, *J. Mol. Biol.* **67**:99–115.

74. Majumdar, C., and Frankel, F. R., 1974, Sequence specific interaction of estradiol receptor with DNA, *Fed. Proc. Fed. Amer. Soc. Exp. Biol.* **33**:1511.

75. Yamamoto, K. R., and Alberts, B., 1974, On the specificity of the binding of the estradiol receptor protein to deoxyribonucleic acid, *J. Biol. Chem.* **249**:7076–7086.

76. Yamamoto, K. R., 1974, Characterization of the 4S and 5S forms of the estradiol receptor protein and their interaction with deoxyribonucleic acid, *J. Biol. Chem.* **249**:7068–7075.

77. Yamamoto, K. R., and Alberts, B. M., 1972, *In vitro* conversion of estradiol-receptor protein to its nuclear form: Dependence on hormone and DNA, *Proc. Nat. Acad. Sci. U.S.A.* **69**:2105–2109.

78. Simons, S. S., Jr., Martinez, H. M., Garcea, R. L., Baxter, J. D., and Tomkins, G. M., 1976, Interactions of glucocorticoid receptor steroid complexes with acceptor sites, *J. Biol. Chem.* **251**:334–343.

79. Puca, G. A., Sica, V., and Nola, E., 1974, Identification of a high affinity nuclear acceptor site for estrogen receptor of calf uterus, *Proc. Nat. Acad. Sci. U.S.A.* **71**:979–983.

80. Spelsberg, T. C., Steggles, A. W., and O'Malley, B. W., 1971, Progesterone-binding components of chick oviduct: III. Chromatin acceptor sites, *J. Biol. Chem.* **246**:4188–4197.

81. O'Malley, B. W., Spelsberg, T. C., Schrader, W. T., Chytil, F., and Steggles, A. W., 1972, Mechanisms of interaction of a hormone–receptor complex with the genome of a eukaryotic target cell, *Nature London* **235**:141–144.

82. Spelsberg, T. C., Steggles, A. W., Chytil, F., and O'Malley, B. W., 1972, Progesterone-binding components of chick oviduct: V. Exchange of progesterone-binding capacity from target to nontarget tissue chromatins, *J. Biol. Chem.* **247**:1368–1374.

83. Elgin, S. C. R., and Bonner, J., 1970, Limited heterogeneity of the major nonhistone chromosomal proteins, *Biochemistry* **9**:4440–4447.

84. Teng, C.-S., and Hamilton, T. H., 1968, The role of chromatin in estrogen action in the uterus, I. The control of template capacity and chemical composition and the binding of H³-estradiol-17β, *Proc. Nat. Acad. Sci. U.S.A.* **60**:1410–1417.

85. Shelton, K. R., and Allfrey, V. G., 1970, Selective synthesis of a nuclear acidic protein in liver cells stimulated by cortisol, *Nature London* **228**:132–134.

86. Tsai, S. Y., Harris, S. E., Tsai, M. J., and O'Malley, B. W., 1976, Effects of estrogen on gene expression in chick oviduct: The role of chromatin proteins in regulating transcription of the ovalbumin gene. *J. Biol. Chem.* **251**:4713–4721.

87. Beato, M., Kalimi, M., Beato, W., and Feigelson, P., 1974, Interaction of glucocorticoids with rat liver nuclei: Effect of adrenalectomy and cortisol administration, *Endocrinology* **94**:377–387.

88. Fang, S., and Liao, S., 1971, Androgen receptors: Steroid and tissue-specific retention of a 17β-hydroxy-5α-androstan-3-one-protein complex by the cell nuclei of ventral prostate, *J. Biol. Chem.* **246**:16–24.

89. Milgrom, E., Atger, M., and Baulieu, E.-E., 1973, Acidophilic activation of steroid hormone receptors, *Biochemistry* **12**:5198–5205.

90. Brumbaugh, P. F., and Haussler, M. R., 1974, 1α,25-Dihydroxycholecalciferol receptors in intestine. II. Temperature-dependent transfer of the hormone to chromatin via a specific cytosol receptor, *J. Biol. Chem.* **249**:1258–1262.

91. Kalimi, M., Beato, M., and Feigelson, P., 1973, Interaction of glucocorticoids with rat liver nuclei. I. Role of the cytosol proteins, *Biochemistry* **12**:3365–3371.

92. Higgins, S. J., Rousseau, G. G., Baxter, J. D., and Tomkins, G. M., 1973, Early events in glucocorticoid action. Activation of the steroid receptor and its subsequent specific nuclear binding studied in a cell-free system, *J. Biol. Chem.* **248**:5866–5872.

93. Kalimi, M., Colman, P., and Feigelson, P., 1975, The "activated" hepatic glucocorticoid-receptor complex: Its generation and properties, *J. Biol. Chem.* **250**:1080–1086.

94. Mainwaring, W. I. P., and Irving, R., 1973, The use of deoxyribonucleic acid-cellulose chromatography and isoelectric focusing for the characterization and partial purification of steroid–receptor complexes, *Biochem. J.* **134**:113–127.

95. Schrader, W. T., Heuer, S. S., and O'Malley, B. W., 1975, Progesterone receptors of chick oviduct: Identification of 6S receptor dimers, *Biol. Reprod.* **12**:134–142.

96. DeSombre, E. R., Mohla, S., and Jensen, E. V., 1972, Estrogen-independent activation of the receptor protein of calf uterine cytosol, *Biochem. Biophys. Res. Commun.* **48**:1601–1608.

97. Notides, A. C., and Nielson, S., 1974, The molecular mechanism of the *in vitro* 4S to 5S transformation of the uterine estrogen receptor, *J. Biol. Chem.* **249**:1866–1873.

98. Rennie, P., and Bruchovsky, N., 1973, Studies on the relationship between androgen receptors and the transport of androgens in rat prostate, *J. Biol. Chem.* **248**:3288–3297.

99. Puca, G. A., Nola, E., Sica, V., and Bresciani, F., 1972, Estrogen-binding proteins of calf uterus. Interrelationship between various forms and identification of a receptor-transforming factor, *Biochemistry* **11**:4157–4165.

100. Notides, A. C., Hamilton, D. E., and Rudolph, J. H., 1973, The action of a human uterine protease on the estrogen receptor, *Endocrinology* **93**:210–216.

101. Sibley, C. H., and Tomkins, G. M., 1974, Isolation of lymphoma cell variants resistant to killing by glucocorticoids, *Cell* **2**:213–220.

102. Iacobelli, S., 1973, Induced protein synthesis and oestradiol binding to the nuclei in the rat uterus, *Nature London New Biol.* **245**:154, 155.

103. Croce, C. M., Koprowski, H., and Litwack, G., 1974, Regulation of the corticosteroid inducibility of tyrosine aminotransferase in interspecific hybrid cells, *Nature London* **249**:839–841.

104. Lippman, M. E., Perry, S., and Thompson, E. B., 1974, Cytoplasmic glucocorticoid-binding proteins in glucocorticoid-unresponsive human and mouse leukemic cell lines, *Cancer Res.* **34**:1572–1576.

105. Gehring, U., Mohit, B., and Tomkins, G. M., 1972, Glucocorticoid action on hybrid clones derived from cultured myeloma and lymphoma cell lines, *Proc. Nat. Acad. Sci. U.S.A.* **69**:3124–3127.

106. Sibley, C. H., and Tomkins, G. M., 1974, Mechanisms of steroid resistance, *Cell* **2**:221–227.
107. Yamamoto, K. R., Stampfer, M. R., and Tomkins, G. M., 1974, Receptors from glucocorticoid-sensitive lymphoma cells and two classes of insensitive clones: Physical and DNA-binding properties, *Proc. Nat. Acad. Sci. U.S.A.* **71**:3901–3905.
108. Liao, S., Leininger, K. R., Sagher, D., and Barton, R. W., 1965, Rapid effect of testosterone on ribonucleic acid polymerase activity of rat ventral prostate, *Endocrinology* **77**:763–765.
109. Bashirelahi, N., Chader, G. J., and Villee, C. A., 1969, Effects of dihydrotestosterone on synthesis of nucleic acid and ATP in prostate nuclei, *Biochem. Biophys. Res. Commun.* **37**:976–981.
110. Davies, P., Fahmy, A. R., Pierrepoint, C. G., and Griffiths, K., 1972, Hormonal effects *in vitro* on prostatic ribonucleic acid polymerase, *Biochem. J.* **129**:1167–1169.
111. Noteboom, W. D., and Gorski, J., 1963, An early effect of estrogen on protein synthesis, *Proc. Nat. Acad. Sci. U.S.A.* **50**:250–255.
112. Gorski, J., 1964, Early estrogen effects on the activity of uterine ribonucleic acid polymerase, *J. Biol. Chem.* **239**:889–892.
113. Raynaud-Jammet, C., Biéri, F., and Baulieu, E.-E., 1971, Effects of oestradiol, α-amanitin and ionic strength on the *in vitro* synthesis of RNA by uterus nuclei, *Biochim. Biophys. Acta* **247**:355–360.
114. Glasser, S. R., Chytil, F., and Spelsberg, T. C., 1972, Early effects of oestradiol-17β on the chromatin and activity of the deoxyribonucleic acid-dependent ribonucleic acid polymerases (I and II) of the rat uterus, *Biochem. J.* **130**:947–957.
115. Hardin, J. W., Clark, J. H., Glasser, S. R., and Peck, E. J., Jr., 1976, RNA polymerase activity and uterine growth: Differential stimulation by estradiol, estriol, and nafoxidine, *Biochemistry* **15**:1370–1374.
116. Dukes, P. P., Sekeris, C. E., and Schmid, W., 1966, On the mechanism of hormone action VI. Increase in template activity of ribonucleic acid from isolated nuclei incubated in the presence of hormone, *Biochim. Biophys. Acta* **123**:126–133.
117. Sajdel, E. M., and Jacob, S. T., 1971, Mechanism of early effect of hydrocortisone on the transcriptional process: Stimulation of the activities of purified rat liver nucleolar RNA polymerase, *Biochem. Biophys. Res. Commun.* **45**:707–715.
118. McGuire, W. L., and O'Malley, B. W., 1968, Ribonucleic acid polymerase activity of the chick oviduct during steroid-induced synthesis of a specific protein, *Biochim. Biophys. Acta* **157**:187–194.
119. Zerwekh, J. E., Haussler, M. R., and Lindell, T. J., 1974, Rapid enhancement of chick intestinal DNA-dependent RNA polymerase II activity by 1α,25-dihydroxyvitamin D_3 *in vivo*, *Proc. Nat. Acad. Sci. U.S.A.* **71**:2337–2341.
120. Davies, P., and Griffiths, K., 1973, Stimulation of ribonucleic acid polymerase activity *in vitro* by prostatic steroid–protein receptor complexes, *Biochem. J.* **136**:611–622.
121. Davies, P., and Griffiths, K., 1974, Further studies on the stimulation of prostatic ribonucleic and polymerase by 5α-dihydrotestosterone-receptor complexes, *J. Endocrinol.* **62**:385–400.
122. Bautz, E. K. F., and Bautz, F. A., 1970, Initiation of RNA synthesis: The function of σ in the binding of RNA polymerase to promoter sites, *Nature London* **226**:1219–1222.

123. Lill, H., Lill, U., Sippel, A., and Hartmann, G., 1970, The inhibition of the RNA polymerase reaction by rifampcin, *in: Lepetit Colloquium on Biology and Medicine. RNA Polymerase and Transcription* (L. G. Silvestri, ed.), pp. 55–64, North Holland Publishing Co., Amsterdam.

124. Tsai, M.-J., Schwartz, R. J., Tsai; S. Y., and O'Malley, B. W., 1975, Effects of estrogen on gene expression in the chick oviduct: IV. Initiation of RNA synthesis on DNA and chromatin, *J. Biol. Chem.* **250**:5165–5174.

125. Tsai, S. Y., Tsai, M.-J., Schwartz, R., Kalimi, M., Clark, J. H., and O'Malley, B. W., 1975, Effects of estrogen on gene expression in chick oviduct: Nuclear receptor levels and initiation of transcription, *Proc. Nat. Acad. Sci. U.S.A.* **72**:4228–4232.

126. Schwartz, R. J., Buller, R. E., Kuhn, R. W., Schrader, W. T., and O'Malley, B. W., 1976, Progesterone-binding components of chick oviduct: *In vitro* effects of purified hormone–receptor complexes on the initiation of RNA synthesis in chromatin, *J. Biol. Chem.* (in press).

127. Schwartz, R. J., Tsai, M.-J., Tsai, S. Y., and O'Malley, B. W., 1975, Effect of estrogen on gene expression in the chick oviduct: V. Changes in the number of RNA polymerase binding and initiation sites in chromatin, *J. Biol. Chem.* **250**:5175–5182.

128. Buller, R. E., Schwartz, R. J., Schrader, W. T., and O'Malley, B. W., 1976, Progesterone binding components of chick oviduct: *In vitro* effect of receptor subunits on gene transcription *in vitro*, *J. Biol. Chem.* (in press).

129. Kalimi, M., Tsai, S. Y., Tsai, M.-J., Clark, J. H., and O'Malley, B. W., 1976, Effect of estrogen on gene expression in the chick oviduct. Correlation between nuclear-bound estrogen receptor and chromatin initiation sites for transcription, *J. Biol. Chem.* **251**:516–523.

130. Harris, S. E., Schwartz, R. J., Tsai, M.-J., O'Malley, B. W., and Roy, A. K., 1976, Effect of estrogen on gene expression in the chick oviduct. *In vitro* transcription of the ovalbumin gene in chromatin, *J. Biol. Chem.* **251**:524–529.

131. Hirose, M., Tsai, M.-J., and O'Malley, B. W., 1976, Effects of estrogen on gene expression in the chick oviduct. VII. Kinetics of initiation of *in vitro* transcription on chromatin, *J. Biol. Chem.* **251**:1137–1146.

132. Tsai, M.-J., Towle, H. C., Harris, S. E., and O'Malley, B. W., 1976, Effect of estrogen on gene expression in the chick oviduct. X. Comparative aspects of RNA chain initiation in chromatin using homologous versus *E. coli* RNA polymerase, *J. Biol. Chem.* **251**:1960–1968.

133. Travers, A., Baillie, D. L., and Pedersen, S., 1973, Effect of DNA conformation on ribosomal RNA synthesis *in vitro*, *Nature London New Biol.* **243**:161–163.

134. Umezawa, H., Mizuno, S., Yamazaki, H., and Nitta, K., 1968, Inhibition of DNA-dependent RNA synthesis by rifamycins, *J. Antibiot.* **21**:234–235.

135. Hartmann, H., Nonikel, K. O., Knüsel, F., and Nüesh, J., 1967, The specific inhibition of the DNA-directed RNA synthesis by rifamycin, *Biochim. Biophys. Acta* **145**:843, 844.

136. O'Malley, B. W., and McGuire, W. L., 1968, Studies on the mechanism of estrogen-mediated tissue differentiation: Regulation of nuclear transcription and induction of new RNA species, *Proc. Nat. Acad. Sci. U.S.A.* **60**:1527–1534.

137. O'Malley, B. W., Woo, S. L. C., Harris, S. E., Rosen, J. M., and Means, A. R., 1975, Steroid hormone regulation of specific messenger RNA and protein synthesis in eucaryotic cells, *J. Cell Physiol.* **85**:343–356.

138. Liarakos, C. D., Rosen, J. M., and O'Malley, B. W., 1973, Effect of estrogen on gene expression in the chick oviduct. II. Transcription of chick tritiated unique deoxyribonucleic acid as measured by hybridization in ribonucleic acid excess, *Biochemistry* **12**:2809–2816.
139. Monahan, J. J., Harris, S. E., and O'Malley, B. W., 1976, Effect of estrogen on gene expression in the chick oviduct: Effect of estrogen on the sequence and population complexity of chick oviduct poly (A) containing RNA, *J. Biol. Chem.* **251**:3738–3748.
140. Harris, S. E., Rosen, J. M., Means, A. R., and O'Malley, B. W., 1975, Use of a specific probe for ovalbumin messenger RNA to quantitate estrogen-induced gene transcripts, *Biochemistry* **14**:2072–2081.
141. Chan, L., Means, A. R., and O'Malley, B. W., 1973, Rate of induction of specific translatable mRNA's for ovalbumin and avidin by steroid hormones, *Proc. Nat. Acad. Sci. U.S.A.* **70**:1870–1874.
142. Palmiter, R. D., and Schimke, R. T., 1973, Regulation of protein synthesis in chick oviduct. III. Mechanism of ovalbumin "superinduction" by actinomycin D, *J. Biol. Chem.* **248**:1502–1512.
143. Palmiter, R. D., 1973, Rate of ovalbumin messenger ribonucleic acid synthesis in the oviduct of estrogen-primed chicks, *J. Biol. Chem.* **248**:8260–8270.
144. McKnight, G. S., Pennequin, P., and Schimke, R. T., 1975, Induction of ovalbumin mRNA sequences by estrogen and progesterone in chick oviduct as measured by hybridization to complementary DNA, *J. Biol. Chem.* **250**:8105–8110.
145. Palmiter, R. D., Catlin, G. H., and Cox, R. F., 1973, Chromatin-associated receptors for estrogen, progesterone, and dihydrotestosterone and the induction of egg white protein synthesis in chick magnum, *Cell Differ.* **2**:163–170.
146. Schrader, W. T., and O'Malley, B. W., 1972, Progesterone-binding components of chick oviduct. IV. Characterization of purified subunits, *J. Biol. Chem.* **247**:51–59.
147. Schrader, W. T., Toft, D. O., and O'Malley, B. W., 1972, Progesterone-binding protein of chick oviduct. VI. Interaction of purified progesterone-receptor components with nuclear constituents, *J. Biol. Chem.* **247**:2401–2407.
148. O'Malley, B. W., and Schrader, W. T., 1972, Progesterone receptor components: Identification of subunits binding to the target-cell genome, *J. Steroid Biochem.* **3**:617–629.
149. Schrader, W. T., Kuhn, R. W., and O'Malley, B. W., 1976, Progesterone-binding proteins of chick oviduct. XI. Receptor B subunit protein purified to apparent homogeneity from laying hen oviduct, *J. Biol. Chem.* (in press).
150. Moudgil, V. K., and Toft, D. O., 1975, Binding of ATP to the progesterone receptor, *Proc. Nat. Acad. Sci. U.S.A.* **72**:901–905.
151. Kuhn, R. W., Schrader, W. T., and O'Malley, B. W., 1976, Progesterone binding components of chick oviduct: XIV. Biochemical characterization of purified oviduct progesterone receptor B subunit. *J. Biol. Chem.* (in press).
152. Coty, W. A., Schrader, W. T., and O'Malley, B. W., 1976, Purification of the progesterone-receptor A subunit, *J. Biol. Chem.* (in press).
153. Britten, R. J., and Davidson, E. H., 1969, A theory. New facts regarding the organization of the genome provide clues to the nature of gene regulation, *Science* **165**:349–357.
154. Buller, R. E., Schwartz, R. J., and O'Malley, B. W., 1976, Steroid hormone receptor fraction stimulation of RNA synthesis: A caution, *Biochem. Biophys. Res. Commun.* **69**:106–113.

155. Milgrom, E., and Atger, M., 1975, Receptor translocation inhibitor and apparent saturability of the nuclear acceptor, *J. Steroid Biochem.* **6**:487–492.
156. Chamness, G. C. Jennings, A. W., and McGuire, W. L., 1974, Estrogen receptor binding to isolated nuclei. A nonsaturable process, *Biochemistry* **13**:327–331.
157. Buller, R. E., Kuhn, R. W., Schrader, W. T., and O'Malley, B. W., 1975, Physiologic function and structure of a steroid hormone receptor purified to homogeneity, *Clin. Res.* **23**:387A.
158. Norris, J. S., and Kohler, P. O., 1976, Steroid receptors in cultured cells: Characterization of the androgen receptor from a Syrian hamster ductus deferens tumor cell line (DDT_1), *Science* **192**:898–900.
159. Toft, D., and Gorski, J., 1966, A receptor molecule for estrogens: Isolation from the rat uterus and preliminary characterization, *Proc. Nat. Acad. Sci. U.S.A.* **55**:1574–1581.
160. Nozu, K., and Tamaoki, B. I., 1975, On the role of the cytosol receptors in the incorporation of androgens into the prostatic nuclei of rat, *J. Steroid Biochem.* **6**:57–63.
161. Hu, A.-L., Loor, R. M., and Wang, T. Y., 1975, Purification of a 3S cytosol androgen receptor from rat prostate that stimulates DNA-dependent RNA synthesis *in vitro*, *Biochem. Biophys. Res. Commun.* **65**:1327–1333.
162. Beatson, G. T., 1896, On the treatment of inoperable cases of carcinoma of the mamma: Suggestions for a new method of treatment with illustrative cases, *Lancet* **2**:104–107.
163. Williams, D. C., 1974, Steroid hormones and breast cancer, *Adv. Steroid Biochem. Pharmacol* **4**:209–231.
164. Jensen, E. V., Block, G. E., Smith, S., Kyser, K., and DeSombre, E. R., 1971, Estrogen receptors and breast cancer response to adrenalectomy, *in: Prediction of Response to Cancer Therapies, National Cancer Institute Monograph No. 34* (T. C. Hall, ed.), pp. 55–70, U.S. Government Printing Office, Washington, D.C.
165. McGuire, W. L., 1973, Estrogen receptors in human breast cancer, *J. Clin. Invest.* **52**:73–77.
166. McGuire, W. L., Chamness, G. C., Costlow, M. E., and Shepherd, R. E., 1974, Progress in endocrinology and metabolism. Hormone dependence in breast cancer, *Metabolism* **23**:75–100.
167. Korenman, S. G., and Dukes, B. A., 1970, Specific estrogen binding by the cytoplasm of human breast carcinoma, *J. Clin. Endocrinol. Metab.* **30**:639–645.
168. Maass, H., Engel, B., Hohmeister, H., Lehmann, F., and Trams, G., 1972, Estrogen receptors in human breast cancer tissue, *Amer. J. Obstet. Gynecol.* **113**:377–382.
169. Engelsman, E., Persijn, J. P., Korsten, C. B., and Cleton, F. J., 1973, Oestrogen receptor in human breast cancer tissue and response to endocrine therapy, *Br. Med. J.* **2**:750–752.
170. Leung, B. S., Manaugh, L. C., and Wood, D. C., 1973, Estradiol receptors in benign and malignant disease of the breast, *Clin. Chim. Acta* **46**:69–76.
171. Savlov, E. D., Wittliff, J. L., Hilf, R., and Hall, T. C., 1974, Correlations between certain biochemical properties of breast cancer and response to therapy: A preliminary report, *Cancer* **33**:303–309.
172. Buller, R. E., 1975, Tumoricidal steroids: Potential cure for advanced breast and prostatic cancer, *Tex. Med.* **71**:86–91.

Index